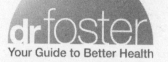

Your Guide to Better Health

GOOD
BIRTH

GUIDE

1 3 5 7 9 10 8 6 4 2

First published 2002 by Vermilion, an imprint of Ebury Press, Random House, 20 Vauxhall Bridge Road, London SW1V 2SA www.randomhouse.co.uk

Random House Australia (Pty) Limited 20 Alfred Street, Milsons Point, Sydney, New South Wales 2061, Australia

Random House New Zealand Limited 18 Poland Road, Glenfield, Auckland 10, New Zealand

Random House South Africa (Pty) Limited Endulini, 5a Jubilee Road, Parktown 2193, South Africa

The Random House Group Limited Reg. No. 954009

Papers used by Vermilion are natural, recyclable products made from wood grown in sustainable forests.

Printed and bound in Great Britain by Bookmarque Ltd,Croydon, Surrey

A CIP catalogue record for this book is available from the British Library.

ISBN 0091883792

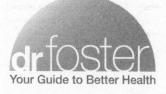
Your Guide to Better Health

GOOD
BIRTH
GUIDE

Data Compiled by Dr Foster
Text by Dr Lorna Gold

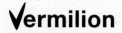

Contents

Who is Dr Foster 6
Preface 7
Introduction 9

Section 1
BEFORE THE BIRTH
Planning Your Pregnancy 20
Antenatal Care 21
Hospital Antenatal Care 27
Scans and Tests 29
Antenatal Appointments 38
Antenatal Classes 40
Miscarriage 46
High Blood Pressure 58

Section 2
GIVING BIRTH
Hospital Birth 66
Home Birth 82
Induction of Labour 90
Assisted Delivery 97
Episiotomy 102
Forceps Delivery 103
Ventouse Delivery 106
Breech Birth 106
Caesarean Section 109
Stillbirth 120
Twins 122

Section 3
AFTER THE BIRTH
Breastfeeding 130
Wound care 137
Postnatal Emotional
   Problems 144
Your New Baby 146
When Things go Wrong 151

Section 4
MATERNITY UNIT PROFILES
The East 152
London 182
The Northwest 220
The North 251
The Southeast 291
The Southwest 338
Trent 372
The West Midlands 393
Scotland 421
Wales 466
Northern Ireland 494

Methodology 509
Index of Hospitals 511
Index 517
Dr Foster Q&A 525

Who is Dr Foster?

Dr Foster provides authoritative information on health services of all kinds in the UK. Our aim is to empower patients with information to help them access the best possible care. We are supervised by an Ethics committee comprising leading figures from the medical profession that has independent legal powers to ensure that guides meet the highest standards.

The ethics committee currently comprises the following membership.

Dr Jack Tinker, dean of the Royal Society of Medicine and chair of the committee

Sir Donald Irvine, president, General Medical Council

Dr Michael Dixon, chair, NHS Alliance

Peter Griffiths, chief executive, Health Quality Service

Dianne Hayter, chief executive, the Pelican Centre, a cancer research charity

Professor Alan Maynard, director health policy unit, York University and chair, York Health Services NHS Trust

Wilma MacPherson, formerly director of nursing and quality, Guy's and Thomas' NHS Trust

Bridget Gill, chair of the Northern and Yorkshire Regional Council of the Institute of Healthcare Management

Kokila Lakhoo, consultant paediatric surgeon, John Radcliffe Hospital

Trevor Campbell Davis, chief executive, Whittington Hospital

Douglas Webb, operations and development director, Friends of the Elderly

Vanessa Bourne, chair, Patients Association

Dr Phillip Davies, medical director, Pontypridd and Rhondda NHS Trust

Professor Charles Gillis, formerly director of the West of Scotland Cancer Surveillance Unit.

Further information about Dr Foster and the independent Ethics committee can be found at www.drfoster.co.uk.

Dr Lorna Gold was born in Kilmarnock, Scotland, and studied medicine at the University of Dundee, graduating in 1986. She worked in hospitals until 1992 and for the past eight years has been a full time GP in Handsworth, Birmingham. She is a regular contributor to medical publications and participates in the community-based undergraduate teaching programme for Birmingham University medical students.

Changing Childbirth

The Good Birth Guide breaks new ground. For someone who has spent the past eight years attempting to spread good practice in maternity care nationwide, this guide and the Dr Foster survey on which it is based mark an important turning point. It clearly sets out how patchy the services that women can expect really are, highlighting both the good, and the bad. For the first time, women will be able to find information that was previously unobtainable to analyse the kinds of services provided in their local hospitals, and to plan accordingly. Changing Childbirth was the report of an expert committee I chaired in 1993, which provided a vision of how maternity services should work – a vision that remains largely unfulfilled. Then, the trend towards older first-time mothers had begun; though the risks were higher for them in childbirth, this group was generally fit, healthy and influential. Having a baby was no longer a duty but an option. My report tried to establish principles that are still relevant today, but, as any service provider knows, practice must move on and take account of social trends. What still holds true is that giving your child a good birth equips them with a head start in life. Childbirth should be both safe, which it is, and sound, which is where we often fail. The criteria set out in the report were threefold. Women should have choice in pregnancy and birth for all services; they should remain in control throughout; they should have continuity of carer, a professional friend and adviser, through pregnancy, delivery and afterwards. Too few mothers will recognize this vision – and worryingly low midwife-staffing levels make this ideal less and less of a real choice. Some women are seen by up to 20 different professionals during pregnancy, left alone during labour and delivered by a stranger. This is unacceptable. This book is an opportunity to demand change, and arms women with the information to do so.

Baroness Cumberlege, junior minister
(Health and Social Services) 1992-97

Introduction

If you are pregnant, you may have some pretty clear ideas about how you want to have your baby. Or perhaps you are still trying to understand what your options are. Either way, you will hear a lot of other people's opinions as your pregnancy develops. The medical professionals who look after you – GP, midwife and perhaps obstetrician – will all offer advice. And friends and family will no doubt offer plenty of anecdotes and old wives' tales.

The truth is, of course, that there is no 'best way' to have a baby. A caesarean delivery can be as fulfilling as a natural delivery and labour can be just as hard with pain relief as without. The most important point for many women is that they feel they are in control of what happens to them.

This book is designed to empower women to take more control over the way they have their children. It doesn't come with any fixed ideas about what is right and what is wrong – it is up to you whether you find the idea of natural childbirth beautiful or horrifying. It is up to you whether you want a pain free birth or would prefer to experience childbirth to the full. The important point is that you need to know what your options are and how to best exercise them.

From the moment you find out you are pregnant, you face some very basic choices over how you have your baby. Do you want to have your baby at home or in a hospital? If a hospital, which hospital should you have your baby in? Who do you want to look after you – a midwife or a doctor? Do you want to try for a natural childbirth? Would you prefer to have a caesarean? Would you prefer something different such as a water birth? Do you want pain relief, and if so, what do you want?

In dealing with these questions, you need to know the issues surrounding them. You also need to know what actually goes on in maternity departments around the country. This book sets out to answer both questions.

You will not find a single midwife, doctor or hospital that does not try to give every woman the type of birth they want. But in busy maternity wards, as often as not, it does not happen that way. What happens to you during labour will probably depend less on what you say you want to happen than on where you choose to have your baby. The simple fact is that between two similar hospitals, you could be twice as likely to be delivered by caesarean section in one than in the other. Your postcode will often determine whether you are more likely to be induced, be assisted in delivery by forceps, or be elected for caesarean section. Your chances of benefiting from the latest antenatal scans and tests, as well as being offered a full range of pain relief also depends on which hospital you go to. Home delivery may be actively promoted in your area, or actively discouraged because of lack of available staff.

This guide is unique. Wherever you are in the UK, it tells you about your local maternity units – what services are offered, and just as importantly, what actually happens to women who give birth there. Whether you want to know which units are short-staffed or overcrowded or which offer alternative therapies for pain relief; which units are most likely to support you if you want to give birth naturally, and which are likely to be sympathetic if you don't, this book can help.

The data about maternity units has been put together with the help of the Faculty of Medicine at Imperial College, London. A statistical team under the direction of Professor Sir Brian Jarman have analysed the raw data for each maternity unit in England and adjusted them to take account of some of the important factors that influence the data. Each unit has been profiled in terms of the age and social background of the women attending it. The data has then been adjusted to take account of this.

To take an example, Queen Charlotte's hospital in London is a specialist referral center looking after many women with more complex pregnancies. It also has a very high rate of caesarean deliveries. But is this just because of the types of people it deals with? After adjusting for the age and social background of the people in the hospital – both of which can be linked to difficulties in pregnancy - it turns out that Queen Charlotte's is slightly more prone to caesarean interventions than other hospitals, but not excessively so. What also emerges, is that the hospital is much more likely to book women in as planned (elective) caesareans and as a result, its rate of emergency caesareans (where a woman is operated on after labour has started) is far lower than in most hospitals.

When you find out you are pregnant, your first stop for advice is most likely to be your GP. Your GP will usually be the best source of advice about local maternity services. But often GPs are quick to recommend the nearest maternity unit and women are usually happy to accept without being aware of the other options available to them. Is there another hospital that might provide a service more in tune with your wishes? Is there a midwife-led unit that might be appropriate? Or is a home birth the right thing for you? This book talks you through how your pregnancy and labour will be managed, who will look after you and what the important decisions are about your care. It provides you with the information you need to help you get the kind of care you want.

Under the law, you are free to give birth wherever you chose. And, by and large, if you decide you would like to have your baby at a particular hospital, the hospital will be happy to look after you. Home birth services can be more restricted. Hospitals are, in theory, expected to offer all women the option of having a home birth. In practice, some maternity services are far more ready to handle a home birth than others. In a hospital, you will be looked after by consultants and midwives jointly, or by midwives alone. Some women prefer to be looked after by midwives and many believe that midwives are better at supporting women to give birth naturally. Other women feel more comfortable under the supervision of a doctor and may regard it as a good thing that doctors are sometimes quicker to intervene in childbirth than midwives. The important thing is for you to know what services are available, where they are offered and how to get the care you want.

With the information contained in this book, you, together with your GP or midwife, can make a more informed choice as to which maternity unit is more likely to meet your needs. Depending on where you live, you can look up the maternity unit nearest to your home and compare its services and facilities with other local units. If your choices of maternity unit are limited, you can still choose between the services and facilities offered by your local unit and can express a preference for your antenatal, delivery and postnatal care.

In the 1992 Changing Childbirth report, Baroness Julia Cumberlege, junior health minister, wrote that there should be choice, control and continuity for women in their maternity care. Women should have choice in pregnancy and birth for all services. Women should remain in control throughout their care, and women should have continuity of care, a professional friend and adviser, through pregnancy, delivery and afterwards. By empowering yourself with the information contained in this Guide, you can demand choice in pregnancy and birth and receive the care that is most appropriate for you and your baby.

How to Use This Book

This guide tells you how maternity care is delivered in the UK and what different maternity units throughout the country do. The idea is that by combining the two, you can get the care that best suits your needs and wishes.

For example:

What do I do if I don't feel happy about the hospital my GP recommended I have my baby in?

On page 20 of this guide we explain about your rights to choose where you have your baby. The fact is that you are pretty much free to say where you want to have your child. But one of the biggest barriers to exercising this choice is not knowing what the options are. At the back of this book we give you a run down on most maternity units in the country – indispensable information for you to exercise this choice.

I want to have a home birth. How do I go about it?

Hospitals and GPs are often reluctant to recommend home births. On page 82 of this guide we explain the issues and the evidence surrounding safety and home births. We also explain your rights with regard to a home birth. Finally, at the back of the guide, you can see which maternity services in your area are actually doing most home births, which is where you will find midwives with most experience in this area.

I want a natural childbirth. How can I make sure I have one?

On page 97 we explain some of the reasons for medical intervention in childbirth and the risks that sometimes mean it is not possible to give birth naturally. We also explain why in many hospitals the rate of intervention in childbirth has been rising rapidly without any clear medical reason. Finally, at the end of the book, we tell you which units have very high intervention rates and which have low intervention rates – and which are therefore more likely to let you give birth naturally. Here you can also find maternity-led units which specialize in helping women with low-risk pregnancies give birth naturally.

I would prefer to have a caesarean. What are my options?

This is a particularly sensitive area with divisions between medical professionals as to the advisability of letting women chose to have caesareans. On page 109, we explain the issues surrounding this debate and why many people regard this as an unwise choice. We also explain why some obstetricians are more willing to go along with maternal choice in this area. At the back of the book you can see which maternity units have high caesarean rates – and in particular which have high elective caesarean rates – and which are therefore more likely to be sympathetic to you.

I want to have full epidural pain relief in labour.
Can I demand this?

This is another issue on which opinion is divided. In France, almost everybody has an epidural. In Holland almost nobody does. In the UK it depends which hospital you go to. Some midwives and doctors counsel against widespread use of epidurals. They can slow down labour and protract the whole process to the point where it might have been less uncomfortable giving birth naturally. Others think women should have one if they want one. Other hospitals simply don't have the resources to give them to everyone who wants one. We explain the issues on pages 76-79. At the back of the book you can see which unit offer epidural services and where epidural and spinal pain relief is most commonly used.

Where to Find What You Need

The first part of this book covers the most common questions asked by pregnant women and gives you straightforward answers. The aim is to avoid taking a view on what is right or what is wrong and to arm you, as far as possible, with the facts.

The second part of the book includes a profile of virtually every maternity unit in the UK. We believe the only units not covered are those in the Hebrides and one small unit in Yorkshire. Units are arranged alphabetically by town by region, with units for low-risk pregnancies (midwife-led) alongside the more familiar consultant-led units in large hospitals.

What We Tell You About Maternity Services

The maternity units are divided into two groups. The biggest group is the traditional hospital based maternity unit staffed with doctors and midwives, which account for the vast majority of births in the UK. These units have consultant obstetricians on staff and are able to deal with both complex and straightforward pregnancies and deliveries. Many will offer a choice of being under the supervision of a doctor or a midwife, although if there are complications you will almost certainly be put under the care of a doctor. These units are capable of carrying out all medical interventions in childbirth and can offer a full anaesthetic service including epidurals.

Consultant units

Each unit has a description and some key facts. In the descriptions we focus on some important issues for pregnant women such as whether the intervention rates are higher or lower than average, whether pain relief services are limited and how midwifery services are organized. A particular issue for women is whether or not they are likely to know the midwife who cares for them in labour. In general women prefer this and statistics show that women who do know their midwife are less likely to require intervention. But many services are organized in such a way that the midwife who delivers you will almost certainly be somebody you meet for the first time when you go into have your baby. A full explanation of different systems of midwifery can be found on page 25.

It is important to remember however, that statistics need to be seen as part of a broader picture. This information should always be used in consultation with your GP and midwife who will often have a good understanding of local services.

Midwife units

There are a large number of maternity units throughout the UK which do not have consultants working in them and are for women who show no signs of having any difficulty giving birth naturally. Most of them are staffed entirely by midwives although in a few, GPs with training in obstetrics also provide care. By and large, these units offer a very different style of care compared with consultant units. In general, there are no anaesthetists to administer epidurals and no surgeons to perform caesarean sections. Interventions are limited or non-existent.

These units tend to provide a friendly, homely environment in which women are given support to give birth without medical intervention or high levels of drugs for pain relief. Often you will get a lot more personal attention, with more midwives around who will get to know you throughout your antenatal care and will then deliver you. It is often argued that the simple fact that there are no doctors around reduces the temptation to intervene. This may result in more women giving birth naturally. That said, if you do get into difficulties at one of these units, you would be quickly transferred to a large hospital. These units also tend to have midwives experienced in home births.

Too often, however, women are unaware of midwife-led units and are therefore not in a position to choose them. This is just one of many areas in which we hope this book will increase awareness of how childbirth is handled in this county and encourage more women to make use of the choices facing them.

The key data for each unit are:

Capacity We tell you how many beds there are, how many births take place in the unit and how many births took place each day for each delivery bed. In some cases there is more than one birth per day per delivery bed. On the one hand, that suggests these units are popular. On the other hand, it suggests they may be a little more crowded than other units.

Staffing levels We tell you the number of births handled each year by each midwife in the hospital. There is a severe midwife shortage in some parts of the country and some units have had to shut down their services from time to time because they do not have the staff to cope with demand. This can involve women in labour being diverted to a different hospital to the one they planned to give birth in. It should be remembered that these figures do not take full account of different staffing patterns and that a unit with, say, 32 births per midwife should not necessarily be regarded as any different from a unit with 35 births. However, where staffing levels fall to 40 births per midwife or more, there is a high likelihood that staffing will be under a great deal of pressure.

Screening We tell you which hospitals offer tests for Down's Syndrome. We tell you where triple testing, the most definitive test for Down's, is routinely offered. If it is not routinely offered and you want this test, you should say. We also tell you which units will arrange for you to have a nuchal fold scan. This is a newer test for Down's which you can have several weeks earlier than a triple test.

Pain relief We tell you which hospitals offer different types of pain relief in labour. We also tell you what percentage of women had an epidural or a spinal as part of their delivery. Epidural or spinal pain relief is the most powerful form of pain relief given to women for delivery. It is used both in labour and also in caesarean deliveries. The figure given is the percentage of all women who had this form of pain relief, not just those in labour. However it gives an indication of the availability of this form of anaesthetic in each hospital.

Intervention rates These figures tell you about the tendency for different hospital departments to intervene in labour either with instruments (forceps or ventouse) or by operating (caesarean section). We also tell you how often labour is artificially induced. The figures for England are adjusted to take account of the types of women going into the hospital. The figures for Wales, Scotland and Northern Ireland are not adjusted, and consequently, hospitals that tend to take higher risk pregnancies will inevitably have higher intervention rates. That said, you can still make comparisons between similar hospitals.

Section One:
Before the Birth

Planning Your Pregnancy

If the world were a logical place, every pregnancy would be planned and every woman would have easy access to good quality information and support to give her the opportunity to maximise her chance of remaining healthy during her pregnancy, carrying the baby to full term, and having a straightforward vaginal delivery.

Women in the developed world today enjoy better reproductive health than at any time in history. This is in part due to good obstetric care, but mainly because we live in an age of plentiful food, good hygiene, and effective contraception. However, where and how you have your baby is something you will want to think very carefully about.

Can I choose which hospital I go to?

Yes. You compare the different hospitals in your area by using the statistics in this guide, by contacting the Information Department of each hospital, or by asking friends who have recently had babies about their experiences. In making your choice, you should consider whether you will feel safer and more relaxed in a large high-tech hospital with all the medical facilities, or a small unit with more individualised care. You might also consider the type of pain relief you would like to have access to, whether high or low-intervention rates are important to you, and whether you would like a water birth.

What are my options regarding where I give birth?

In hospital Under the care of a consultant obstetrician. This does not mean that you will be delivered by the consultant, nor does it mean that you will necessarily have a high-tech delivery. Most hospitals offer a wide range of options, including low-tech rooms and water births, and all deliveries are attended by midwives.

In a midwifery unit Sometimes called a birth centre, this is a low-tech unit, run by community midwives, sometimes with input from GPs, independent of the main hospital, but attached to it so that you can be transferred quickly if problems arise. Not every area has a midwifery unit, for example, in Northern Ireland, there is only one.

At home A home birth takes place under the care of the community midwifery team or an independent midwife.

If I don't like the hospital I'm referred to, can I change my mind and go elsewhere?
Yes. You can ask your GP to write to your preferred hospital. Transfer of information is rarely a problem, as you will be carrying your own antenatal records.

Can I be referred to a female obstetrician?
Currently the majority of consultant and trainee obstetricians are male, although this looks set to change. It is impossible to guarantee that you will see only female doctors during your pregnancy and labour but your GP can refer you to a female consultant. Ask for it to be recorded on your notes that you want to see female doctors whenever possible. Alternatively, think about having midwife-led care as most midwives are women.

Antenatal Care

'Antenatal' means 'before birth', and antenatal care is the health care you receive during pregnancy. It includes regular check-ups for you and your developing baby – a process that normally involves midwives, your GP, and a consultant or trainee obstetrician (a doctor who specialises in childbirth). Most antenatal care is done in the community, in that you will visit your midwife at your antenatal clinic, or she will visit you at home. However, almost every woman attends hospital as an outpatient at least twice during her pregnancy (usually for scans), and if problems arise she may need an in-patient stay on the antenatal ward. Some hospitals now offer drop-in antenatal clinics and day care facilities which avoid the need for an overnight stay.

Routine antenatal care for women in the UK now includes blood tests and ultrasound scans. Antenatal care also includes health advice and preparation for the later stages of pregnancy, the process of giving birth, and caring for a newborn baby. Antenatal and

Birth Story Dawn Howarth

Twelve weeks is a big turning point in pregnancy. Not only does the chance of early miscarriage plummet dramatically, but with luck any nausea and exhaustion comes to an end. It is when you know your baby's main organs are formed, and it is when your antenatal care really gets going, beginning with the ultrasound scan which allows you to see your baby for the first time

It was at this stage of my pregnancy that my husband, Patrick, and I moved to Cornwall. I had a long first appointment with my midwife – there was no need to see my new GP – filling in forms and having various tests. She was patient, unhurried and kind, and answered all our questions. I was told about the NCT classes and about the local midwife-run parentcraft classes, and she also explained what the options were regarding where to have the baby. As in many rural areas, home births are very popular in Cornwall, but as this was my first baby, a hospital delivery was recommended. Sadly there is not enough funding in the area for a domino system. I was disappointed about this, as I had hoped that I would get to know and bond with the midwife who would deliver my baby.

The 12 week scan was a wonderful experience, carried out by a midwife who was again able to answer all our questions, and an appointment was then made to see the consultant and have a further scan at 20 weeks. The midwives at my practice understood that waiting for results of Down's Syndrome and other tests can be a scary time, and I was phoned at home within days of having these done, the results were clearly explained and my mind set at rest.

At this point antenatal care went quiet for a few months and I turned my attention to my health, contacting the Active Birth Centre who organize weekly yoga classes nearby. These classes have been the most important aspect of my antenatal care, as we not only do yoga exercises, but also practice labour positions and discuss different kinds of labour.

Suddenly it seemed very important to think about what sort of birth I wanted and where to have it, and I learned that Derriford Hospital in Plymouth has an excellent low rate for emergency caesarians, good midwife-per-mother figures and a low epidural rate. Through conversations with other women, I was also able to start work on my birth plan. I am requesting that fetal monitoring is done using a hand-held monitor, and not one which requires me to be lying flat on my back, as the ability to move about freely is top of my list of priorities. I have also asked that there are no students or other observers present. I want as little interference as possible, and the final delivery of the baby is, especially, to be hands-free. Things may not go according to plan, of course, but I now feel empowered to make decisions on the spot if necessary.

As I write, we have ten more weeks to go and my midwifery care is now fortnightly. I still haven't seen my GP, and my brush with the consultant was very brief as I had no complications. I have kept my antenatal care almost exclusively among women which seems entirely natural and comfortable, and I am hoping that the birth goes along the same lines.

parentcraft classes are available through the NHS, and many women seek further advice from organisations such as the National Childbirth Trust and from the vast resources available in bookshops and on the internet. Nearly 40 per cent of units offer parent education classes and antenatal classes at weekends. Ninety per cent offer them in the evening and more than half offer women-only classes. Some units offer aquanatal classes. Other classes include those aimed at teenagers, grandparents and minority ethnic groups.

Getting the right antenatal care and advice is an essential part of making your pregnancy and birth go as smoothly as possible. You need to make sure that you get the right level of care whether that is a midwife, GP or obstetrician. It is also good if you can be looked after throughout your pregnancy and birth by the same person. Women who are looked after in labour by a midwife they have got to know during their pregnancy tend to feel more confident about giving birth and have a better experience. In addition to supporting you throughout your pregnancy, your service should prepare you for the birth itself and the postnatal period. Research indicates that if you know what to expect and feel in control going into labour, you are less likely to suffer from stress or require medical intervention.

What are my options for antenatal care?
Shared Care Most women's antenatal care is shared between their GP, the community midwives and the hospital. If you choose to have this arrangement, see your GP and tell them that you are pregnant and, if possible, the date of the first day of your last period. They will arrange for you to attend the antenatal clinic at the surgery, and write to a consultant obstetrician at the hospital to ask them to share your care – this is called booking. Both your midwife and GP will usually take a medical history, looking for specific risk factors. In the majority of cases, however, women will be fit and well. Shared care involves visits to both your GP surgery and hospital-based midwives. Both groups of professionals will be involved in ensuring your pregnancy goes smoothly but the midwives will be more intimately involved with the labour and delivery.

Midwife-led Care If you would like all of your antenatal care provided by midwives, contact your GP's surgery and ask for an appointment with the midwife at the antenatal clinic. If your GP does not have a midwife-led antenatal clinic, contact the Director of Midwifery Services for your area. The health authority will be able to tell you how to do this. There are several forms of midwife care:

- **Community based midwifery** You will receive antenatal and postnatal care in the community (either at home or in your local clinic or surgery) from the one or a number of midwives. However, you are more likely to be delivered by a midwife who is available on the labour ward than by one known to you.

- **A domino (DOMiciliary IN and Out) delivery** Your community midwife will look after you at home for most of your labour then accompany you to the hospital or maternity unit for delivery. If all goes smoothly, you will return home with your baby after a few hours.

- **Team midwifery** A team of midwives look after a large group of women between them. You will get the opportunity to meet all midwives in the team and will usually see one of these midwives for your antenatal care, labour and postnatal care.

- **Group practice/caseload midwifery** Midwives work in pairs. All antenatal, delivery and postnatal care is provided by one midwife with her 'buddy' acting as backup if she is sick or on leave. This ensures continuity of care and greatly increases the chances that you will know the midwife who delivers you, but is not very common. One study has shown that caseload midwifery reduces the need for medical intervention and the use of epidurals.

- **Independent midwife** For a fee of around £2,500 a private midwife provides continuity of care and offers a convenient service at home, 24 hours a day. You can deliver at home under the midwife's care or in a hospital that the midwife has a contract with. Antenatal and postnatal care is more intense, with midwives making between 14-16 antenatal visits and daily visits for the first week following pregnancy and regular visits for up to six weeks afterwards. Independent midwives are fully trained and are bound by the same code of practice as NHS midwives. If you have a private midwife the arrangements for scans and blood tests may vary and they will discuss these with you. You will, however, still have a formal booking and assessment. Unfortunately, few independent midwives practise outside London and the Home Counties. For more information, contact: Independent Midwives Association, Tel 01483 821104, www.independentmidwives.org.uk

Private Care You can have all of your antenatal care carried out privately by an obstetrician. Some NHS hospitals have a private wing but there are very few private hospitals outside of London that cater for private obstetric care (48 out of 245 private hospitals employ obstetricians). If you choose to have this type of care, expect to pay at least £5,000.

Obstetrician-led Care You can also choose to have your care led by an obstetrician in an NHS hospital although you will rarely see the obstetrician.

I have private medical insurance. Will it pay for my antenatal care?

Most private medical insurance policies exclude pregnancy and normal delivery, although they may provide cover if you have to have a caesarean section for a reason that could not be foreseen when you took out the policy. Check with your insurer.

Should I make a birth plan?

It is a good idea to prepare yourself for the birth by thinking about what you would like to happen – where you want to give birth, whom you would like to be there, how you are going to manage pain and what you would rather avoid. Even apparently minor details like whether or not you want to be the first to touch and pick up your baby can be important. If you decide to make a written birth plan, make sure one copy is filed in your notes and keep a copy for your own reference.

However, an excessively detailed and restrictive birth plan can be a recipe for disappointment, as some women find their expectations of childbirth are very different from reality – in particular, it may be more painful than anticipated. It's a good idea to think through what you would like to happen if you need pain relief, or if you need forceps or a caesarean section.

Who is the birth plan for?

Above all, it's for you. The act of writing down your birth plan makes you focus on what you really want during labour, and can turn vague objectives such as 'I want the birth to be as calm as possible' into something more specific. For example, 'I want the baby to be placed on my stomach as soon as it is born, and only moved if resuscitation is necessary.'

Your birth plan is also intended to let those looking after you know your wishes. You should discuss its contents with your community midwife, and it is essential that you ask the midwife looking after you in labour to read it.

Your birth partner should know and understand your plan so that he can ensure that everyone who attends you in labour knows your wishes. However, they should be careful not to take the plan too literally, for instance, if a woman is screaming for an epidural while her husband insists that she only wants aromatherapy for the pain.

What will my birth plan look like?

Many patient-held maternity records include a section where you can write your birth plan, with helpful pointers to the issues you might want to consider. (see page 41)

Hospital Antenatal Care

When will I have my first appointment at the hospital?

For the first three months of your pregnancy you are unlikely to need to see your GP or midwife a great deal, unless you experience problems such as severe vomiting, bleeding or a urine infection. Your first hospital appointment will usually be booked for when you are around three months pregnant. At this appointment, you will see a midwife and an obstetrician and usually an ultrasound scan will be arranged. The main reason for this scan is to confirm your estimated date of delivery, although some problems can be detected at this stage.

What information will I be asked to provide?
At the first hospital appointment, you will be asked questions about yourself and your health and previous pregnancies. It will help if you are ready with the following facts:

- **Your personal details** such as your date of birth, your address, the name you want to be known by, your religion and the language you prefer to speak.
- **Details of health professionals involved with your care** such as your GP, community midwife, social worker or community psychiatric nurse.
- **Your next of kin.** This will usually be your partner or your parents; This person would have to give consent on your or your baby's care if you are incapacitated.
- **Your partner's details** and whether or not they are a blood relation.
- **Your LMP (last menstrual period)** and whether your cycle is normally regular. The date you had a positive pregnancy test, if relevant.
- **Whether you conceived while using contraception.**
- **Any previous significant illnesses or operations you have had.** Particularly relevant are high blood pressure, heart disease, thrombosis (blood clots in your legs or lungs), diabetes, epilepsy, thyroid disease, kidney disease, hepatitis B or C, HIV infection, psychiatric illness such as schizophrenia or depression, and fractures of the bones of your pelvis.
- **Any allergies you have,** especially to medication.
- **Any problems during the early part of this pregnancy,** such as vaginal bleeding, urinary infections, or severe vomiting.
- **Diseases that run in your family,** particularly high blood pressure, diabetes, puerperal psychosis and inherited conditions such as cystic fibrosis.
- **Details of your previous pregnancies.** For each, you will be asked the date the pregnancy ended, the gestation (the length of

the pregnancy), the length of labour, the type of delivery, whether you had a tear or episiotomy, the weight, sex and state of health of the baby, whether the baby was breastfed (and for how long), and whether you or the baby had any problems in the first six weeks after your delivery. Remember to include miscarriages and terminations.

Scans and Tests

Antenatal testing allows early detection of problems that pose health risks to you or your baby, some of which can be treated before birth. However it is a complex area that can create difficult emotional and moral dilemmas as tests may reveal abnormalities in the fetus that may lead you to have to consider the possibility of terminating the pregnancy. It is important to consider the implications of any test before you have it.

There are a range of different tests ranging from the booking ultrasound scan – a usually straightforward ultrasound scan at around 12 weeks designed principally to establish the age of the fetus, the viability of the pregnancy and to exclude the possibility of twins – to more complex screens and tests for abnormalities such as Spina Bifida and Down's Syndrome.

Down's Syndrome testing illustrates the issues that testing can create. As women get older the likelihood of having a child with Down's Syndrome increases. There are a number of screening tests that can be done to look for signs of this. They include the nuchal fold scan – an ultrasound scan that can be performed between 12 and 14 weeks – or a blood test, commonly known as the triple test or double test usually performed at 16 weeks.

In both cases, these tests cannot determine whether you will or will not have a child with Down's Syndrome – they can only tell you if you are at higher risk of having one. Two tests – amniocentesis and chorionic villus sampling – allow a more certain diagnosis to be made.

Usually, if the risks appear to be greater than 1 in 250 (for example, 1 in 100) you will be offered the option of an amniocentesis – a test which involves taking some fluid from the amniotic sac for genetic testing. This test should establish with a high degree of certainty whether or not your child has Down's Syndrome. Unfortunately it also carries with it a 1 in 100 chance of causing a miscarriage.

So if you are told your child has a 1 in 200 chance of having Down's, does it make sense to have a test which carries a 1 in a 100 chance of ending the pregnancy? That will depend on whether you feel you would rather have a child with Down's Syndrome than not at all.

Plainly the ethical and emotional issues involved are difficult and it is important to remember some key points.

- You do not have to have any tests at all. In Ireland, where abortion is illegal, no one has any diagnostic tests during pregnancy. If you are sure you want to go through with the pregnancy whatever and would rather not know if there are problems, then you can refuse all tests. On the other hand, you may feel you will carry on with the pregnancy regardless, but would like to know as early as possible if there are any problems.

- If a screening test shows a high probability of Down's Syndrome you are free to refuse further tests – although you may sometimes find people put you under pressure to proceed. If you decide you would rather take the risk of having a child with Down's Syndrome than the risk of losing the baby, that is your choice.

- Even if the fetus is diagnosed as having Down's Syndrome, you are not obliged to terminate the pregnancy. Again this is your choice. If you do decide not to have the child, most hospitals have midwifes and other professionals experienced in providing counselling.

- The availability of tests varies greatly between hospitals. Most hospitals do offer the triple test (see p34) although some only do double tests, which provide a less certain result. A growing number can also provide nuchal fold scans. A great advantage of the nuchal fold scan is that it can be done earlier than the triple tests. However, you may not be automatically offered these scans. Many hospitals do not routinely offer testing and may only offer it to women over a certain age. Nuchal fold scans may also only be offered to certain groups. You can, however, request testing if you are worried. The unit profiles at the end of the book tell you which units routinely offer triple testing and which are able to arrange nuchal fold scans.

What is an Early Pregnancy Ultrasound scan?

Early pregnancy ultrasound scans, performed between 8 and 14 weeks, can give a reliable indication of fetal age and location. As well as giving an indication of your delivery date and revealing whether you are expecting twins, this information provides early warning of conditions such as placenta praevia. However, this diagnosis should not cause undue concern as a definite diagnosis cannot be made until between 32-34 weeks. Around 70 per cent of maternity units offer this scan.

What is a Nuchal Fold Scan?

A nuchal fold, or nuchal translucency, measurement may be done during the booking (or twelve week) scan in some hospitals. The thickness of the small pool of fluid at the back of the baby's neck is measured. If it is thicker than normal, the risk of Down's Syndrome, other chromosomal abnormalities, and congenital heart disease, is increased. Although only 60 per cent of hospitals offer it, the advantages of the nuchal fold scan are that it can be done earlier in pregnancy than amniocentesis (see p36) or blood tests. However, it is only a screening test – it will only detect three out of every four babies with a chromosomal abnormality, and very rarely, a normal baby will have an abnormal nuchal fold scan. It would be unusual for you to be advised to terminate your pregnancy on the basis of a nuchal fold scan alone. Further tests such as a detailed scan of the heart, amniocentesis, or chorionic villus sampling are normally carried out to find out exactly what is wrong with the baby unless you decide that you do not want any more tests. Almost every maternity unit offers amniocentesis testing and 70% offer chorionic villus sampling. However, there are risks associated with these tests and you need to discuss these thoroughly with your obstetrician.

What is an Abnormality Ultrasound Scan

The abnormality ultrasound scan, performed between 20 and 23 weeks, can reliably diagnose many structural abnormalities in the fetus including spina bifida (abnormal development of the spinal cord) and anencephaly (abnormal development of the brain). Around 90 per cent of maternity units offer this scan. 90 per cent of units offer an abnormality ultrasound scan between 20-23 weeks. At around 20 weeks, you will also be offered a detailed scan which can show whether your baby's important organs are developing normally. The brain, heart, lungs, liver, kidneys, bowel and bones are examined closely, as are the placenta and umbilical cord. At this stage you can even see your baby's facial features, fingers and toes. If you want to know the sex of your baby in advance, this is the time to ask, although a few hospitals still have a policy of not disclosing this.

What detailed information can an ultrasound scan provide?

An ultrasound scan can give the following information on:

Gestation How far your pregnancy is advanced and when your baby is expected to be born. In the first 4 months of pregnancy, there is very little variation in size between babies, so measurements of the biparietal diameter (the width of the baby's head), head circumference (the measurement around the baby's head), and femoral length (the length of the baby's thigh bone) give an accurate assessment of the baby's age. Before twelve weeks gestation, the width of the gestation sac or the crown-rump length (the distance from the top part of the baby's head to the point of its bottom) are used instead.

How many babies are in your womb Twins and higher multiples are usually detected at an early scan.

The position of the placenta Usually the placenta is at the top of the womb, well away from the birth canal. If it is close to the cervix, you will need further scans and special care, possibly including observation as an in-patient, later in your pregnancy. An ultrasound scan to locate the placenta is also essential for chorionic villus sampling.

Whether your womb is a normal shape Occasionally, some women have a partially divided womb, or even two separate wombs side by side. In most cases this does not cause any problems, but it can lead to an increased risk of miscarriage and caesarean section which may be something you would need to consider.

Fibroids These are very common benign tumours of the muscle wall of the womb. They do not normally cause problems, but occasionally they can cause pain during pregnancy, premature labour, or they can, very rarely, block the birth canal.

Abnormalities in the baby Conditions such as spina bifida and cysts in the kidneys, can be detected on a routine ultrasound scan. Approximately 50 per cent of heart defects can also be detected this way.

How well the baby is growing in the third trimester of pregnancy This is especially useful if you have a multiple pregnancy, as it is impossible for doctors and midwives to assess the growth of each individual baby just by examining your abdomen.

The volume of the amniotic fluid It is possible to estimate the amount of amniotic fluid present using ultrasound – if there is too much or too little fluid, there may be a problem with the baby. Should amniocentesis be necessary ultrasound can help locate the biggest pools of amniotic fluid.

What does an ultrasound scan not show?

An ultrasound scan cannot show up disorders caused by abnormalities of the body chemistry, such as cystic fibrosis, phenylketonuria, or sickle cell disease. Many of these conditions only become obvious after the baby is born. It may not show up minor problems such as fused or extra fingers or toes, cleft lip, or hypospadias (an abnormality of the shape of the penis in baby boys).

Can I choose not to have any ultrasound scans?

Yes. Although you will be counselled about your decision to decline what professionals believe to be a safe and informative test, ultimately the decision is yours.

If I have all of my antenatal care from the community midwives, does that mean I won't be able to have scans?

No, community midwives are able to organise routine ultrasound scans. However, if the scan shows any problems which need to be followed up, you will need to be referred to a consultant obstetrician for this part of your care. This will be organised by either your community midwife or your GP. You can still have most of your antenatal checks by your community midwife, and hospital booking does not commit you to giving birth in hospital. Maternity services are organised to allow you to make choices about your care at every stage of your pregnancy.

What is Triple Testing?

The most widely used screen to see if CVS or amniocentisis is appropriate is alpha-feto protein testing, a maternal blood test. This test can give an indication of the risk of neural tube disorders, such as spina bifida, and also of the risk of Down's Syndrome. To get a more reliable indication for Down's Syndrome, one or two maternal hormone tests can be performed at the same time. This is known as double, triple or even quadruple testing. Triple testing is the most widely available screen for Down's Syndrome. Once you have undergone a screening you will be told the likelihood of serious abnormalities in the fetus. If the risk is sufficiently high, you may be advised to have an amniocentesis or chorionic villus sampling test (see below), however you are free to refuse at any stage.

What are the blood tests at 16 weeks for?

At around 16 weeks into your pregnancy, you will be offered the following blood tests:

A test to find out your blood group, and whether you are rhesus positive or negative.

In the UK, about one person in six is rhesus negative, and if you are a blood donor this information will be on your donor card. It is a harmless genetic variation under most circumstances. However, it becomes important if you need to have a blood transfusion (when it is important that you are given only rhesus negative blood) or when you are pregnant. If your baby is rhesus positive and a few of its blood cells get into your circulation, your body will recognise that they are not yours and make antibodies against them. This is called iso-immunisation. These antibodies can get across the placenta into your baby's circulation and break down your baby's blood cells, causing severe anaemia and even death. In addition, once you have made rhesus antibodies they are permanent, so future rhesus positive babies will also be affected. However, this can be prevented from happening by the routine administration by injection of a substance called anti-D at 28 and 34 weeks gestation. Anti-D may also be given at various other times during your pregnancy, including:

- If you have any vaginal bleeding.
- If you have chorionic villus sampling, amniocentesis, or external cephalic version.
- If you have a miscarriage or termination.
- When your baby is born, a blood sample will be taken from the umbilical cord to check your baby's blood group and rhesus factor. If the baby is also rhesus negative, you do not need to have another dose of anti-D. If he is rhesus positive, you will be given a dose of anti-D within 72 hours of delivery.
- If the father of your baby is also rhesus negative, your baby will definitely be rhesus negative. However, you will still be offered anti-D routinely. In this situation, if you are absolutely sure of your baby's paternity, you can safely decide not to have anti-D.
- In the reverse situation, where you are rhesus positive and your baby is rhesus negative, iso-immunisation does not occur, so you will not need anti-D if you are rhesus positive.

A test for anaemia. If you are anaemic due to lack of iron, you may be prescribed iron tablets. Looking pale and feeling tired or faint do not necessarily indicate anaemia. If you are not anaemic, you will not benefit from iron tablets, and they can make any pregnancy-induced indigestion and constipation you may already be suffering from worse.

In some areas, a test to see whether you are a carrier of an inherited blood condition called sickle cell disease. If you are of African, Caribbean, Asian or Mediterranean descent and are not offered this test, ask for it. Your partner should arrange to be tested too.

A test for immunity to rubella (German measles).
A test to see if you are carrying any infections which might be passed to your baby. These include syphilis and, in some areas, hepatitis B and HIV. Testing for HIV is offered to all pregnant women as the risk of fetal infection is significantly reduced if diagnosed and treated effectively.

AFP and HCG levels, to assess your risk of having a baby with Down's Syndrome, spina bifida, or several other less common problems.

Rather than giving me anti-D which I might not need, wouldn't it be better to find out the baby's blood group in advance?

No. Finding out the blood group of an unborn baby involves invasive tests such as chorionic villus sampling, which can actually cause iso-immunisation and carries the risk of miscarriage, whereas it is safe to have anti-D even if you discover later that your baby was rhesus negative.

Can I choose not to have these blood tests?

Yes. Although most of the tests are uncontroversial and have the potential to benefit you and your baby, a significant minority of parents have ethical doubts about the AFP and HCG test and choose not to have it. If you are not sure whether you want this test, discuss it with your GP or midwife, or ask for an information leaflet when you attend the hospital.

What if the blood tests show that my baby is at high risk of Down's Syndrome or spina bifida?

The blood tests cannot diagnose these conditions, they can only indicate whether or not your baby is at high risk. If this is the case, you will be offered an amniocentesis. This is a test in which the specialist, guided by an ultrasound scan, puts a needle through your abdomen and takes a sample of the amniotic fluid that surrounds the baby. Testing this fluid provides more definitive information than the blood tests. An amniocentesis is a relatively safe test in expert hands, although it will cause a miscarriage in around one woman in 100.

Can I refuse to have an amniocentesis even if I'm at high risk?

Most maternity units recognise that parents find it difficult to decide whether or not to have an amniocentesis, and offer counselling and support. They may suggest that, even if you would not terminate an affected pregnancy, you might want to know in advance whether there is a problem, and the reassurance of a normal amniocentesis may help you to relax and enjoy the rest of your pregnancy. If you do decide not to have an amniocentesis, however, you should not be put in the position of feeling that the professionals looking after you disapprove of your decision. Your care will not be compromised in any way.

Why are all mothers aged over 35 offered an amniocentesis?

The risk of Down's Syndrome and some other conditions affecting the baby's development rise as the mother's age increases. The 'cut off' for 'high risk' will vary from one hospital to another, depending on the laboratory and the particular procedures being performed. Those in the high risk category (roughly 5 per cent of those having the tests) will be offered an amniocentesis. It is entirely the mother's choice to have this test or not.

My blood test shows that I have a one in 200 risk of having a baby with Down's Syndrome. What does that mean?

This is higher than the usual cut-off level of one in 275 and places you in the high risk category, but it still means that your baby has a 99.5 per cent chance of not having Down's Syndrome.

When might I be offered chorionic villus sampling instead of amniocentesis?

Chorionic villus sampling (CVS), like amniocentesis, is used to diagnose abnormalities in the unborn baby. It involves putting a thin tube into your womb, either through your abdomen or through your cervix, and taking a sample of cells from the baby's side of the placenta. These can be tested for chromosomal abnormalities.

The advantage of CVS is that it can be done very early in pregnancy, although not before 11 weeks to avoid damaging the fetus. You are only likely to be offered this test if you already know that you are at high risk of having a baby with a genetic disorder such as Down's Syndrome. It is of no value in testing for conditions in which the chromosomes are normal, such as spina bifida.

Like amniocentesis, CVS causes a miscarriage in about one pregnancy in 100. Although a higher number of pregnancies – 2-3 in 100 – will miscarry after CVS, most of these would have happened anyway. Genetic mapping is allowing an ever increasing number of diseases to be identified by examining the chromosomes, so the potential uses of amniocentesis and CVS, and the resultant ethical questions, will increase over the next few years.

Antenatal Clinic Appointments

From about 20 weeks, you will start to make regular visits to your midwife or GP. The pattern varies slightly from hospital to hospital but will typically involve a visit every four weeks until 32 or 34 weeks, two weekly until 38 or 39 weeks and weekly thereafter.

What is the midwife looking at when they examine me at the antenatal clinic?
Your general condition Whether you look in good health, or fragile and tired.
Your blood pressure This will be measured every time you attend the antenatal clinic to detect pregnancy-induced hypertension (abnormally high blood pressure).
Your urine The midwife will ask you to do a urine dipstick test to check for two things:
Protein in your urine This can indicate a urinary tract infection (which can be confirmed by sending a urine sample to be examined in the microbiology laboratory), or can occur with pregnancy-induced hypertension. A trace of protein in the urine may, however, simply be due to contamination with a drop of vaginal discharge.

Glucose in your urine It is not unusual for a pregnant woman to have a trace of glucose in her urine, as glucose is more likely to leak through the kidneys into the urine during pregnancy. If glucose is present in the urine on two separate occasions, a glucose tolerance test is necessary to check for gestational diabetes.

The size and position of the baby The midwife will measure the height of your bump in inches or centimetres and compare it with the normal range. If you are more than 24 weeks pregnant, she will feel around your bump to try to work out the baby's position and, in particular, which part is pointing downwards towards your pelvis. Later in pregnancy, she will check your baby's head (or bottom) quite firmly to determine whether it is moving down into the pelvis (engaging).

The baby's heartbeat During the abdominal examination, the midwife will also listen to your baby's heartbeat with a trumpet-like stethoscope (pinard stethoscope) or a hand-held electronic machine called a doppler or Sonicaid.

Your legs The midwife will examine your legs for fluid retention and varicose veins.

When might I have an internal examination?

In some countries, women are still examined internally at every antenatal check. This is purely traditional and does not contribute any useful information about the health of the woman or her baby. Routine internal examination has never been a feature of antenatal care in the UK.

You might be asked to consent to an internal examination in the following circumstances for which you should be asked your consent:

To take a smear test If you have never had one before. However, it is usually best to defer a smear test until you are no longer pregnant provided your previous smear tests are normal.

If you bleed during pregnancy If you are more than 24 weeks pregnant, this will be investigated by a speculum examination, although you should not consent to a digital examination until you have had an ultrasound scan to check the position of the placenta.

If an ectopic (outside the womb) pregnancy is suspected
Although a transvaginal ultrasound scan is safer and more accurate.
If an ovarian cyst or a pelvic abscess is suspected Again, an
ultrasound scan is more reliable.

**If you have had a late miscarriage or termination in the past,
or if you have had an operation on your cervix following an
abnormal smear test** In these circumstances, the obstetrician will
need to assess whether it is worth putting a stitch into your cervix
to help support the weight of your pregnancy.
**If you think your waters have broken, but you are not in
labour** A speculum examination under sterile conditions can help
to distinguish between ruptured membranes and the much more
common leakage of urine.
**To check whether you are ready to go into labour or whether
induction of labour is likely to be successful**.

Antenatal Classes

What happens at antenatal classes?
Antenatal classes are normally organised and facilitated by midwives
by the National Childbirth Trust (NCT). All hospital maternity units
run antenatal classes, and in many areas it is possible to attend
classes run by community midwives in GPs' surgeries or health
centres. These are free of charge. If you would like to attend
antenatal classes, let your hospital or community midwife know as
early as possible, as they may not be offered automatically, especially
if this is not your first pregnancy.

Antenatal classes will cover what to expect as your pregnancy
progresses, during labour, and how to look after your new baby. They
normally include a tour of the delivery suite and tend to be lively
and interactive, giving you an opportunity to meet other women
who will have babies similar in age to your own. Antenatal classes
often hold reunions after all the babies are born, and can give rise to
lasting friendships.

Paula White's birth plan

I want to go into labour by myself if possible, but if induction is medically necessary I will accept it.

I would like to stay at home for as long as possible during labour, and to have a community midwife (Helen if possible) visit me. If she says I'm really in labour, I'll call Mum and ask her to come over and look after the children.

I want Richard to take me to hospital and stay with me during the birth. If he's not available, my friend Nasreen (mobile no. 0845 787546) will take me and stay with me until Richard can be contacted.

I want to try to cope without pain relief. If I'm really distressed, encourage me to use gas and air. On no account give me pethidine – it gave me hallucinations last time. If I need a caesarean section, I'd rather be put to sleep than have an epidural.

I don't mind a student (medical or midwifery) doing my delivery, as long as it's not their first time and they're supervised by a senior midwife. I also don't mind students observing. Everyone's got to learn.

I'd rather tear than have an episiotomy. If I do tear, I don't want it stitched unless it's enormous.

When the baby's head crowns, don't try to put my hand on it.

As soon as the baby is born, it should be held below the level of the placenta until the cord has stopped pulsating. And under no account put the baby on my tummy before the cord is cut.

I do not want to be told the sex of the baby – I want to discover it for myself.

I want Richard to take me home as soon as I've had a shower. It doesn't matter if the paediatrician hasn't been. My GP has promised to visit me and the baby at home and do the necessary check-ups.

Birth Story   Heidi Lawrence

I decided to attend antenatal classes because I wanted to meet other pregnant women; and I wanted to be prepared and informed about birth and postnatal care; and to continue to exercise and stay fit during pregnancy.

The midwife told me about my choices. I could attend free midwife-run parentcraft classes, which took place locally during the day, and included a session for partners and visits from a breastfeeding counselor and an aromatherapist. Or I could attend the classes run for a fee by the local branch of the NCT in the evenings. Evening classes meant my husband Patrick would be able to attend, and feeling that to be very important, we opted for the NCT.

The other couples in the classes were of a similar age to us and we all quickly got on well. Focusing on labour and birth can be daunting, especially for fathers who tend not to have read the books or talked to friends about their experiences, so to be with other first-time fathers eased some of the fear and apprehension. Indeed, the men seemed to bond better than the women, as they joked about taking gameboys in to the delivery room to while away the time, and worried about whether or not their cars would start.

The NCT classes were frank about the realities of labour and our instructor constantly sought ways to include the men in the discussions and to encourage them to talk about their roles. Patrick and I have drawn up a birth plan, and as a result of the classes Patrick now understands that it will be his job to make sure that it is adhered to as far as possible. There may be times when I won't be able to communicate with the hospital staff, and for him to be certain about the sort of intervention and pain relief I want is really crucial.

The early stages of labour are most likely to take place at home and the NCT classes have helped us prepare for that. We have bought lots more cushions as most of the labour positions suggested seem to involve plenty! We also learned that you only tend to get into those positions which you have practiced beforehand, and have been doing our 'homework', focusing on the general advice of staying active and allowing gravity to help labour along. Almost all the positions include a supporting role for the man or birth companion.

There is so much more that partners can do to help than either of us realized. We have learnt about massage and breathing, and the importance of encouragement and emotional support. On the way home from the classes we seem to find even more to talk about each week, and I feel that, although I will be the one experiencing the birth and the pain first-hand, my husband is now informed enough to be sympathetic, supportive and practical.

I have also been attending a local antenatal swimming class, which has been great for exercise and for meeting people – and means that only fellow whales can see you in your swimsuit. In addition, I have found the yoga classes run locally by the Active Birth Centre really useful for learning relaxation techniques to ease labour.

I really hope that we will see the people from some of these classes again after the baby is born, especially as we have only recently moved to Cornwall from London.

What is the NCT?

The National Childbirth Trust (NCT) is a UK wide self –
help charity run by parents for parents and its services
and support are open to all. For many new parents the
most important thing the NCT does is put them in touch
with other new parents. The NCT has always played an
important role in campaigning for improvements in
maternity services and parents' rights. Changes in health
care practice can be attributable to the NCT. For example,
the presence of fathers/partners at birth, babies being
given to mothers straight after birth and the fact that
enemas and shaving are no longer considered necessary
preparation for birth. The NCT is currently actively
campaigning for a midwife to be present for every woman
in labour, for an increase in availability of home births
and birth center births and for improvements to hospital
conditions to increase a woman's likelihood of a
straightforward vaginal birth.

Joining the NCT or contacting your local branch will
give you the opportunity to meet lots of other pregnant
women and their partners in your community. Most
branches can offer childbirth classes, new baby groups,

Can my partner come to antenatal classes with me?

Most classes welcome partners, and you should certainly encourage
your partner to attend with you as it will help him to feel more
closely involved with your pregnancy, to prepare him for the birth,
and to have the confidence to handle your newborn baby.
Although you are entitled to time off work to attend antenatal
classes, you partner isn't. Recognising this, 90 per cent of maternity
units hold classes in the evenings and 38 per cent hold classes at
weekends.

open house get-togethers, support for fathers, working parents' groups, nearly new sales of baby clothes and equipment, postnatal courses and drop-in sessions and a regular neighbourhood newsletter.

In addition to the local branch work the NCT provides:
- Trained antenatal teachers for you and your partner/birth helper
- Trained breastfeeding counsellors and a national breastfeeding phone line 0870 440 8708
- Useful goods e.g., specialist pregnancy bras, books, toys, baby goods
- A comprehensive information website
- A national New Generations magazine published quarterly for members

You can contact the NCT for an information pack by phoning 0870 444 8707 or 0870 990 8040 to join, alternatively email enquiries@national-childbirth-trust.co.uk. or visit www.nctpregnancyandbabycare.com, or www.nctms.co.uk

I'd feel uncomfortable in a class with other women's partners.
You're not the only woman who feels like this. Around 55 per cent of maternity units offer women-only classes so ask your midwife if there are any in your area. If you belong to an ethnic minority group, are expecting twins or are a teenager, there may also be a special class to suit your needs.

Miscarriage and Ectopic Pregnancy

What is a miscarriage?

A miscarriage occurs when a pregnancy ends spontaneously before the baby is mature enough to survive outside the womb. The earliest age at which a fetus can be considered capable of survival is 24 weeks gestation. Four out of five diagnosed miscarriages happen in the first 13 weeks of pregnancy.

Is it common?

At least one in five diagnosed pregnancies ends in miscarriage, and if we include the many pregnancies which fail to establish properly and are dismissed as 'late periods', the figure could be much higher.

Why do miscarriages happen?

Most miscarriages happen before 14 weeks gestation and are known as early miscarriages. These occur for the following reasons:

Abnormalities in the embryo. These account for 50-90 per cent of early miscarriages in different studies, and most are due to chromosomal abnormalities such as Down's Syndrome. The most extreme example of this is a blighted ovum, where the embryo dies and disintegrates, leaving a sac containing only placenta.

Some medical conditions in the mother such as diabetes, thyroid disease and SLE.

Infection with a wide range of bacteria and viruses, including food poisoning bacteria and influenza viruses.

Abnormalities in the shape of the inside of the womb which may be hereditary, or can result from the womb being distorted by fibroids.

Older mothers are at higher risk of miscarriage, possibly because their eggs are more likely to have chromosomal abnormalities.

Women who smoke are at increased risk of losing their baby at all stages of pregnancy, including by early miscarriage.

Poisons such as some prescribed drugs, herbal preparations (including certain aromatherapy oils) and x-rays.

How will I know if I'm having a miscarriage?

The commonest early sign is vaginal bleeding, which can vary from a light brownish discharge to very heavy bleeding with clots. The bleeding may be accompanied by period-like cramps.

What should I do if I discover that I'm bleeding?

Try not to panic. Fewer than half of bleeds in early pregnancy are followed by a miscarriage, although all episodes of bleeding are described as threatened miscarriages unless another diagnosis is obvious. If the bleeding is very heavy and accompanied by a lot of pain, you should go straight to the nearest accident and emergency department. It is possible to lose a great deal of blood with a miscarriage. Call an ambulance if you feel very unwell or if you do not have transport immediately available. On no account should you drive by yourself or try to travel by public transport. If the bleeding is light, with little or no pain, attend your GP's surgery (or have a telephone consultation with your GP) at the next available opportunity. If it happens at the weekend when the surgery is closed, you can safely wait until Monday morning provided the bleeding does not become heavier. If in doubt about what to do, telephone NHS Direct (0845 4647), where a trained nurse will be able to offer you advice and, if appropriate, reassurance.

Once you have seen your GP, they will offer you an ultrasound scan within 24-48 hours. Even if the bleeding is quite light, you are unlikely to be able to relax or stop worrying until you have had a scan and seen the baby's heartbeat.

If you suddenly develop very severe pain on one side of your lower abdomen, with little or no bleeding, call an ambulance – you may have an ectopic pregnancy.

After one miscarriage, am I at greater risk of having another?

Not significantly. Even after three consecutive miscarriages, there is still a 75 per cent chance that your next pregnancy will be successful.

What is an Early Pregnancy Assessment Unit (EPAU)?

This is a special clinic where women with problems in early

pregnancy can be seen and assessed quickly – often within hours of seeing their GP and being referred. Most maternity units have one, usually attached to the antenatal clinic. At the EPAU, you can expect to see a doctor or specially trained midwife, have a urine pregnancy test and an ultrasound scan performed, and, if necessary, have blood tests. If you are definitely having a miscarriage and it is not appropriate to let you go home, you will be admitted to hospital – either to an antenatal day case unit or to a gynaecology ward.

How long should I stay off work after a miscarriage?
You should be physically able to resume all of your normal activities – including work, sport, driving and sex – within two weeks. However, you might find it psychologically difficult to come to terms with the loss of your baby. If this is a major problem and is stopping you from carrying out your normal daily routine, ask your GP if you could be referred for counselling.

Why did my doctor tell me not to become pregnant for three months after my miscarriage?
This advice is commonly given, and may date back to the days when women were poorly nourished, often miscarried without medical support and lost a lot of blood. For most women nowadays, it is unnecessary. Your first period after the miscarriage is a sign that your hormone cycle has resumed and that your body is ready to cope with another pregnancy. It is less easy to predict when you will be psychologically ready. Some couples want to conceive again at the earliest opportunity, while others feel the need to grieve for several months for the baby they have lost before moving on.

Will I have tests to find out why I had the miscarriage?
Having one or two miscarriages is very common and does not increase the risk of future miscarriages so tests are not usually offered after a first or second early miscarriage. If you have three consecutive miscarriages, tests will be done to ensure that neither you nor your partner has a medical problem. In most women who

have had three or more consecutive miscarriages, all the tests are normal and they go on to have a successful pregnancy.

What is an ectopic pregnancy?

Ectopic pregnancy occurs when the fertilised egg implants somewhere other than in the womb. Most commonly this occurs in the fallopian tube; very rarely it is in the ovary or on the lining of the abdominal cavity.

Why is this so dangerous?

The womb is uniquely designed to expand to hold a full-term baby, and its blood vessels can enlarge to deliver an adequate blood supply to the growing baby and placenta. The fallopian tube is a tiny structure – inside, it is no wider than a drinking straw – and by 6-8 weeks gestation the embryo in its sac is big enough to stretch, and then to break through, its thin walls. This process is accompanied by bleeding into the abdominal cavity. Several litres of blood can easily be lost this way.

How will I know if I have an ectopic pregnancy?

The levels of pregnancy hormones tend to be lower, so you may have few early pregnancy symptoms – however, these vary so much from one woman – and one pregnancy – to another, that this is an unreliable way of making the diagnosis. The usual first symptom is pain to one side of your lower abdomen. At first this might come and go, or be quite mild. Alternatively, if the fallopian tube bursts you will suddenly develop very severe pain and feel faint and sick. Vaginal bleeding may occur, but is rarely heavy.

What should I do if I suspect I have an ectopic pregnancy?

If your pain is mild, see your GP as soon as possible (use the out of hours service or go to the accident and emergency department on weekends and public holidays). He will ask for the date of your last period and whether you have had a positive pregnancy test, and will examine your abdomen. He may also give you an internal examination, but many doctors believe that internal examinations are risky when an ectopic pregnancy is suspected. Unless he is confident that you do not have an ectopic pregnancy, he will refer you immediately to the EPAU or the duty gynaecologist.

If you have sudden, severe pain, call an ambulance and get someone to stay with you in case you become unconscious.

Will I need an operation?

Not necessarily. Some early ectopic pregnancies are broken down and reabsorbed by the body, and close observation with repeated ultrasound scans and blood tests to measure hormone levels may be sufficient. However, in most cases, an operation is needed. If the fallopian tube is still intact, the sac can be removed through a small incision or injected with a substance which will destroy it – either a strong salt or glucose solution or a drug called methotrexate. This may be done by keyhole surgery. If the fallopian tube has burst, an operation will be done to remove the part of the fallopian tube which contains the ectopic pregnancy. The gynaecologist will always try to save as much of the fallopian tube as possible, and your ovary will not normally be removed. You will have a 10-15cm horizontal cut just within the top margin of your pubic hair, and will need 3-5 days in hospital and up to 6 weeks off work.

Will I have more difficulty becoming pregnant again after an ectopic pregnancy?

It is more likely that you will have difficulty getting pregnant naturally after an ectopic pregnancy, especially if you needed an operation or if there is damage to both fallopian tubes. However, many women do go on to have a normal pregnancy without medical intervention. As the risk of a further ectopic pregnancy is quite high (one in ten), you should ask your GP to refer you to the early pregnancy assessment unit for a scan as soon as you know that you are pregnant – ideally within six weeks of the first day of your last period.

Late Miscarriages

Why do late miscarriages happen?

Late miscarriages – miscarriages occurring between 15 and 24 weeks gestation – are much less common than early miscarriages. They occur for the following reasons:

The contents of the womb become too heavy and force the cervix to open This happens very rarely in cases of large multiple pregnancy or if you have had surgery on your cervix in the past – the most common reasons for this would be to remove precancerous cells (an operation called a cone biopsy) or to perform a late termination of pregnancy. In this situation, the weakened cervix cannot support the growing weight of the fetus(es), placenta and fluid sac, and responds by dilating. There is no evidence that early termination of pregnancy (before 14 weeks gestation) increases the likelihood of miscarriage in future pregnancies.

Infections including severe urinary tract infections, gastroenteritis, and viruses which damage the baby and placenta. A condition called bacterial vaginosis, which results from overgrowth of a range of bowel bacteria in the vagina and which is normally harmless although inclined to cause a smelly discharge, increases the risk of late miscarriage.

Foetal abnormalities, although chromosomal abnormalities are less common in second trimester miscarriages than in first trimester miscarriages.

Placental failure Sometimes in the second trimester the placenta becomes incapable of carrying enough oxygen and food to the fetus, which is effectively starved to death. A tight knot which prevents the flow of blood through the umbilical cord can have the same effect.

Smoking, excessive alcohol intake and use of narcotics all increase the risk of late miscarriage.

Injury Although the fetus is very well protected by its fluid sac and the bony shell of the mother's pelvis, there have been occasional cases of late miscarriage following falls (typically downstairs or from a height), car crashes and even sudden severe psychological shocks.

Birth Story Sarah Arden

MISCARRIAGE is no fun at all. It may be sudden and painful, as my first one was. Or it may be slow and painless, as with my second. Both occurred at 10 weeks.

When you have one, you find no context in which to place your emotions. There is a miscarriage support group which your GP can put you in touch with, but you may not feel that this private sorrow is something you want to share with others. There may be very few people in your life who even knew you were pregnant. Those whom you have told are embarrassed and clumsy in their responses to your bad news.

Is it something to mourn about ? After all, this is the death of a baby. Already, even in a couple of months, you and your family have made plans and adjusted relationships in anticipation of its arrival. There was such hopeful optimism in the air, now turned to misery. But that baby was much younger in its stage of development than the age acceptable for deliberate abortion.

Is it something 'Nature intended'? This is what the doctor will probably reassure you with – the statistic of 1 in 5 pregnancies ending in miscarriage. Nature flushes out the damaged or weak embryos. You are somehow relieved that this one went now, rather than later when you loved it even more.

Should you worry that there is something wrong with you rather than the child ? With my second miscarriage they scanned me carefully and revealed some sort of kink at the top of my womb –'look, your womb is heart-shaped !' the radiographer announced. For me it might be a reason for my failure to retain my embryos, perhaps even a reason that I don't get pregnant more easily. 'Opinions differ' said the registrar.

The fact is that out of three pregnancies, one of mine has been supremely successful – a happy, healthy 40-week pregnancy, an exciting delivery and an adorable, sunny daughter to enjoy. My statistic ups the average – mine, so far, is 2 in 3 pregnancies ending in miscarriage. But I know someone who has had 6 miscarriages. My grandmother had seven, and two children. Some people seem to be prone to them. I have now met people with this same strangely shaped uterus, both of whom suffered miscarriages and both of whom had operations to flatten out the kink. One of them is now expecting her second child. I think I will wait for one more miscarriage at least before I will plead for the operation. For me, miscarriage is the greatest mystery around the miracle of birth. Being fit and happy and retaining hopeful optimism is the only way to deal with it.

Uterine abnormality Rarely, exceptionally large fibroids are associated with late miscarriage, as are recurrent episodes of vaginal bleeding, even if the cause of the bleeding has not been determind.

How will I know if I'm having a late miscarriage?

The symptoms can be very variable, and you may not bleed in the early stages, although you should seek urgent medical attention if you have any vaginal bleeding during the second trimester of your pregnancy. You may stop 'feeling pregnant' and your bump may become a little smaller. Some women do not realise that they are miscarrying until their waters suddenly break and they pass a tiny but recognisable fetus attached to its umbilical cord. You may have pain – early in the second trimester this takes the form of period-like cramps – but from about 18 weeks you can have recognisable contractions. You may notice a watery discharge which can be pink, brown, or bloodstained.

Will the miscarriage be complete?

Probably not. In the second trimester, the placenta is not ready to separate from the wall of the womb. This means that the womb cannot contract properly and there is a serious risk of heavy bleeding. Most women will need an operation under general or epidural anaesthetic to remove the placenta after a second trimester miscarriage.

What should I do if I have a late miscarriage at home?

Seek medical attention urgently – call an ambulance or ask for a visit from your GP or midwife. Lie down and do not have anything to eat or drink.

If I have bleeding in the second trimester, should I go to the EPAU?

Ask your midwife for advice. In many hospitals, women who are more than 20 weeks into their pregnancy and are at risk of miscarriage are assessed on the labour ward rather than in the EPAU.

Why is this? I didn't think babies could survive if they were born before 24 weeks.

Between 20 and 23 weeks, a baby is not mature enough to be kept alive even with access to the full range of high-tech medical intervention in the Neonatal Intensive Care Unit (NICU). However, from the mother's point of view the labour ward, with access to operating theatres, good pain relief (including epidural anaesthesia) and regular attention from midwives and obstetricians, is the safest place to be.

I'd get very upset being on the labour ward and hearing other babies crying while I was losing mine. Is there any alternative?

If you cannot cope with being on the labour ward, ask if you could be offered a side room or even an amenity bed on the general gynaecology ward. Having a late miscarriage is unspeakably distressing, and the staff should make every effort to ensure that you have privacy and do not have to share a room with women who are in normal term labour or are looking after their babies.

Will tests be done to find out why I had the miscarriage?

In all second trimester miscarriages, tests are carried out on both the mother and the fetus to try to find a reason for the miscarriage. These include:

Blood tests to see whether you might have rhesus antibodies or had an infection such as listeria, toxoplasmosis, cytomegalovirus or rubella – all of which cause no symptoms at all or a minor flu-like illness in a healthy adult, but which can damage the fetus and placenta so severely that miscarriage results.

A detailed post-mortem examination on the fetus and placenta. Often, however, no explanation for the miscarriage is discovered.

Will I be able to see and hold my baby after a late miscarriage?

Yes. In fact, you will normally be encouraged to do so. Distressing though it might be, seeing and holding the baby helps you to give it a real identity and to know who you are grieving for.

Birth Story Cathy Lawrence

I had my first baby in the United Sates, followed by two very different pregnancy experiences in the UK. The first (a miscarriage at a London hospital) was frustrating and frightening and engendered a feeling of powerlessness. The second (a complicated pregnancy and planned caesarean as a private patient) was characterized at all times by a dialogue with the doctors which kept me feeling involved, informed and calm during my pregnancy and delivery.

When I rang my local hospital one morning to say that I was newly pregnant and experiencing heavy bleeding, the registrar told me to come in immediately. However, I wasn't seen by a doctor until the evening, and then he couldn't tell me what was happening, only that I needed to stay in for observation. I went into the ward, sat on the bed and immediately stepped in a puddle of unidentified liquid. Alongside it under the bed were two bloody bandages, several dead bugs and some rubbish. Although this was distressing, what was worse was not knowing what was happening.

Over the next three days, I saw three different doctors, none of whom appeared to be communicating. When I asked questions, they seemed slightly surprised, and generally gave me simplistic, unsatisfactory answers. They finally decided on keyhole surgery to determine whether or not the pregnancy was ectopic, but were not able to do it for three more days. After all this uncertainty and waiting, I broke down in tears and said to the doctor, 'I can't wait. I need this surgery right away. I have to get home.' To which he replied, 'Why, what do you do?' I explained that I was a wife and mother and needed to get back to my family. He sighed and said 'Oh, that.' Astonished at this dismissal of my distress, I insisted that there must be a way to be seen more quickly, and as a result had the procedure done privately the following day. The (non-ectopic) miscarriage occurred without any further incident, but the whole experience left me feeling exhausted, depressed, and very uncomfortable with the care that I had received.

When I became pregnant again, I went to a private consultant at a private hospital in London who had been recommended by a friend. I was seen regularly, and when complications arose, we were kept informed in a thorough, non-patronizing fashion, and invited to discuss available options. When my baby was found to be in a particularly difficult breech position, the consultant spent weeks helping us consider all the options, and together we decided to go for a planned caesarean.

When the day came, I knew exactly what to expect. My consultant had explained the operation in detail, and I had been on a tour of the spotless labour ward and operating theatre, and been told where it was in relation to the NICU should the baby need emergency care. As a consequence of this open channel of communication, I was absolutely confident that we were doing the best thing possible for our baby.

I know there must be many reasons why the doctors and staff at my local hospital didn't have the time or resources to answer my queries properly, or to clean under the bed. But surely this communication between doctor and patient should be a priority for the medical community at large, not just those treating the ones who have access to private care.

Can I have a religious burial service for my baby?

Although a baby born dead before 24 weeks is not legally entitled to a burial, you will almost certainly find that your local church, mosque or temple has encountered this situation before and can offer an appropriate formal burial ceremony.

After a late miscarriage, can I have maternity leave?

No. However, you may not feel ready to return to work for several weeks afterwards and you should ask your GP to give you a sick note. For information and support you can contact The Miscarriage Association, tel 01924 200799.

High Blood Pressure in Pregnancy

Why do I have my blood pressure checked every time I go to the antenatal clinic?

High blood pressure develops in about one pregnancy in ten and is more common in first pregnancies. If not diagnosed early and managed properly, the consequences for both mother and baby can be very serious.

Why does high blood pressure develop in pregnancy?

Over the years, many theories have been suggested. It is currently thought that if the placenta fails to embed properly into the muscular wall of the womb, a cascade of abnormalities follow which leads to high blood pressure and other features such as protein in the urine, fluid retention, and sometimes abnormal liver and kidney function and a low platelet count in the blood. This collection of symptoms and signs is sometimes called pre-eclampsia or pre-eclamptic toxaemia. High blood pressure in pregnancy is not caused by stress, going out to work, taking insufficient rest, or anything else that you might have done. The process begins in the first few weeks after conception, and nobody knows the underlying cause.

If that's pre-eclampsia, what is eclampsia?

Eclampsia is a very dangerous condition which may follow pre-eclampsia, although high blood pressure in pregnancy is now treated so seriously that eclampsia is most likely to occur without warning after delivery, or in women who have not had antenatal care. Eclampsia occurs when a woman has a convulsion due to high blood pressure during, or immediately after, pregnancy.

Who is at risk of pre-eclampsia?

The risk is highest in the following situations:

First ever pregnancy, or first pregnancy with a new partner. Even a previous early miscarriage or termination offers protection against pre-eclampsia.

Extreme age range for childbearing – mothers in their teens and in their forties, although women of any age can be affected.

High blood pressure (hypertension) that was present before pregnancy.

Multiple pregnancy.

Diabetes, either gestational diabetes or diabetes which predates the pregnancy.

Sickle cell disease.

Pre-eclampsia in a previous pregnancy There is about a one in five risk of recurrence in the next pregnancy, although it is likely to develop later in the pregnancy and to be less severe. Women who did not have pre-eclampsia in their first pregnancy are very unlikely to develop the condition in subsequent pregnancies fathered by the same partner.

Is it possible to tell early in pregnancy whether I am at risk of pre-eclampsia?

There is no reliable screening test and there are no known interventions that can prevent pre-eclampsia from developing. In women at high risk, ultrasound scanning of the uterine artery may be beneficial.

What will happen if I develop pre-eclampsia?

The only effective treatment for pre-eclampsia is to deliver you, but

Birth Story   Emma Field

I had a normal pregnancy up until 38 weeks, when routine antenatal tests revealed raised blood pressure and traces of protein in my urine, both symptoms of pre-eclampsia. I went to hospital to be monitored.

I was allowed home, but told to return that afternoon as my blood tests showed definite protein, and my increasing blood pressure was making my face, hands and legs swell. The registrar examined me and we decided to induce labour. By 6pm I was in the delivery suite and realising that I wouldn't be having the active birth I'd planned, as I had to be closely monitored. I was calm and understood what was happening, thanks to my NCT classes. I was given a pessary to induce labour, but by late evening nothing had happened so we waited until morning to try again, and I was given a sleeping tablet (which didn't help, and probably slowed the baby down).

At 8am the next day they gave me a second pessary, which didn't work either, so they decided to induce me by drip. I was given an epidural to keep my blood pressure down and ease what could be a fast and therefore painful labour. Then after an internal examination, my waters were broken, and I was put on an oxytocin drip and surrounded by equipment. But by 3pm, 20 hours after the induction started, I was still only 2cm dilated, so we decided on a caesarean. Again, I was fairly calm, as I knew what was going on, but my husband was very anxious.

The operation was quick and my husband took photographs, which I found helpful later, especially one of the cord being cut. There was a frightening moment when I was expecting to hear her cry but didn't. I later learned that the cord was around her neck and she had swallowed meconium, so she was very distressed. Her initial Apgar score was 2, (her second score was much higher), and she weighed 5lb 12oz, low, but not too low – typical of pre-eclampsia. I saw her briefly before she went to special care for examination, and she and my husband were in the delivery suite when I returned.

The next 24 hours were painful, my body was in shock, and I did not get out of bed, which made breastfeeding a dazed baby impossible. Eventually, I was moved to the maternity ward, but breastfeeding was still a struggle, as Isabel slept a lot, and wouldn't latch on. So, as well as breastfeeding, I expressed colostrum and then milk, feeding her with a syringe and then with bottles. I found it all very confusing, as each shift brought a different midwife with different ideas, and I didn't know what to believe. I wanted to learn how to breastfeed Isabel, and needed to stick at it to sustain and increase my milk flow, but it was difficult as my milk production was hindered both by the blood pressure drug and the fact that I hadn't experienced the milk-producing stimulus of labour.

On leaving hospital Isabel's weight dropped to 5lb 4oz, and under pressure from the visiting midwives, I gave her formula, which didn't help, so I continued breastfeeding and expressing. After four weeks she regained her birth weight. I felt under constant pressure about her weight, although she thrived, and at six weeks began topping her up with a bottle after breastfeeding, and managed to keep this up for eight months.

if you are less than 34 weeks pregnant this has to be balanced against the risks to your baby of being born prematurely.

Symptoms such as headache, vomiting and abdominal pain are worrying. Your blood will be tested to check liver, kidney and clotting factors. You may be given medication and steroids to help mature your baby's lungs if premature delivery is being considered. If delivery is required, a decision will be made as to whether attempted vaginal delivery or caesarean section is best, depending on the circumstances.

In most instances, pre-eclampsia is less severe than this, and the high blood pressure is treated with bedrest (often at home, although if you cannot rest at home you may be admitted to hospital), regular blood pressure measurements, urine tests, scans and CTGs, and possibly medication such as methyldopa or labetalol. If your blood pressure does not settle down, if you pass increasing amounts of protein in your urine, or if your baby stops growing, you will be delivered urgently.

Can I have an epidural in labour?

Yes, provided your blood clotting tests are normal. Most obstetricians advise women with pre-eclampsia to consider epidural anaesthesia as it can help to lower the blood pressure.

I suffer from high blood pressure when I'm not pregnant. What should I do?

Ideally, see your GP or specialist before becoming pregnant. Some of the drugs used to treat high blood pressure should not be taken during pregnancy, so your medication may need to be changed.

Once you are pregnant, you will be monitored very carefully because you are at increased risk of developing pregnancy-induced hypertension and having a small baby, especially if your high blood pressure is due to an underlying problem such as kidney disease. You may be seen jointly by a physician and obstetrician when you attend the antenatal clinic.

If I need medication for high blood pressure after my baby is born, will I be able to breastfeed?

Yes. The amount of blood pressure medication that is passed into the breast milk is insufficient to harm your baby.

Section Two:
Giving Birth

Hospital Birth

When should I go into hospital?

When you are sure you are in labour – this generally means when your contractions become stronger and more frequent, maybe lasting 20 to 40 seconds every 5 to 10 minutes. For a time you may feel unsure. Time the contractions occasionally. At the start of the first stage of labour your contractions may last 10 to 40 seconds every 20 to 30 minutes. You can call your midwife or the hospital at any time for information and advice. If your waters break but contractions have not become established within four hours, or if you have fresh red bleeding with or without pain, you should also go to hospital. You will usually have been advised to telephone the hospital in advance to confirm that you really should come in and to let them know when you are arriving.

If I call an ambulance because I have a pregnancy-related problem, will I be taken to the hospital where I am booked?

Not necessarily. If you are booked at a hospital which is a long way from where you live, the ambulance crew will take you to the unit closest to the address from which they pick you up. If you decide to book at a hospital which is not your local one, you will need to be able to provide your own transport.

Can I go to hospital by taxi?

Yes. It is safe to travel by taxi provided you are able to walk, your waters have not broken, and you are not bleeding. If your waters have broken, you are at increased risk of infection. It is worth checking with local taxi firms in advance to find out which ones are happy to transport a woman in labour.

My partner plans to take me to the hospital by car. What do we need to find out in advance?

You should familiarise yourself with the quickest route to the hospital – and an alternative route in case there are road-works. Find out where parking spaces are most reliably available in the hospital grounds. This may not always be in the main car park.

Most hospitals now charge for parking, so find out the cost and keep a supply of coins with your hospital bag. Many units will allow your partner to stop briefly outside the maternity unit, so that you do not have to walk too far, and then go and park the car once you are in the care of a midwife.

What will happen if it's a false alarm?
If you arrive at the hospital and your contractions stop, you will have a CTG (a trace of the baby's heartbeat) and, if this is normal, you may choose to go home. In late pregnancy, you may have runs of Braxton-Hicks ('practice') contractions, and these can be quite painful, so false alarms are not uncommon. If in doubt, it is better to present unnecessarily to the labour ward than to have an unplanned home birth. An alternative course of action if you are not sure whether or not you are in labour is to contact your community midwife. Check whether she provides this service before you go into labour, but she may be able to visit you and do an internal examination to assess the condition of your cervix (whether or not it is beginning to dilate). In some areas it is considered preferable for the midwife to visit you at home during early labour.

What will happen when I am admitted to hospital in labour?
You will be seen by a midwife, who will ask when your contractions started, and/or when your waters broke, and if the waters are clear. She will quickly check your notes to see if any problems are anticipated and examine your abdomen and perform a vaginal examination. She will want to check your baby's heartbeat and the strength and frequency of your contractions. This can be done with a hand-held stethoscope (Pinard) or sonicaid. If you decide to have any continuous electronic monitoring, ensure that you are in an upright position when it is done. If all is not well, or problems have been identified antenatally, she will call the duty obstetrician. If you are only in the earliest stages of labour you may be much more comfortable at home. However, if you cannot or do not want to go home, you will be admitted to the antenatal ward until your labour is established.

Sometimes, if your labour has progressed particularly quickly, there will be no time to do any more than examine you, ask if you need gas and air pain relief, listen to the baby's heartbeat, and tell you to push.

If I am admitted to the antenatal ward, will my partner be allowed to stay with me?

Around 50 per cent or maternity units allow your partner to stay with you on the antenatal ward. In other units however, your partner will only be permitted on the ward during set visiting hours except in special circumstances in which you might need his support as having partners in the ward at all times may upset other women. If you are in labour and likely to be transferred to the labour ward in the next hour or two, the antenatal ward staff will usually exercise discretion and allow your partner to stay with you.

What is an amenity room?

An amenity room is a private room on the main antenatal or postnatal ward of the hospital. It is a single room usually with its own toilet and bath or shower, and may be equipped to a higher standard than other rooms – for example, you may have your own television. For nursing and medical care, you are treated as an NHS patient, however, you will need to pay for the room. Charges vary between hospitals, but an amenity room typically costs less than an equivalent room in a private hospital. The average price is £45 but prices vary from £15 to £525. If you stay in an amenity room, your family will be subject to the same visiting restrictions as the rest of the ward.

How do I arrange to stay in an amenity room?

First, ensure that you book at a hospital which has amenity rooms – 61 per cent of maternity units have them. Look up your local hospitals in this guide, or contact the hospitals directly. Your community midwife may be able to give you more information.

If you know when your baby will be born – if you are having an elective caesarean section or induction of labour – book an amenity

Giving Birth in Hospital

Pros

- You have the reassurance of easy access to high-tech intervention, should you need it.
- Specialists in obstetrics, paediatrics and anaesthetics are always available in the hospital.
- The hospital may have a neonatal unit on the same site.
- Most consultant-led units can offer a wide range of birth choices, from waterbirth and moxibustion through to caesarean section.
- If you have a multiple pregnancy, a breech baby or a serious medical problem of your own, a consultant-led unit is the best option.

Cons

- You may not have the same midwife throughout your delivery.
- Decisions may sometimes be made by relatively junior obstetricians rather than by experienced midwives.
- You may be more likely to have interventions such as having your waters broken, being monitored continuously and having forceps or a caesarean section.
- You will give birth in an environment which is likely to be completely alien to you. Your partner may not be able to stay with you at all times during early labour.

room as soon as possible. If you are admitted to the antenatal ward as an emergency and would like an amenity bed, tell the midwife in charge.

It is rarely possible to guarantee that an amenity room will be available when you want one. If a woman with a medical reason for needing a single room is admitted at the same time as you, she will be given priority.

Birth Story Josie Mathews

I was six days overdue with my second child when, having had no sign of impending labour, I sensed that things might be about to happen. Although to begin with my contractions were only mild, by the morning of the next day, they seemed to be getting stronger, and at about 8am we went to the hospital. I had opted for GP/midwife shared care, and was also pretty familiar with the hospital as my son had been born there.

The midwife who examined me said that I was only 1cm dilated and that with any luck my baby would be born that evening. She suggested that we'd be better off at home. Back at home, the labour seemed to be progressing, and although the pain was bearable, the contractions were coming fairly regularly every ten minutes. At midday I called the hospital, but was told to stay at home. An hour later I called again, but was told that it still did not sound as if I was in proper labour. By 1.30, the contractions were coming every five minutes and I called the hospital saying that I wanted to come in, even if I still had a long way to go.

I can remember the 20 minute car journey vividly, as by now the contractions were really quite painful. We got to the hospital, and after searching desperately for a space in the underground car park, my husband stopped the car. By now, the pain had reached its height and I said to him, 'I am definitely getting an epidural if it's going to be like this.' I climbed out of the car, and as I did so, my waters broke. Instantly, I knew that the baby was coming. My husband started calling for help, and trying to find the lift, but I refused to move. I put my hands between my legs, felt that the baby's head had crowned, and had the most overwhelming urge to push.

Meanwhile, a couple of passers-by had gathered, and one man who was fixing a car threw a dirty old rug beneath me. I could not lie down, however, and the urge to push was too much, so I pushed out the baby's head, and then, remembering vaguely that the rest would slither out of its own accord, I tried to pant and not push too fast. Nevertheless, the rest of her shot out pretty quickly, fortunately landing, on the old car rug (not the tarmac) and on her back, whereupon the cord snapped. She gave the most almighty yell, and I had a gut feeling that she was fine. In fact, I had remained remarkably calm throughout, and I remember picking her up, discovering to my delight that she was a girl and standing, rather dazed, with my trousers around my ankles for about five minutes, until a security guard who had seen the whole thing on CCTV, turned up with a wheelchair, closely followed by a midwife.

All in all, the experience turned out to be a positive one, if a little strange. The labour was only really painful for the last 20 minutes. If I have another child, however, I think I'm going to have a home birth. I love hospitals, and have no theories about invasive or non-invasive, drugs or no drugs, water, joss sticks or ambient music. I just don't want to risk having my next one in the car.

What are the three stages of labour?

Labour is traditionally divided into three stages, although it is rarely possible to identify the exact time at which the first stage and the second stage begin.

- **First stage** This is the longest part of labour, lasting from 6 to 20 hours in a normal first delivery. It starts when labour begins – usually with the onset of regular painful contractions, although sometimes the waters break first. During this first stage, your cervix will gradually become softer and thinner, and the small hole in the middle will open up until it is impossible to feel the cervix on an internal examination. This is called full dilatation and means that the opening out of the womb is 10cm in diameter and big enough to allow the baby's head to pass through.

- **Second stage** This lasts from the time the cervix becomes fully dilated until the baby is born – it can last from 10 minutes to 2 hours although this takes longer with an epidural. During the second stage, the contractions become stronger and push the baby's head downwards. As the head moves down, it stretches the pelvic floor and, unless you have had an epidural, causes an urge to bear down (to push) which is impossible to resist. Bearing down in sync with your contractions helps the baby to be born. After the head has emerged, the pain caused by its head stretching the perineum is suddenly relieved, and the rest of the baby's body normally slips out without any difficulty. Most midwives and obstetricians will put your baby straight on to your abdomen before cutting the umbilical cord. If you do not want this, include it in your birth plan, and ask your birth companion to mention it in the delivery room. After the cord is cut, if your baby is well (usually indicated by vigorous crying) she will be handed to you or your partner.

- **Third stage** This is when the placenta is delivered. As your baby's body is being born the midwife can give you an injection of a drug called syntometrine in your thigh. Whether or not you want this injection should be discussed before you go into labour. There are a few cases where you will be strongly advised to have it, e.g. if you are having twins or you have a previous history of bleeding. The injection is thought to reduce blood loss and in some cases will help your womb to contract and push out the placenta more quickly. The midwife will wait for a few minutes with her hand on your abdomen until she feels the top of your womb rise up and become firm. She will then gently pull on the cut end of the umbilical cord and the placenta will come away. She will check it all over to ensure it is complete. If your placenta does not come away by itself, it may have to be removed under anaesthetic.

Syntometrine does carry possible side effects, for instance raised blood pressure and more pain. If you have planned not to have the injection, being upright will help your body to expel the placenta.

What are my options for pain relief in labour?
Breathing exercises, using different positions, and the support of your partner or other birth companion The pain of labour is certainly more bearable if you feel that you are in control, and there is evidence that labour progresses more quickly and smoothly if you have a supportive birth companion.
Using the birthing pool or getting into a warm deep bath as long as someone is there who can help you to get back out. Many women find this very effective, especially if there is a supportive midwife involved. In some units, you may have to book the birthing pool in advance – a tricky matter given the difficulty of predicting when labour will start. Sixty-nine per cent of units offer water birth but of these, only 82 per cent have their own birth pool and only 65 per cent have a midwife trained in waterbirth available 24 hours a day. You may need to bring your own pool and it worth checking whether a midwife will be available when you need one.
TENS machine transcutaneous electrical nerve stimulation. This is a little machine which attaches to your back with small sticky pads. It can be used to stimulate the small skin nerves to boost the body's natural endorphins and so reduce the deep pain sensation caused by contractions. Some maternity units will let you borrow or hire a TENS machine, or you can hire one from a commercial organisation – your community midwife will be able to put you in

Birth Story Emily Dynan

I always thought that I would probably end up having an epidural for the birth of my first child, and I did. But as I result, I was determined not to have one the second time round.

I went through the early stages of my first labour overnight on my own in an empty 8-bed room on an antenatal ward staffed by a single (busy) night nurse. I had been admitted the evening before as my waters had broken, but as I wasn't having any noticeable contractions, my husband had been sent home. The contractions started around midnight, and by the following morning I was ready to go down to the delivery suite. By this time I was very tired and in a lot of pain, and had been vomiting all night (quite common apparently). I was also feeling a bit defeated, as I hadn't had anyone with me to urge me on. So when I got to the delivery suite, where my husband joined me, and found the gas and air to be of no help (in retrospect, because I wasn't shown how to use the mouthpiece), I was soon asking for, and given, an epidural.

I now wish they'd reminded me that it could slow everything down, but there was no discussion. At this stage I hadn't been assigned a midwife, they were changing shifts, so there was no one person to run through the pros and cons with me, and anyway, I was a very tired first-timer (first labours are usually the longest), without a written birth plan, begging for an epidural. And I certainly hadn't briefed my husband to try to talk me out of it.

The relief the epidural brought was wonderful. The pain went, I was numb from the waist down although I could occasionally feel some faint discomfort, and I could at last rest. However, I didn't like not being able to move around at all, and unfortunately the epidural caused my contractions to weaken to the extent that I had to be induced by drip. I did then have a go at pushing, but I never felt 'the urge', and after an hour or so they gave up on me. The room filled with people (three midwives, two doctors and a student), out came the ventouse, stirrups, screens, episiotomy knife, and eventually at half-past three, a 7lb baby girl.

I don't think any of us were traumatized by this delivery, nor do I feel, as some might, that I had missed out on the 'proper', natural birth experience. However, I wasn't keen to go through the same thing when the time came for my second child to be born. This time the whole process was much faster. I arrived at hospital at 3am and had my son at 6.30am. The midwife showed me how to use the gas and air, which I found very effective for a while, and when I asked for something else, suggested pethidine, which was wonderful. This time I did experience the extraordinary urge to push, and yes it was very painful, as, although I was still using gas and air, pethidine wears off. The baby's shoulders were difficult to deliver and he was a hefty 9lb 4oz. To say I screamed a bit would be an understatement, however, it was very quick, unclinical and intimate (a second midwife joined us for the last stage), and certainly the better of the two deliveries.

contact with a supplier of TENS machines in your area. The effect of TENS on labour pain is unpredictable – some women find it extremely effective, while others do not feel it makes any difference or even that it makes the pain worse.

Entonox, or 'gas and air' This is a mixture of 50 per cent nitrous oxide and 50 per cent oxygen which you breathe in through a mask or a mouthpiece. The mouthpiece is particularly useful if you cannot tolerate the rubbery smell of the mask. The advantage of gas and air is that it needs to be used only during contractions and quickly disappears from your body when you stop using it so it does not affect your baby.

The technique for using gas and air effectively needs a little practice. As it takes about 20 seconds to start working, you should start inhaling it in deep, slow breaths as soon as each contraction starts, and stop inhaling it when your contraction reaches its peak. If you do this, you should not have too many problems with side-effects – typically, feeling nauseated, spaced-out or giggly.

Gas and air can be used in addition to other forms of pain relief. Every maternity unit offers entonox. It will not take your pain away completely, but it can make it bearable.

Pethidine This is a drug related to morphine which the midwife can give you by injection. It can be quite effective in relieving the pain of the first stage of labour, but should not be given when the second stage is approaching because it passes through the placenta into your baby's circulation and can make your baby sleepy and reluctant to breathe after birth.

Some women tolerate pethidine extremely well and need no other pain relief in the first stage of labour. Others find that it does not work very well, and a minority suffer side effects such as sleepiness, hallucinations, or nausea and vomiting (if you know that pethidine makes you sick, but would like to use it, ask the midwife to give you an anti-sickness injection at the same time).

You can use pethidine in addition to gas and air, but you should not get into the birthing pool after having pethidine. Most maternity units offer this, but a few midwife-led only units do not.

Giving birth in a midwife-led unit

Pros:

- It can be the best of both worlds – a friendly, low-tech unit with the reassurance that you can be transferred quickly to the consultant-led unit if necessary.
- Decisions are made by senior midwives who are experienced in managing labour in a relaxed setting.
- You may already know your midwives before you go into labour.
- You will be encouraged to stay mobile and have intermittent monitoring.

Cons:

- It could be seen as the worst of both worlds – a hospital, but without lifesaving machinery. This is especially true if the unit is not attached to a consultant-led unit.
- You may have to travel to the unit while in labour.
- You will not be able to have epidural or spinal anaesthesia.
- If you need a drip to speed up your contractions, you will need to be transferred to a consultant-led unit.

Epidural or spinal anaesthesia If you want to have a pain-free labour, this is your best option, and 69 per cent of maternity units now offer women in labour an epidural on request (if it is appropriate) without any need to book it in advance. However, you may be refused an epidural if the anaesthetist is too busy or there are medical reasons why you should not have one (see p79).

The midwife or obstetrician will call an anaesthetist, who will check that there are no reasons not to give you an epidural and that you are not allergic to iodine, local anaesthetics, or elastoplast. They will then put up a drip and run clear fluid from a bag into your vein – this is called preloading, and its purpose is to stop your blood pressure dropping too low, which is a recognised complication of epidural anaesthesia. They will then clean your lower back with an antiseptic solution to prevent germs from your skin from being carried into the injection site, give you a small injection of local anaesthetic (this will sting for a minute or two), and pass a thin plastic tube into the space around your spinal cord and inject anaesthetic into it. You will have a warm feeling in your back, then your abdomen, bottom and legs will gradually become numb over a period of 5-10 minutes.

Once the epidural is in place, you will continue to have fluids through the drip and your blood pressure will be checked regularly. When your bladder fills up, it may need to be emptied with a catheter. Someone should stay with you at all times. If you have a long labour, the epidural will start to wear off and will have to be topped up one or more times (the midwife can do this). When the second stage of labour is approaching, you will have to decide whether to have the epidural topped up to avoid pain, increasing the risk of assisted delivery, or to let the epidural wear off, which may make it easier for you to push effectively but exposes you suddenly to the pain of advanced labour.

After an epidural, you may develop a headache or have difficulty in emptying your bladder for a day or two. There is also a risk of backache – this is probably not caused by the epidural itself, but by the fact that you may get into awkward positions during labour without realising it at the time, and suffer the consequences later.

On average, 31 per cent of women in England choose epidural pain relief. The eastern region has a higher than average epidural rate along with the north where a third of women receive one. In contrast, the southwest and northwest have a below average rate. Wales has the fewest epidurals in the UK overall.

Mobile epidural This is similar to an epidural, but a different mix of anaesthetic is used so that your legs do not become numb and, after the initial 30 minutes of intensive monitoring, you may be able to stand up and walk about. This type of epidural is less reliable in providing total freedom from pain, but you are less likely to need a forceps delivery than if you had a full epidural. Around a quarter of maternity units offer mobile epidurals.

I don't understand the difference between an epidural and spinal anaesthesia.

Both involve injections into the spine – but the spinal anaesthetic is put into a deeper layer of the membranes covering the spinal cord. This gives it a quicker onset of action and it wears off more quickly so it is particularly useful for elective caesarean, but it has a slightly higher risk of a 'spinal tap', where the fluid which bathes the brain and spinal cord can leak out, causing changes in the pressure in the fluid-filled spaces around the brain, and an almighty headache. In these circumstances, if the leaking persists the hole in the membrane has to be closed.

When might I be advised not to have an epidural?

If your blood is not clotting properly This can occur in pregnancy-induced hypertension. If you have this condition and would like an epidural you will need to have a blood test first.

If you are likely to give birth within an hour By the time the epidural is working, you will be ready to have your baby (fully dilated and ready to push). In this situation, gas and air is a far better choice.

If you have an infection in the skin of your back such as impetigo or infected eczema.

If you are allergic to any of the components of the anaesthetic.

If the labour ward is particularly busy and it will be impossible to guarantee that a trained midwife will be able to stay with you throughout your labour.

Can I insist on having an epidural?

Ultimately, no. The anaesthetist will not take the risk of doing a complicated procedure such as an epidural when, for whatever reason, it is not safe to do so.

Do I have a right to have a trained midwife with me throughout labour?

This is certainly desirable, and whenever possible the same midwife will stay with you throughout labour. Most units cannot guarantee one-on-one midwife care if the labour ward is particularly busy or staffing levels are low due to unpredictable factors such as illness, and you may have to share a midwife with another woman who is at a different stage of her labour. In addition, hospital midwives work shifts, and if you are still a long way from delivery when your midwife's shift ends she will hand your care over to a colleague before she goes off duty. In the 1992 Changing Childbirth report, an objective was set that all women should know their midwife during labour. However, almost ten years later, over 50 per cent of maternity units do not record whether women know their midwife in delivery, and of those units that do, few mothers end up knowing their midwife. If you give birth at home or if your community midwife comes into hospital to deliver you (as in a domino delivery), it is far more likely that the same midwife will be with you until your baby is born.

Will I see my obstetrician when I am in labour?
Not necessarily. Even in consultant-led maternity units, most women give birth without needing the involvement of an obstetrician. Normal deliveries are managed by midwives, leaving the obstetric team free to attend to women whose labours are not running smoothly.

When will the obstetrician become involved?
If you have previously had a caesarean section or extensive perineal damage.
If your labour is progressing too slowly When you are admitted in labour, your midwife may draw up a chart called a partogram on which she will record your progress. If your cervix is not dilating as quickly as expected and the baby's head is not coming down your birth canal properly, she will alert the duty obstetrician.
If there are signs of fetal distress such as an abnormal fetal heart trace on the CTG or meconium-stained amniotic fluid.
If you become unwell with, for example, a fever, high blood pressure, or dehydration.
If you start to bleed heavily.

Domino delivery

Pros:

- You will be accompanied throughout by a midwife you already know.
- You can stay at home for most of your labour. If your labour is proceeding well, the midwife can advise you on whether you should consider staying at home instead of going to hospital.
- You can give birth in a consultant-led unit with all of the associated advantages, but your midwife will act as your advocate if intervention is suggested.
- You will be able to go home as soon as you and your baby are well enough.

Cons:

- You may need to travel to hospital in advanced labour, and travel home again when you are exhausted after giving birth.
- You cannot have epidural or spinal anaesthesia if you want to go home within 6 hours of delivery.
- If you need forceps or a caesarean section, you will have a longer hospital stay for which you may not be prepared.

If your cervix has been fully dilated for over an hour and your baby has not been born.

In all of these situations, you may need some form of intervention – a Syntocinon drip to strengthen your contractions, fetal blood sampling, an instrumental vaginal delivery, or a caesarean section. At present these procedures can only be performed by an obstetrician, but they should be performed in consultation with the midwife and your wishes taken into account.

Will I see the obstetrician with whom I am booked?

Not necessarily. The obstetric teams cover the labour ward on a rota, and your own consultant's team may not be on duty when you go into labour. In most units, the consultant obstetrician is on call from home and only comes to the labour ward to do ward rounds at set times and to deal with particularly difficult problems. Most obstetric interventions are performed by trainee obstetricians who have reached a suitable level of competence.

I've heard that I should make sure my baby is tagged. Why is this?

The abduction of a baby from a hospital in the English Midlands three years ago led to measures such as video surveillance and entry phones to internal doors in maternity wards. Many hospitals have increased security by installing closed circuit television cameras and restricting access. An electronic tagging system for babies has also been introduced in some hospitals. The system involves a tag being put around a baby's ankle which responds to sensor panels located at hospital exits. If the baby is taken through the sensor an alarm goes off and the hospital's security team is alerted.

If my baby is not tagged, should I be worried?

Tagging is a good security measure but not the sole factor of effective security. Vigilance by staff and parents make the most secure system complete. Parents should be vigilant and not allow any midwife, nurse or doctor, to take their baby away from their bedside unless she or he is wearing a hospital name badge, and you should challenge staff who are not wearing a form of identity.

Home Birth

What are the advantages of home birth?

Having a baby at home means that you are in familiar surroundings and may feel more relaxed and in control of pain. You will not be faced with the decision about when to admit yourself to hospital and your labour will not be interrupted by travel and a possible wait

at hospital. You are also more likely to have got to know the
midwife or midwife team that care for you during the labour.

I asked about home birth, and my GP said I couldn't have one.
It is your choice to give birth wherever you want. If your GP does not
have the confidence or expertise to deliver a baby or deal with any
complications that might arise they may not have to agree to be
involved with home births. However your community midwife has a
professional duty to provide you with the help you need, or to refer
you to a colleague who will do so. The hospital profiles in this guide
tell you which units do most home births. Alternatively, contact the
Director of Midwifery Services through a hospital or health authority
for information about the procedure in your area.

Can anyone choose to have a home birth?

Anyone can choose to have a home birth, but some women will be
advised that it is not a good option for them because of their
individual circumstances. The risks associated with home birth are
no greater than those associated with delivery in hospital.
However, there are some circumstances in which it is advisable to
have your baby in hospital:

- If you are having twins.
- If your baby is not in the head-down position with the head
  engaging in the pelvis.
- If you have had four or more previous babies. This increases
  your risk of haemorrhage after delivery.
- If you have any difficult domestic circumstances, such as
  someone at home whose behaviour is unpredictable, or if you do
  not have basic facilities like electricity, hot water and a telephone.
- If you go into labour before 37 weeks gestation.
- If you have pregnancy-induced hypertension.
- If your baby has been identified as being small for dates.
- If your previous babies have been small for dates or have needed
  resuscitation at birth.
- If your last baby was born by caesarean section, forceps or
  ventouse.
- If you want an epidural for pain relief.

Birth Story Sharon Morris

I have two children, both of whom were delivered at home, and I always knew that I wanted home births, as I wasn't keen on doctors or hospitals. During my first pregnancy, I waited three months before going to see the GP, who then expressed reluctance to supervise a home birth and signed me over to the community midwifery service. I did have an appointment to see a consultant at my local hospital where my wish not to have any medical intervention at all, including scans and checkups, met with resistance, but in the end my decisions were respected.

My midwife was a specialist in home birth, but because of the shortage of midwives at the service, I was told that I would not always be able to see her at each appointment. In the end, I was able to see the same midwife most of the time (although I had visits from others in between), and was lucky enough to be delivered by her. Nevertheless I was aware that the midwives' visits were kept as short as possible because the service was so understaffed.

I got through both pregnancies with a combination of physical and breathing exercises, careful nutrition, and a great deal of research, which I undertook myself. I was told that the main problem with giving birth at home was fatigue, so I knew I would have to make myself as strong as possible in order to cope, particularly because I was also adamant that I didn't want any pain relief. I was able to keep up a positive outlook through my supportive network of family and friends, and my determination to be in control of my own situation as far as possible.

My first labour was quite protracted. I started my 'practice' contractions (Braxton-Hicks) on a Monday, and by Thursday I felt the soft plug of my cervix giving way. By Friday my contractions were well underway, but I waited until Sunday to call the midwife. She was not at all happy that my labour had already gone on for so long, and she called the hospital who advised her to send me in, but I resisted. What was worrying her was that I was only 3cm dilated, and the baby had already moved part of the way down the birth canal and then stopped. I persuaded her to give me more time, and eventually things began to happen more quickly. That extra time was crucial. I think the reason that so many home births fail is due to pressure from the midwife or the hospital to abandon them the minute things look even a little unusual.

I was relieved that I had made such an effort to work on my breathing exercises, as these really helped to control the pain, and I also used hot baths. The whole home birth experience felt comfortable and intimate, and my husband and sister felt fully included.

I think that there are a number of factors putting women off home births. The level of care at community midwife level is not sufficient to make women confident that they can do it, and when they do decide on home birth, they can find their choice easily undermined by a service fearful of litigation. I think that more women would opt for home births if community midwifery were better funded and staffed, because very few can afford the security of private care.

Home Birth

Pros:

- You have the reassurance and comfort of being in your own environment.
- Unlike a hospital, your home is not likely to be harbouring dangerous bacteria such as MRSA and Pseudomonas, even if you have let the housework lapse.
- You do not have to travel while in labour – that journey to hospital can be extremely stressful.
- You will be attended throughout by experienced community midwives, and will have the same midwife throughout your labour.
- For healthy women with uncomplicated pregnancies, home birth is as safe as hospital birth.

Cons:

- If problems arise, you may have to travel to hospital, possibly in advanced labour.
- Pain relief choices are very limited. You can't have an epidural, for example.
- If you want a water birth, you need to make your own arrangements for hiring and filling the pool.
- You may need to go to your GP's surgery to have the baby checked after birth.Home birth is not the best choice if you are at high risk of complications – if you have diabetes or if your baby is small for gestational age, for example.

What will happen when I tell the midwife that I want a home birth?

The midwife will visit you a few weeks before your baby is due and will ensure that you have everything you need. They will give you a list of equipment that you will need to provide (such as waterproof bed covers, a thermometer, and blankets for your baby), and leave a delivery pack and a cylinder of gas and air. The delivery pack will contain sterile towels, a large plastic or stainless steel bowl, cotton wool and forceps, a cord clamp and scissors to cut the cord. They will also ensure that you are aware that you may need to be transferred to hospital in labour if problems arise. However, midwives are under no obligation to guarantee that they will be available to deliver you at home, especially if there is a shortage of midwives in your area.

What pain relief can I have at home?

You can have gas and air, pethidine injections (which many community midwives do not carry with them, so you may need to get them on prescription from your GP), and/or a TENS machine, which you may need to hire in advance and pay for yourself. You will also benefit from the pain-relieving properties of being in your own home with familiar people and being able to occupy yourself with domestic tasks during early labour.

Can I have a water birth at home?

Yes, if your house is suitable, bearing in mind the weight of a pool full of water. You will need to supply and pay for the pool yourself. They can be hired – check your local telephone directory for details, or ask your community midwife.

When should I call the midwife?

When you are sure that labour has started, either because you are having regular painful contractions or because your waters have broken. Normally one midwife stays with you for most of your labour then calls a second midwife to join her when you are ready to give birth.

What will happen about my postnatal care?

The midwife will visit regularly until your baby is ten days old. Your GP may visit to check your baby as you will not have an opportunity to have your baby examined by a paediatrician in hospital. Alternatively, since you are likely to be up and about very quickly after delivery, you could take your baby to see your GP at the surgery. Increasingly, midwives are performing this examination.

Birth Story Ruth Stone

My first labour was a very long, drawn out affair,
primarily, I now believe, because my labour symptoms
were misinterpreted. On the Friday morning two days
before my due date, I experienced a sensation that made
me think that my waters had broken, and I took myself
off to the labour ward where this was confirmed. Looking
back, and having experienced a second labour, I don't
think my full waters had in fact broken, and I was
therefore probably at a much earlier stage of labour than
they assumed at the time. Nevertheless, I was told I was in
mild labour, and was monitored all day because the fetal
heartbeat did not sound strong. That evening I was sent
home to pack, and I then returned to the ward as
instructed, but nothing further happened during the
night.

On the Saturday morning, I was given the first of the
pessaries needed to induce me, but still nothing
happened, despite my walking up and down Chiswick
High Street with my husband in a vain attempt to speed
up the process. In the evening I was given another
pessary, and at last felt my first labour pains, but, much to
my distress, these were dismissed by the midwife as 'false
contractions'.

On the Sunday morning, concerned that it was now
forty-eight hours since my waters had broken, they
decided to place me on a full drip to induce me
immediately. I was also given an epidural, as the sudden
onset of labour that the drip causes can be very painful.
When the obstetrician came to examine me, however, she
discovered that it was only my hind waters that had

broken, and it became necessary to break my full waters with an amnihook. I got the impression that this doctor was surprised that I had been given the full inducement and consequently the epidural, but nothing was ever said.

At midnight on the Sunday, I was finally found to be 10cm dilated and was immediately told to start pushing by the student midwife in attendance, even though I had no strong urge to push. I now feel that I should have been allowed to wait until that urge arrived. As it was, I pushed for an hour and a half straight, and made very little headway. I was exhausted and upset, and, remembering that the antenatal classes had stressed that we were not to push for more than an hour and a half in one session, I refused to push further, despite the midwife's insistence that I 'try harder'. In the end, they delivered my daughter using a ventouse, and I strongly believe that she was traumatized by this method of birth, as she cried continuously for the first two months of her life.

After the delivery, I was given a catheter, because I had haemorrhaged, and was kept in hospital for a further three days, and my baby was given antibiotics to ward of any infection she might have caught after the protective waters had broken. Once home, I was visited by the district midwife every day for five days, but remember feeling that she was interfering and yet ineffectual, as I struggled with a baby who wouldn't latch on and who screamed all the time. The health visitor who took over, however, had a much more commonsense approach, and helped us a great deal in those early rather difficult days.

Where can I find out more about home birth?

Angela Horn, Home Birth Co-ordinator for the National Childbirth Trust, provides lots of useful information including summaries of scientific research papers, advice on the practical aspects of home birth, and women's accounts of their experiences of home birth, on www.homebirth.org.uk

Induction of Labour

Induction of labour is a controversial issue. There have been accusations that it is done more for the benefit of doctors than patients in order to speed up a slow labour. Whereas NICE guidelines on induction state that women should be offered induction of labour beyond 41 weeks and from 42 weeks, women who decline induction should be offered increased antenatal visiting consisting of twice-weekly CTG and ultrasound examinations. Whereas a lot of women feel that they would rather have their labour progress naturally, some women would prefer to be induced if it means that they can have their baby when they planned.

Why might I decide to have my labour induced artificially?

In the UK, around one labour in five is induced. However, induction may be offered if you are not showing signs of going into labour spontaneously, and there is a risk of either you or your baby suffering problems if your pregnancy is allowed to continue. Situations in which this might apply include:

Your pregnancy has already lasted 42 weeks, or two weeks past your EDD (estimated delivery date). Babies who remain in the womb longer than this are at increased risk of being stillborn or becoming distressed, as the placenta becomes less effective at transferring nutrients to the baby.

Your baby has stopped growing If scans show that your baby is not growing, this means that your placenta is no longer working properly and there is nothing to be gained by delaying delivery any longer, even if it means that your baby will be born very prematurely.

Your waters have broken but contractions have not started
There is a risk of infection if you are not delivered quickly.

If you have previously had a caesarean section or extensive perineal damage and your baby is very large.

If your labour is progressing too slowly. When you are admitted in labour. If your cervix is not dilating as quickly as expected and the baby's head is not coming down your birth canal properly, the midwife will alert the duty obstetrician.

If there are signs of fetal distress such as an abnormal fetal heart trace on the CTG or meconium stained amniotic fluid.

If you become unwell with, for example, a fever, high blood pressure, or dehydration.

If you start to bleed heavily.

If your cervix has been fully dilated for over an hour and your baby has not been born.

If you have diabetes, especially if it is poorly controlled and your baby is likely to be very large.

If a part of the placenta has separated from the womb – a painful and potentially very dangerous condition for both mother and baby. The medical term for this is placental abruption.

If your baby has died in the womb, or has been found to have abnormalities which mean that it will not survive.
In all of these situations, you may need some form of intervention – a Syntocinon drip to strengthen your contractions, fetal blood sampling, an instrumental vaginal delivery, or a caesarean section. At present these procedures can only be performed by an obstetrician, although they should certainly take your wishes and the midwife's view into account.

I feel as if I've been pregnant for ever, and I'm only 36 weeks. Can I be induced early?
If you are nearing 40 weeks and you are exhausted and anaemic and carrying a 4kg baby, few obstetricians would refuse to try to help you into labour. If, however, you have not reached your EDD it would depend on your own obstetrician's views. Some are quite liberal about induction on request, others feel that the timing of labour should not be interfered with unless there is a sound

Birth Story Rebecca Lowe

My pregnancy was made up of a series of highs and lows.
I had several complications, beginning with a large cyst
on one of my ovaries which was discovered at my 12 week
scan. I was immediately referred to a consultant for an
operation which I had at 17 weeks, and had to face the
very real danger of losing my baby, my ovary, or both.
Happily the operation went well, but after this experience
I decided to opt for a water birth with little active medical
intervention.

At my 20 week scan, I discovered a second problem.
My placenta was very low, and although it wasn't
blocking the cervix, it still presented a problem, and could
have meant that I had to have a caesarean section at 38
weeks. But luckily, by my 34 week scan the placenta had
moved. Although it was hard at times, I tried to keep a
positive outlook for myself and the baby throughout these
complications, and once I had the all clear again, I
attended a number of water birth and breastfeeding
workshops at the hospital.

When I finally went into labour the midwife on duty
delegated responsibility for attending the water birth to
another, as she didn't feel sufficiently comfortable with the
idea of it. The midwife who took over was an expert in
home births, which was very reassuring, but I wasn't
allowed into the pool until a doctor had checked my ovary
scar and ensured that I was fit enough to undergo a water
birth. At last, almost twelve hours after my first contractions
had started, I entered the pool. Up until that point, I'd kept
the pain at bay using a TENS machine, but it was getting less
effective with the onset of strong contractions.

During the UCH water birth workshops, I'd been warned that I would face huge opposition to my wish to actually deliver the baby in the pool, in case complications arose with its breathing. But at the hospital itself, the community midwives turned out to be quite happy to let me give birth in the pool, as they had had plenty of experience dealing with water births at home. There were some things however, that the midwives were very particular about: one was that I should not go into the pool until I was at least 6cm dilated, as it could slow down labour, and the other was that I should be either completely in the water or completely out of it during the delivery itself, rather than moving about between the two. Nor would they allow my partner to be in the water with me, in case there were complications and I had to be lifted out suddenly.

The pool was like a jacuzzi, large enough for four or five people, and the water was quite deep. It was also kept at a constant temperature, in line with the temperature of the baby inside the womb. During the labour the midwife intervened only to monitor the baby's heartbeat and feel the baby's head, but in the last stages, there were four midwives assisting the delivery.

I believe that having a water birth has had a profoundly beneficial effect on my baby's development. My daughter is calm and relaxed, crying only when hungry, and another mother I know who also had a water birth says the same thing about her baby. Significantly both babies love water.

medical reason to do so. However, there is a strong association between induction before 41 weeks and an increased risk of caesarean section.

How might labour be induced?
Using a drug called a prostaglandin, which helps to make the cervix soften and open up. This can be given as a gel or pessary. It can make you have contractions which are painful enough to require pain relief – you will be offered a mild analgesic initially, then pethidine or gas and air.

By breaking your waters and putting up a Syntocinon drip This can only be done if it is possible to reach the membranes through your cervix. A little barbed device rather like a crochet hook is used to rupture the sac of waters, and the Syntocinon will encourage your womb to contract.

What if attempts to induce labour aren't successful?
There is an escalating scale of medical intervention starting with Prostaglandins through to rupturing membranes and to the use of Syntocinon. Sometimes any or all of these techniques will fail to achieve vaginal delivery and therefore caesarean section will be recommended.

I'm 42 weeks pregnant, and I would prefer my labour to start naturally. Do I have to be induced?
No. If you feel strongly that you do not want your labour induced, your wishes will be respected. The obstetrician has a professional duty to tell you about the risks your baby faces by remaining in your womb beyond 42 weeks, but the final decision is yours. If you do not have your labour induced, you should attend hospital every day or two to be monitored to make sure your baby's heartbeat is all right. Statistically, you will probably go into labour before reaching 43 weeks.

Why might my labour not progress properly?
If your contractions are not strong enough Breaking your waters and giving you Syntocinon through a drip may help.

If your contractions are strong but not well co-ordinated
This is more likely in your first labour, or if you are anxious.
Having an epidural anaesthetic will help the muscular wall of your
womb to relax properly between contractions, and you can be
given a Syntocinon drip to give you strong, regular, productive
contractions.

If the opening in or out of your pelvis is too small In the past,
a contracted pelvis was a common consequence of rickets. This
disease has been very rare in the UK for several generations,
although its effects are occasionally seen in women who have come
to the UK from South Asia. If you are less than 150cm in height,
your pelvis may be an appropriate size for you, but too small to
allow an average sized baby to pass through.

If your pelvis is an unusual shape If the bones of your pelvis are
flatter, or more funnel-shaped, than normal, it may be difficult for
your baby's head to get into a good position for birth, resulting in
delay in labour.

If there is an obstruction caused by your soft tissues for
example, if your cervix is scarred from a previous cone biopsy and
cannot dilate, or if there is a fibroid (a benign tumour of the
muscle of the womb) blocking your cervix.

If your baby's head is in an unusual position Your baby's head,
just like your own, is not a perfect sphere – it is larger in some
dimensions than in others. The best position of the baby's head for
birth is flexed (bent forward with its chin on its chest) and facing
your back. This gives a presenting diameter of around 9.5cm,
which can pass easily through a normal pelvis. If your baby is
facing forward, or if its head is not fully flexed, the presenting
diameter is larger and labour may be difficult or prolonged. In
some positions – if the head is stuck facing sideways, or if the
presenting part is the baby's forehead – vaginal delivery is
impossible and a caesarean section will be needed even in the
presence of a fully dilated cervix and good contractions.

What is meconium, and what does its presence in the amniotic fluid signify?

Meconium is a slimy greenish-brown substance which is present in the bowel of the unborn baby. It does not resemble faeces at all – it is sterile and virtually odourless. Most babies pass meconium in the first 24 hours after birth, but a baby who is distressed during labour may pass meconium before birth. This changes the colour of the amniotic fluid. If the baby's heartbeat is normal and labour is progressing well, the presence of meconium need not cause concern, but in the presence of other signs that the baby is stressed it may be the factor that tips the decision in favour of caesarean section.

What does fetal blood sampling involve?

If the CTG suggests that your baby might be distressed, the obstetrician may advise fetal blood sampling – taking blood from your baby while it is in the womb.

Either your legs will be put up in stirrups, or you will be helped to lie on your left side with your right leg raised and supported. The obstetrician will put the narrow end of a long funnel-shaped instrument called an amnioscope into your vagina and place it firmly against your baby's scalp (or buttock if your baby is breech). He will then clean the area with a sterile swab so that the sample is not contaminated with amniotic fluid, meconium, or your blood. He will make a cut in your baby's skin with a tiny blade on a long handle, and collect less than a millilitre of blood in a capillary tube. The blood sample will be put into a machine which gives a printout within a few minutes. The machine analyses the acidity and oxygen content of your baby's blood. If your baby's blood is becoming more acidic than normal, this is a reliable indication of distress. If your baby's blood is normal but the CTG remains abnormal, fetal blood sampling will need to be repeated at least every hour.

Is fetal blood sampling dangerous?

There is no risk to you, and your baby should suffer nothing worse than a tiny wound on its head. The blade used has a guard so that it cannot puncture your baby's skull, even over the soft spot.

There is a risk that decisions may be made on the basis of a blood sample which has accidentally become contaminated with alkaline amniotic fluid. This is rare, however, as the rest of the results on the printout are usually so bizarre following contamination, that it is obvious that the sample contained something other than fetal blood. If your baby has a very hairy scalp, it may prove impossible to get an uncontaminated fetal blood sample. In this case, decisions will have to be based on the CTG and your progress in labour.

What will happen when labour is over?
You may have an attack of shivering, and you may feel sick or even vomit. Don't worry – these are normal reactions to the physical stress of giving birth, and will not last long. You will be given an opportunity to wash. The midwife will help you if you are too exhausted to wash yourself. Then you and your partner will be offered something to eat and drink before being transferred to the postnatal ward. Provided the baby is well and the initial check by your midwife is normal, the baby will normally be seen the following morning by a paediatrician. If there are any immediate concerns at all about the baby, the paediatrician will be called immediately to review the situation.

Assisted Delivery

One of the factors responsible for making childbirth safer for both mothers and babies over the last century has been the development of safe and effective ways to assist delivery when problems arise. Although many authorities now suggest that the pendulum has swung too far in favour of intervention.

Assisted vaginal delivery using forceps or ventouse occurred in 11.3 per cent of deliveries in 1999, up from 10.5 per cent in 1997. The Royal College of Obstetricians and Gynaecologists has suggested that a rate of 8.5 per cent would be more acceptable. There is a wide variation between hospitals – in a few units, one in four babies is born by assisted vaginal delivery.

The rate of caesarean section is also increasing. The World Health Organisation has stated that no more than 15 per cent of babies in

Birth Story Lucy Collins

My first child was delivered by emergency caesarean when I was two weeks overdue. Up until that point my pregnancy, monitored by the community midwifery service and my GP, had been normal, and I had decided to aim for as natural a birth as possible, and even hoped to make use of the hospital pool. As it turned out, none of this was possible.

On the day the doctors decided to induce me, I was given my first dose of prostaglandin gel in the morning. Nothing happened, so I was given a second dose that evening, and began to have my first labour pains during the night. At 5.30 the next morning my waters broke, and I was taken for a check-up. It was only at this point that the doctor discovered that my baby was facing the wrong way, and that it would be a breech birth unless I had a caesarean. I was extremely shocked at this news, having been completely unprepared for it, and also very alarmed because I had been induced. To make matters worse, I had just eaten, so I had to wait six hours for the operation.

I was finally taken into theatre at 10pm and given an epidural, so that I could be awake throughout the operation. I could feel the pressure, but not the pain. The caesarean took about ten minutes, the stitching required afterwards, much longer. Once my daughter was born, my husband joined me in the theatre, and I was then transferred to the High Dependency Unit where they monitored my temperature and blood pressure and inserted a catheter. A midwife bathed my daughter, and then give her to me to feed.

The next morning the doctors examined me, removed the catheter, and gave me an oral painkiller before transferring me to the maternity unit. There were noticeably fewer staff on this ward, and they seemed to be extremely busy. I had hoped to see the community midwives throughout my hospital stay, but due to staff shortages, this was not always possible. I was kept in hospital for five days, longer than I would have liked, because my daughter had lost 11 per cent of her birth weight, and this is slightly over the average amount.

After the birth I needed antibiotics for an infection in my wound, and was visited by the community midwives once I was discharged. It was difficult to resume normal activities for five or six days after the birth. I couldn't walk to the shops or push the pram, but I had a supportive family network to help me.

Looking back, I never felt pressurized into having a caesarean. I simply felt that there was no other option. My first concern was the safe delivery of the baby, and I trusted the doctors to have our best interests at heart. Only later did I begin to wonder whether the decision had been right, but after some research, I discovered that breech births are often only performed vaginally if the baby is under eight pounds. As my baby was over this weight, a caesarean was the only option.

With my second pregnancy, I was again two weeks overdue. The hospital was reluctant to induce the birth as there was a chance of rupturing the scar, so I had another caesarean, but this time it was easier to prepare for because it was planned.

developed countries should be born by caesarean section. In 1997-98, 18.2 per cent of babies in the UK were born by caesarean section – almost double the rate of a decade earlier – and the figure for 1999-2000 is over 20 per cent. Over half of these caesarean sections are elective (planned) operations.

The Royal College of Obstetricians and Gynaecologists is currently investigating the reasons for the rising caesarean section rate. It is unlikely that a genuine increase in the number of women needing a caesarean section is responsible. Explanations include defensive obstetrics (an obstetrician is unlikely to face litigation for performing a caesarean section which, with hindsight, proves to have been unnecessary), increasing evidence that caesarean section is the preferred mode of delivery for breech babies, and the mistaken belief that caesarean section is safer for mother and baby.

Another factor may be maternal choice. Women expressing a wish for elective caesarean may have found previous experiences of natural childbirth 'traumatic' or may have a deep psychological fear of natural childbirth. Others may find the idea of vaginal examination distressing and would prefer simply to have an operation. Alternatively, they may want to have a pain-free delivery, or wish to avoid the risk of tearing and other damage resulting from childbirth which could lead to problems such as incontinence and the need for surgical repair.

Many doctors will take the view that it should be up to the woman whether she wants a caesarean. Others, however, will be less sympathetic. The figures in this guide show which hospitals are more likely to give a to a woman requesting an elective caesarean, and which ones are most likely to deliver by emergency caesarean. For more information about assisted vaginal delivery, The Royal College of Obstetricians and Gynaecologists has an excellent, although slightly technical, summary of the scientific evidence on www.rcog.org.uk/guidelines/guideline26.html.

What is an obstetric operating theatre?
An obstetric operating theatre is no different from any other operating theatre except that it has facilities for resuscitating a newborn baby. In the UK, 72 per cent of maternity units have an

obstetric operating theatre attached – in large teaching hospitals, there may be a whole suite of obstetric operating theatres. The unit used for resuscitating babies is portable, so you can safely have a caesarean section or other obstetric operation in an ordinary operating theatre. The main advantage of a dedicated obstetric theatre is that it allows obstetric operations to be done urgently.

Midwife-led birthing centres do not have an operating theatre, so you will be advised to give birth in the main obstetric unit if you are known to be at risk of complications during delivery.

Is the obstetric operating theatre just for caesarean sections?
No, although caesarean sections are the most common operation performed in them. Procedures which may lead to emergency caesarean section, such as breaking the waters when the baby's head is high in the pelvis or attempting to turn the baby's head using forceps, are often carried out in an operating theatre set up for an immediate caesarean section. If the placenta does not come away after the baby is born, or if you bleed heavily during labour or after delivery, you will be taken to the obstetric operating theatre.

Is it safe to give birth without an operating theatre nearby?
The majority of women will not need operating facilities – seven out of every ten births are uncomplicated vaginal deliveries. If you are at low risk of complications, it is safe to give birth at home or in a birthing unit with basic resuscitation equipment which the midwives are trained to use. Even if problems do arise, there is usually time for you to be moved safely to a unit which has an operating theatre.

If I have a caesarean section, can my partner stay with me?
If you have an epidural or spinal anaesthetic, your partner or birth companion can come into the operating theatre to support you. If you have a general anaesthetic, he may not be allowed to be present, but the baby will be taken out for him to hold as soon as possible.

Episiotomy

What is an episiotomy, and why might I have one?

An episiotomy is a cut which is made in the skin between the vaginal opening and the anus (the perineum) to make the vaginal opening wider and help the baby to come out. It is usually performed where there is a risk of a large tear extending into the anus and causing muscle damage.

The use of episiotomy became popular early in the 20th century, and from the 1960s until around the mid-1980s it was rare for a woman having her first baby not to have an episiotomy. Now, episiotomy is used less commonly and it is accepted that a small tear in the midline will cause less pain and will heal more quickly. Increasingly, small tears are left to heal on their own without stitches. The average episiotomy rate for England is 15 per cent, but in some units, up to 30 per cent of women may have an episiotomy during labour. The rest of England has some of the highest episiotomy rates in one country.

The reasons for which an episiotomy may be needed are:

- **A previous operation on the perineum or pelvic floor** Many women who have had a prolapse or extensive perineal tears repaired in the past will be advised to have a caesarean section, and those who give birth vaginally may need an episiotomy to prevent the scar tissue from tearing.
- **Instrumental delivery using forceps** Ventouse delivery does not always require an episiotomy. .
- **Breech delivery** The baby's bottom is less effective than the head at stretching the perineum.
- **If the baby is distressed** If the head is nearly born, an episiotomy can speed up the process of birth and gain valuable minutes.
- **If the baby's shoulders get stuck after the head is born**

How can I increase my chances of avoiding an episiotomy?

Choose a hospital which has a stated policy of minimising episiotomy rates. Ideally, the episiotomy rate for the unit should not exceed 20 per cent.

- Include your wish to avoid an episiotomy in your birth plan. Small tears can be left to heal on their own naturally and you may prefer to be allowed to allowed to tear rather than be given an episiotomy.
- Choose a more upright position such as kneeling in which to give birth. It is difficult for the perineum to stretch properly if you are lying on your back. Think of gravity as a factor which you can use to your advantage. Try to relax you mouth, as this relaxes your vagina.
- Raspberry leaf extract to tone the uterus and massaging the perineum is popular as a 'natural' way of making the perineum more stretchy.

If I have an episiotomy, who will repair it?

Most trained midwives are able to suture an episiotomy; if they cannot, and the episiotomy (or tear) is small and straight, one of the junior obstetricians will suture it. If the episiotomy has enlarged by tearing further, or has been cut too far to the side (as occasionally happens), or if a tear extends to the anus, it should be repaired by an experienced obstetrician. This is extremely important. If perineal damage is not repaired properly and the tissues do not heal in the correct position, you may develop problems in the future with a painful lumpy scar, painful intercourse, or loss of bowel control.

Forceps Delivery

What are forceps?

A set of obstetric forceps consists of two metal instruments about the same shape as a large pair of serving spoons, with interlocking handles. They are designed to allow the obstetrician to assist delivery when the cervix is fully dilated and the baby's head is well down the birth canal, but the baby is distressed or the mother is too exhausted to continue pushing. Epidural anaesthesia reduces the mother's ability to push effectively against the pelvic floor, and women who have had an epidural are at greatly increased risk of needing a forceps delivery. The average forceps rate of England is 4 per cent but the rate varies from 0.2 per cent to 13 per cent in other hospitals. In the north of England forceps are used with more frequency than the ventouse and Trent also has a high usage. Northern Ireland's forceps rate is double that of England.

What will happen if I have a forceps delivery?
The midwife looking after you will call the duty obstetrician – usually the registrar or an experienced senior house officer – and they will discuss your situation with you and your partner. You and your companion should be involved in the discussion and you should be asked to give your consent to forceps delivery. If you have an epidural, it will be topped up with extra anaesthetic medication to ensure that the pain is minimised. If you do not already have an epidural, the obstetrician will inject local anaesthetic into your vagina to make it numb before putting the forceps in place. If your contractions are weak, you may be given a drug called Syntocinon through a drip to make them stronger.

Your legs will be put up in obstetric stirrups and the end of the bed removed so that your bottom is at the edge of the bed with your legs held out of the way. Your perineum will be cleaned with antiseptic solution and the area will be covered with sterile drapes. Your bladder will be emptied using a catheter and the obstetrician will feel your abdomen to make sure the baby's head is far enough down the birth canal for forceps to be used safely. He will then examine you internally to check the position of the baby's head before slipping one of the forceps blades on to each side, locking the handles together, and pulling downwards while you push with each contraction. If your epidural is so effective that you cannot feel your contractions, the midwife will put her hand on your abdomen and tell you when to push. The baby should be born within two or three contractions, and an episiotomy will be cut as the head comes out.

From there, everything is exactly like a normal delivery. Once the placenta has come away and been checked to ensure it is complete, the obstetrician or midwife will repair the episiotomy. Then your legs will be taken down from the stirrups and you will be able to rest.

What are the risks of forceps delivery?

Perineal damage After delivery you will have stitches inside your vagina. These may be very uncomfortable for a week or two after delivery, although you will be given regular pain relief that is safe to use while you are breastfeeding.

Long term problems with bowel control In some cases, this includes incontinence of faeces, although this is uncommon. Many more women have less severe but nonetheless troublesome problems such as painful splits in the skin around the anus, or loss of the ability to distinguish between flatus and faeces in the rectum.

Injuries to the baby's scalp This is less likely to occur with forceps than with the ventouse. Brain damage resulting from forceps delivery is extremely rare if the forceps are used correctly.

What can I do to avoid having a forceps delivery?

- Early in labour, keep up your strength by resting and by taking fluids and a light meal unless you are nauseated.
- Be prepared to try alternative positions in labour, particularly upright positions.
- The presence of a supportive companion (particularly one-to-one midwifery) during labour will help you to relax and stay calm, and reduce the likelihood that you will need a forceps delivery.
- State in your birth plan that you are keen to avoid having a forceps delivery. If you would rather have a caesarean section than an assisted vaginal delivery, discuss this with your obstetrician in advance.
- If you are having a hospital birth, choose a hospital that does not limit the amount of time you can take for the second stage of pregnancy. If the baby is slow to descend, standing, walking, stepping up and down steps can help shift the baby.
- Choose pain relief that does not involve epidural or spinal anaesthesia. Other forms of pain relief in labour do not increase the likelihood of needing a forceps delivery.
- Choose a hospital which is committed to minimising the rate of forceps delivery by allowing the second stage of labour to last as long as is needed provided the baby is not distressed and the mother is not exhausted.

Ventouse Delivery

What is a ventouse?

A ventouse, or vacuum device, is a metal or silicone rubber cup rather like a sink plunger. It is placed over the baby's head and controlled suction is applied using a machine. In the hands of an experienced obstetrician, it is possible to have a ventouse delivery without using stirrups, an episiotomy, or additional pain relief. Recent evidence suggests that ventouse is no better or worse than forceps for the baby, but less traumatic for the mother. The average ventouse rate in England is 7 per cent, but the rate varies between hospitals from 0.4 per cent to 14 per cent.

Will my baby's head be misshaped after forceps or ventouse delivery?

Most babies who are born vaginally have a slightly squashed head because the skull bones mould to the shape of the birth canal and fluid collects under the scalp of the part of the head that is born first. The baby's head will return to its normal shape within a few days. After a forceps delivery, your baby will have marks shaped like part of the forceps blades on one or both sides of his head, and these may bruise. They will disappear in a few days. After a ventouse delivery, your baby will have a soft lump called a chignon on his scalp where the cup was applied. This normally disappears in a few days. Occasionally there is a bleed into the layers of the baby's scalp – a cephalhaematoma. In this case, the lump will be present for weeks or months but will disappear eventually. Very rarely, so much blood is lost into a cephalhaematoma that the baby becomes anaemic.

Breech Birth

I've been told my baby is breech. What does that mean?

Breech is the obstetric term for the baby's bottom, and a breech presentation means that instead of lying with its head pointing down towards the birth canal, your baby is effectively sitting on its bottom in your womb. At 28 weeks of pregnancy, one baby in four presents by the breech, but most of these babies turn themselves round so that only one full-term baby in thirty is a breech presentation.

Giving birth to a breech baby carries more risks to the baby if the baby presents head-first. The breech, being softer than the head, is less effective at dilating the cervix. In a breech birth, the largest part of the baby – the head – is born last, which means that it is possible to discover that the pelvis is too small for the head only after the body has been born.

Can my baby be turned round?

If your baby is still breech after 36 weeks, a procedure called external cephalic version (ECV) should be offered to try to turn the baby round. Sixty-three per cent of maternity units use this procedure. It is always done in hospital, as a planned procedure, and by an experienced obstetrician. In expert hands, more than half of breech babies can be turned round to become head-first.

You may be given a drug such as ritodrine through a drip to relax the muscle wall of your womb. Then, using ultrasound scans to check the baby's position, the obstetrician will gently try to work the baby round to the head-down position by pressing on your abdomen. It is a little uncomfortable, but should not cause severe pain.

Although rare, there are some risks associated with ECV including the risk of pulling part of the placenta away from the wall of the womb or starting off labour. ECV may also cause some of the baby's blood cells to enter the mother's bloodstream, so if you are rhesus negative you will be given an injection of anti-D.

What if my baby does not turn round?

In most units, especially if it is your first baby, you will be advised to have a caesarean section.

Is a caesarean section really necessary for the delivery of all breech babies?

Not always. A well-planned and well-conducted vaginal breech delivery can be immensely satisfying for everyone involved.

However, although vaginal breech delivery is safer than caesarean section for the mother, it is probably more hazardous for the baby. Studies show a higher mortality rate for breech babies born vaginally rather than by caesarean section. For this reason, some hospitals will now only deliver breech babies in this way. Unfortunately, the move towards routinely recommending caesarean section for breech presentation at term means that midwives and obstetricians may not have done enough vaginal breech deliveries to gain expertise. The number of breech presentations identified before the onset of labour that resulted in vaginal delivery vary between hospitals from 0.1 per cent to 50 per cent.

If you fulfil the following conditions, it is worth considering a trial of vaginal breech delivery:

- **You are carrying an average sized baby** This can be assessed by ultrasound.
- **You have had at least one previous vaginal delivery of a normal sized baby** This is the best indication that your pelvis is big enough.
- **There are no known risk factors for fetal distress** such as high blood pressure or heavy smoking.
- **Your baby's head is flexed (bent forward on the chest) and there are no spinal deformities.**
- **The breech is descending into the pelvis** If the breech does not engage properly, there is a risk that the baby's foot or the umbilical cord might fall through your cervix when it starts to open up.
- **You are willing to accept the possibility that you might need an emergency caesarean section** This is the outcome in about 50 per cent of attempted vaginal breech deliveries.
- **The staff in your obstetric unit are familiar with vaginal breech delivery** If not you can ask for your care to be transferred to a different unit, even if your pregnancy is very advanced.

How does a breech delivery differ from a normal delivery?
Vaginal breech delivery should be carried out in hospital in view of the high probability that intervention will be needed. During early

labour, you should stay as upright and mobile as possible. When the second stage is approaching, you will be monitored very closely (probably using an external cardiotocograph, although an electrode to measure the heart rate may be attached to the baby's buttock), and will be encouraged to have an epidural. As the breech is not as good as the head at dilating the cervix, you may need a Syntocinon drip to make your contractions stronger.

The techniques used by the midwife and obstetrician to deliver you of a breech baby are different from those used in a normal delivery, and your baby's head may need to be helped out with forceps. There will be a lot of people in the delivery room. You may be asked whether you would be willing to let midwifery or obstetric trainees, or even a medical student, watch your baby being born.

Just before your baby is born, a paediatrician will come into the delivery room and set up resuscitation equipment in case your baby needs oxygen immediately after birth.

Will my baby need any special tests after birth?
Breech babies are at increased risk of a condition called congenital dislocation of the hip, or CDH. Your baby will have an ultrasound scan of his hip joints in the few days after birth to check for this condition.

Caesarean Section

Caesarean sections are without doubt the most talked about and controversial issue in childbirth today. Some regard the rising rate of caesarean sections as evidence that doctors are taking away from women the right to give birth naturally. Many doctors agree that it is the safest way to deliver a child. Some women feel strongly that they would prefer to give birth by caesarean, others that they would try to avoid it at all costs. Some obstetricians would refuse to perform a caesarean section even if you were set on having one. Others are much more ready to listen to women who want one. This is reflected in the varying rate of elective caesareans at different hospitals. Some deliver as few as 4 per cent of babies this way, others as many as 14 per cent. Hospitals with higher elective caesarean rates are more likely to be sympathetic to women who want a caesarean. The unit profiles at the end of this book give elective and emergency caesarean rates for each maternity unit.

What is a caesarean section?

A caesarean section is an operation used to bring your baby into the world through a cut in your lower abdomen, just where your pubic hair begins. It can be performed under epidural or spinal anaesthesia, allowing you to stay awake, or under general anaesthetic. Afterwards you will have a 15cm horizontal wound held together by stitches or clips, and on average will stay in hospital for 4-5 days. In England, an average of over 20 per cent of women deliver their babies by caesarean section. The highest caesarean rate in England with 22 per cent of babies being born this way is the West Midlands. In contrast, the southwest of England has the lowest rate of caesarean sections, followed closely by the northwest. Northern Ireland has an average of 25 per cent, which is higher than England, Wales and Scotland.

Why might I be advised to have a caesarean section?

An elective caesarean section is one that is planned before you go into labour. The average elective caesarean rate for England is 8 per cent, but this varies between units from 3 per cent to 16 per cent. It may be offered in the following situations:
- If you have had two or more caesarean sections in the past.
- If your baby is lying in the wrong position – breech, for example.
- If your placenta is lying across the cervix (placenta praevia).
- If you are having a multiple birth. Triplets and higher multiples are almost always born by caesarean section.
- If you had extensive perineal damage (a third- or fourth-degree tear) in a previous labour.
- If you have a health problem of your own which might make it hazardous for you to labour.
- If you have active genital herpes when your baby is due, as there is a risk that your baby may become infected during birth and develop a dangerous form of meningitis.

- If you are HIV positive, as your baby is less likely to become infected if you have a caesarean section.
- An emergency caesarean section is carried out after labour has started. On average, 12 per cent of women give birth by emergency caesarean, but this figure varies between units from 1 per cent to 21 per cent. It may be necessary for the following reasons:
- Your cervix does not dilate effectively.
- Your baby starts to become distressed before your cervix is fully dilated.
- You start to bleed heavily.
- You are scheduled to have an elective caesarean section but go into labour early.
- Your baby is unexpectedly found to be breech and there is nobody available who is experienced in vaginal breech delivery.
- The umbilical cord, or the baby's hand or foot, comes through the cervix first.

The thought of giving birth terrifies me. Can I choose to have a caesarean section even if none of the above reasons apply to me?

Most obstetricians are seeing an increasing number of women requesting an elective caesarean section in preference to a normal vaginal delivery. Caesarean section rates are as high as 30 per cent of all deliveries in some hospitals and are continuing to rise – a figure which cannot be due entirely to an increase in the number of women for whom vaginal delivery would be unacceptably hazardous.

A study performed a few years ago showed that around one in three female obstetricians would choose to give birth by caesarean section. In another study, a group of midwives voted overwhelmingly in favour of giving birth by the traditional route. This may reflect the fact that midwives attend to normal deliveries while obstetricians only become involved when there is a problem and therefore perceive vaginal delivery to be more dangerous than it really is. If you feel strongly that you want a caesarean section, discuss the matter with your midwife or obstetrician. They will take your concerns seriously.

Birth Story Louise Sheppard

Before I became pregnant, I fully expected that childbirth would see my body 'opening like a flower', as the natural birth gurus say. I'd read the books on water birth and aromatherapy, but my friends' experiences of labour did not bear out the propaganda. Though all of them had wanted a natural birth, most had 'given in' and opted for epidurals, either sooner (at the first contraction) or later (after many hours of labour), some ending up with forceps deliveries and stitches. Lucy, who tried for a water birth, ended up with an emergency caesarean 48 hours later. Only Laura had managed the perfect 5 hour drug-free labour. Neither woman's pregnancy had given any indication of the birth ahead. Everyone knows horror stories. But my own pregnancy made me hunger for hard information that would show my chances of ending up like Laura or Lucy. I couldn't find it in the birth books or the pregnancy magazines. What I did find was an article in Vogue on the phenomenon of caesareans as a matter of maternal choice. These were the women who were 'too posh to push'. The gist of the argument was that birth needn't be a lottery, and that somewhere out there were surgeons who believed that for a healthy woman with a healthy pregnancy, elective caesareans were the safest option for both mother and child. This was the first article I had read that questioned the ideal of natural birth. It was also the first I had read where women who'd had caesareans did not feel as though they had somehow 'failed'. My local hospital was a 'push 'em out and send 'em home' place. If things went 'wrong', then you could have pain relief – or surgery – but only then. Luckily one midwife gave me the name of a consultant in the neighbouring health authority who believed in maternal choice as an absolute. I dug out medical journals, followed the pro- and anti- debate, and learned about the differences between sections performed at 38 and 39 weeks gestation. I learned about post-operative infection, about fetal oxygen deprivation, and, sure enough, when I finally met my consultant, it was like sitting a university viva. As he later put it, you have to understand that you are exchanging one set of risks for another. When the day came – we were offered a choice of two – I felt both calm and frightened. I walked into the theatre with my partner, exchanged a few wobbly jokes with the anaesthetists as they inserted the epidural, said good morning to my obstetrician and waited for ten of the strangest minutes of my life before hearing my son angrily greet the world. No, it wasn't entirely straightforward – my son's head was briefly stuck and I lost too much blood – but it was as intimate an experience as the very different one I had first imagined. The next few days were less blissful. Moving was tough, dealing with this strange little being was tough. The morphine drip was removed with stunning alacrity and most of my pain relief came from over-the-counter analgesics my partner smuggled in. But I recovered quickly, as do most mothers who get the birth that they wanted. The reactions of my friends varied. Some said they wished that they had had the courage to 'opt out', most simply didn't know that one could, and some wondered how I could 'miss out' on the experience of labour. But as the condemnation of us 'posh' girls gets harsher and harsher, I'm glad I fought for my right to the birth method of my choice.

Although some doctors may regard caesarean section as safer or less painful than vaginal delivery, you will lose more blood and are at greater risk of all types of infection and of blood clots in the legs and lungs. You will also have more pain in the days after delivery, and will take much longer to become fit to do everyday activities than after a normal delivery – for example, you will be unable to drive until your doctor considers you fit (on average, four weeks). Nor is caesarean section a completely safe option for your baby. Transient tachypnoea of the newborn is a condition in which babies become breathless in the first few hours of life. It is usually mild and settles down in a few days, but some babies need to be taken to the neonatal unit to have help with their breathing. This condition occurs almost exclusively in babies born by caesarean section and is thought to be due to the fact that these babies do not have the excess fluid in their lungs squeezed out during birth.

Can I be made to have a caesarean if the obstetrician thinks I should?

Almost certainly not. This has been the subject of a legal test case. Although the obstetrician could theoretically obtain a court order to carry out a caesarean section, by carrying out an operation against your wishes he would be open to a charge of assault. The survival of your unborn baby does not take priority over your wishes. If you have strong feelings about this, it is worth ensuring that you write down your wishes – and the reasons for them – before you go into labour, so that there can be no doubt about your intentions.

What can I expect to happen during a caesarean section under epidural?

An obstetrician – probably a senior house officer – will examine you and ask you to sign a consent form. If it is an elective caesarean section, you will be asked to stop eating 6 hours before the operation, and to stop taking fluids four hours before. This is to ensure that you do not vomit. You will be given a drink of medicine to neutralise your abdomen acid. Premedication with a sedative drug is not usually given because there is a risk that it will

Elective Caesarean Section

Pros:

- It is the only way to have a short, genuinely pain-free delivery.
- The risk of damage to the muscles of the pelvis is reduced.
- You can plan for your baby's birth in advance – you may even be able to choose the date.
- You can stay awake throughout using epidural or spinal anaesthesia.
- If you have had two or more previous caesarean sections, if you are having triplets, or if your baby is breech, an elective caesarean section is, on balance, the safest choice.

Cons:

- Even an uncomplicated caesarean section can leave you with severe pain around the wound for days afterwards.
- You are at increased risk from many types of infection – about 30% of women will have an infection in the womb, bladder or chest after a caesarean section.
- You are at increased risk of developing a blood clot in your leg or lung.
- You will not be able to drive for a month afterwards.
- It is more difficult to get your abdominal muscles back into shape after a caesarean section than after a vaginal delivery.
- Although your baby will have a beautiful rounded head, it will also be at increased risk of breathing difficulties in the first few days of its life.

interfere with your baby's ability to breathe in the first few hours of life. At the time of delivery you may be given an antibiotic to reduce the risk of infection and after the delivery, an injection of heparin to help prevent thrombosis.

Birth Story Lorna Gold

Doctors have a reputation for being difficult obstetric patients, and I was no exception. My first baby was born by elective caesarean section for breech. With my second baby, I was completely unprepared for how painful a labour can be. I started off under the care of a midwife who wanted to send me to the antenatal ward before she went off duty, while my only thought was to get an epidural in place quickly. I was given a dose of pethidine which I did not want and which was ineffective. When the shift changed, I had my epidural and excellent care from a midwife with whom I had worked in the past. I was delivered using forceps, bled so heavily that I became anaemic, and could not sit properly for several weeks afterwards due to pain in the wound.

When my third baby was on the way, I was not worried about the pregnancy itself, but felt convinced that I was incapable of giving birth normally. My bowel had not recovered after my previous delivery, and I was afraid that any more perineal damage would make me incontinent. I therefore chose to book at a different hospital under the care of an obstetrician who had a reputation among my patients for being particularly good at handling anxious mothers-to-be, and stated from the outset that I wanted an elective caesarean section. The obstetrician did not dismiss my concerns, but suggested postponing the final decision about the mode of delivery until after an ultrasound scan at around 38 weeks to assess the likely size of the baby.

The baby was predicted to weigh around 3kg, and the obstetrician suggest I try to give birth vaginally. I agreed, on the understanding that if I ran into difficulty I should have an immediate caesarean section rather than another forceps delivery. The obstetrician wrote in my notes that she should be contacted as soon as I was admitted in labour, even if it was the middle of the night.

Two days after my due date, I woke up in labour in the early hours of the morning, and within an hour was almost immobilised by a succession of painful contractions. Somehow my husband managed to get me into the car. When I crawled, howling like a hyena with a thorn in its paw, into the maternity unit, I apologised for making so much fuss so early in labour. The midwife took one look and told me that she thought I was in the second stage already. She was right. There was no time for pain relief (I was in too much pain to use the Entonox properly), and I can remember thinking that I would rather die that suffer one more contraction. Half an hour after I arrived at the hospital, Elizabeth was born, weighing 3.1kg. I had only a tiny tear which was not worth stitching. There had been no time – and no need – to disturb the obstetrician.

I was surprised how much more quickly I recovered from a normal delivery. I took Elizabeth home within a few hours, and was able to drive the following day. Less than two years later, my fourth baby was born at home – a wonderful experience, which I might not have had, had I not been encouraged to try for a natural birth with Elizabeth.

The top part of your pubic hair will be shaved. You will be taken to the operating theatre and moved on to a table which may be tilted so that your right side is a little higher than your left. You will have a drip in your arm, and the anaesthetist will put a thin plastic tube into the layers of tissue around your spinal cord and inject a test dose of anaesthetic. This should give you a warm feeling in your back and make your legs start to go numb. If this happens, he will inject the rest of the dose of anaesthetic.

Your skin will be cleaned with an antiseptic solution (if you are allergic to iodine, tell the theatre staff in case they use an iodine-based antiseptic), and your bladder will be emptied using a catheter. After testing to ensure that your abdomen is numb, the obstetricians will put sterile drapes from your chest to your feet, exposing only the place where the cut will be made. Meanwhile, the anaesthetist will be keeping an eye on your pulse and blood pressure. If your partner is present, he will be encouraged to sit near the head end of the operating table.

There will be several people present – two obstetricians and one midwife scrubbed up for the operation, at least one other midwife to look after the baby, an operating department assistant, a paediatrician and an anaesthetist. With your consent, medical or midwifery students may be present as observers.

Once the operation starts, your baby will be born within two or three minutes, then wrapped up and handed to you or your partner if all is well. It then takes around 20-30 minutes to suture all the layers of the wound. At most, you will have a sensation of someone rummaging around in your abdomen a long way away.

After your abdomen has been stitched back together, you will be taken to the recovery room. The midwife will check your vital signs and help you to put your baby to the breast, and you should be given an injection of a strong painkiller like morphine before the epidural wears off. If you are not offered this, consider asking for it, as the pain could come as a big shock when the epidural stops working.

You will go back to the postnatal ward within a few hours, and the drip will be taken out if you are well and your blood pressure is normal. Once the feeling has returned to your legs, you will be encouraged to start getting up to the toilet and to look after your baby. The catheter will be removed after about 12 hours.

How long will I be in pain?

Everyone recovers at different rates, but it will be three or four days before you can stand up straight without bracing yourself first. After that, the pain will settle quite quickly and within a couple of weeks you should no longer need painkillers, but it is not uncommon to feel pain for weeks or months afterwards.

Will I be fit to look after my baby?

Realistically, you will need help. Nobody would dream of telling a woman to get up and look after a newborn baby after having, for example, a hysterectomy – yet a caesarean section is just as big an operation. For the first few days, you will not safely be able to give your baby a bath unaided, and you may need help to find a comfortable position in which to feed your baby. Don't be afraid to ask the midwives for help. Now is also an ideal time for your partner to get involved in the practical aspects of caring for the baby.

When will I be able to go home?

If you are making an uneventful recovery, you will be discharged after 4-5 days – earlier in some units. You will still need help with your baby at this stage, so if you will not have anyone at home to help you, it is worth asking if you can stay in hospital for a few more days.

Will I have my postnatal examination in hospital?

Until recently, a woman who had had a caesarean section would be given an appointment to have her postnatal check-up at the hospital by the obstetrician. Now, even after a caesarean section, your postnatal examination will be done by your GP or practice nurse six weeks after delivery. If you have not received an appointment by the time your baby is four weeks old, contact your GP.

Stillbirth

What is a stillbirth, and how common is it?
A baby is stillborn if it is born after 24 weeks gestation without showing any signs of life. About one baby in 200 in the UK is stillborn.

What causes stillbirth?
Only one in ten stillbirths is due to problems arising during birth. Another one in ten is caused by abnormalities in the baby, and in the remainder the baby is normal but dies before the beginning of labour. In many of these cases no cause is found, but placental insufficiency, in which the placenta becomes incapable of carrying enough food or oxygen to the baby, may be at least partly responsible. Smoking and pregnancy-induced hypertension both cause the blood vessels of the placenta to harden and stop working properly and increase the risk of stillbirth. They also increase the risk of placental abruption, in which part or all of the placenta is torn away from the wall of the womb and which is often fatal for the baby and sometimes for the mother too.

Babies born prematurely are more likely to be stillborn, especially if they are born before 28 weeks gestation. Babies born after 42 weeks gestation are also more likely to be stillborn than those born between 37 and 42 weeks, which is why most obstetricians advise inducing labour before 42 weeks.

How can I reduce the risk of my baby being stillborn?
Stop smoking before conceiving, or as early as possible in your pregnancy, and if your partner lives with you he should stop smoking too.
Don't drink a lot of alcohol during pregnancy There is no 'safe' limit – the best approach is to avoid alcohol altogether.
Minimise your risk of coming into contact with infections which can cause stillbirth These are the same as for second trimester miscarriage – listeria (found in chilled food and unpasteurised soft cheeses), toxoplasma (found in cat faeces and, therefore, in the soil of most gardens), cytomegalovirus, and rubella.

Always call the hospital if you notice any change in the pattern of movements of your baby.

What are the signs that a baby may have died in the womb?
In most women, absence of movements is the main sign. Some women stop 'feeling pregnant' and the bump may shrink as the amount of fluid around the baby decreases.

What tests will be done to find out whether my baby is still alive or not?
The first test is likely to be a CTG (cardiotocograph). If a trace of your baby's heartbeat can be obtained, your baby is alive, although the pattern of the trace will be studied carefully because it may show if your baby is becoming distressed and you need to be delivered urgently.

If no fetal heart trace can be recorded, you will have an ultrasound scan. If your baby's heart is seen and is not beating, this is definite evidence of death.

What will happen if my baby is dead?
You will need to be delivered promptly. Many women go into labour by themselves soon after the baby's death, but if you do not then labour will be induced within 48 hours of the diagnosis.

Will I be able to see and hold my baby afterwards?
Yes. You will be encouraged to do so for as long as you wish.

Can I wait for my labour to start naturally instead of having it induced?
Up to a point. If you are well with no evidence of infection and your waters have not broken, it is reasonable to take 12-24 hours to come to terms with the death of your baby and await the start of labour. However, the longer the baby stays in your womb, the greater the risk that you will develop a severe infection in the fluid around the baby. This can lead to blood poisoning, haemorrhage and collapse, and can be fatal within hours. If your waters have broken or if you have a vaginal discharge, you should accept induction immediately.

Am I entitled to maternity leave after a stillbirth?

Yes, provided your baby is born no more than 11 weeks before its due date.

What will happen in my next pregnancy?

If your baby was stillborn because it was abnormal in some way, you will be offered detailed scans and, if appropriate, CVS or amniocentesis, in your next pregnancy. In most cases the abnormality has arisen by chance and the next baby is fine, but occasionally there is a genetic problem which means that future babies are at risk.

If you had an unexplained stillbirth, you will probably be seen regularly in the consultant unit during your next pregnancy and will be offered extra scans, tests of placental function, and CTGs as your pregnancy progresses.

After a stillbirth caused by problems arising during birth, many women choose to have an elective caesarean section in future pregnancies although the chance of another stillbirth during vaginal delivery is very low.

Where can I find further information and support?
The national organisation for support after stillbirth is the Stillbirth and Neonatal Death Society (SANDS), Helpline 020 7436, www.uk-sands.org

Twins

About one pregnancy in 80 in the UK is a twin pregnancy. The rate is higher in some populations, particularly women of African descent, women who are over 35 or who have had several babies already, and women who have had assisted conception. Higher multiples are rare, especially now the number of embryos that can be replaced during each cycle of assisted conception has been limited to two by law. Triplets occur in around one pregnancy in 6,400, and quadruplets in one pregnancy in 500,000 – about one set a year in the UK.

How will I know if I'm having twins?

Often, you will suspect early in pregnancy that something is different, especially if this is not your first pregnancy. The higher hormone levels in a twin pregnancy can make early pregnancy symptoms such as nausea and tiredness worse, and you may develop an obvious bump earlier than expected. However, most women who have a twin pregnancy find out unexpectedly when two babies show up on a routine ultrasound scan.

Can the scan show whether or not my twins are identical?

Sometimes. If both twins are in the same sac of amniotic fluid, they are definitely identical. However, if they are different sexes they are definitely not identical. Twins of the same sex who are in separate sacs can be either identical or non-identical.

What can I expect during a twin pregnancy?

You will be seen more frequently in the hospital antenatal clinic, and will have more scans. This is because it is more difficult to assess the growth of each baby in a multiple pregnancy by feeling the size of the bump, and because twins are at greater risk of being small for dates.

Although each baby in a pair of twins is normally smaller than a singleton baby, the presence of two babies and their placentas and amniotic fluid means that your bump will become very large quite quickly. You will need a lot of rest during pregnancy, and will probably be more than ready to start your maternity leave at the earliest possible opportunity – currently 11 weeks before the babies are due.

You are more likely to become anaemic, and your midwife or obstetrician may advise you to take an iron supplement to try to prevent this.

Twins are at higher risk than singletons of being born prematurely. On average, twins are born at 37 weeks gestation rather than 40 weeks (the figure is 34 weeks for triplets and 30 weeks for quadruplets). Until around 20 years ago, women carrying twins were routinely admitted to hospital for bedrest between 28 and 32 weeks to try to prevent premature labour. This practice has now been discontinued as it did not reduce the rate of premature labour and bedrest vastly increases the risk of blood clots developing in your legs or lungs. The outlook for a baby born at 28 weeks has improved considerably in the past few decades – most will survive without any permanent handicap.

Will I have to have a caesarean section?

Not necessarily. If the twin to be born first is in the head-down position and there are no other problems, you have a good prospect of being able to have a vaginal delivery. If you are having triplets or a higher multiple, you will almost certainly need to have a caesarean section.

What does a twin delivery involve?

There is a risk of problems arising unexpectedly with the second twin, and there is a greater chance that you will haemorrhage after delivery because the raw area left after the placenta has come away is bigger and the overstretched muscle of your womb is less able to contract and stop blood loss. You might prefer therefore to choose a hospital delivery.

In early labour, you should be able to move around and have intermittent monitoring. As the second stage of labour approaches, you will be advised to have a drip (so that fluids and medication to stop blood loss can be given quickly) and possibly an epidural. Both twins will be monitored continuously. The delivery room will be full of people – two obstetricians (of whom one should be a consultant or senior registrar), three midwives (one for you and one for each baby), two paediatricians, an anaesthetist, and an ultrasonographer with a portable ultrasound scanner. If you consent, medical or midwifery students may be there as observers. In some units, all twin deliveries take place in the operating theatre so that a caesarean section can be performed promptly if problems arise.

After the first twin is born, the obstetrician or midwife will examine your abdomen to check the position of the second twin, and an ultrasound scan may be done. If the second twin is presenting by the head or breech, delivery should be straightforward. If not, the obstetrician may put a hand into your womb, pull down the baby's foot and perform a breech delivery (a technique called internal podalic version). Occasionally it is necessary to deliver you of the second twin by emergency caesarean section.

Afterwards, you may be given Syntocinon through the drip for a few hours to make sure your womb contracts properly. Cross-matched blood will have been prepared in advance in case you bleed heavily and need a transfusion.

What is selective fetal reduction?
If you are carrying four or more fetuses, your obstetrician may suggest that you consider having selective fetal reduction performed. This involves killing one or more of the fetuses early in pregnancy by injecting potassium chloride (a type of salt) into the heart. The dead fetuses are absorbed and the remaining babies are less likely to be born prematurely and therefore at lower risk of being significantly handicapped.

Selective fetal reduction can also be performed in twin or triplet pregnancies if an early scan shows that one of the fetuses has a major abnormality.

Apart from the emotional implications of consenting to sacrifice one or more fetuses for the benefit of the others, selective fetal reduction carries a one in ten risk of causing the entire pregnancy to miscarry. It is an option worth considering in certain circumstances, but one that requires counselling and reference to your own moral and religious beliefs.

If I have twins, am I entitled to any extra maternity leave or benefits?
You are not entitled to a longer period of maternity leave or to a higher rate of maternity benefit, but you can claim child benefit for each baby.

What about extra help with the babies?
As soon as you know you are having a multiple birth and are unable to afford a private nurse qualified in child care for the first three weeks, it is worth looking into the possibility of providing a

placement for a student doing a nursery nursing course. You can either discuss this with your health visitor – who may have links with the course tutors – or make a direct approach to the further education colleges in your area.

Nursery nursing students are able to help with practical aspects of caring for your baby under your supervision, but you cannot use them as childminders or babysitters.

If I have twins, will I be able to breastfeed?
Twins can be breastfed very successfully. The best approach to breastfeeding twins is to feed them at the same time, with each twin latched on to a breast. You will be shown a special way of holding your twins for breastfeeding, with their bodies tucked under your arms. You can choose to feed twins separately, but if you do this you may end up feeling as if you are never without a baby attached to your breast. Breastfeeding triplets is much more difficult, and you are more likely to need to give supplementary bottles.

Where can I find out more?
Most hospitals have a support group for women who are pregnant with twins or higher multiples. Details should be available from the antenatal clinic. You can also contact the national Twins and Multiple Births Association at TAMBA, tel 0870 121 4000 or 0151 348 0020, www.tamba.org.uk

Section Three:
After the Birth

The responsibilities of your maternity service do not end at birth. The first weeks and months after delivery can be a very stressful time, and your service should be supportive as you take on the enormous responsibility of having a new baby to care for. Postnatal care begins at the maternity unit as you recover from the birth and extends to your home, where community midwives should be available to visit you. You may also be given access to a postnatal support helpline.

One key objective of postnatal care is the establishment of successful breastfeeding. Breastfeeding reduces the risk of babies developing many illnesses, and is thought to lower the incidence of illnesses later in childhood as well. Breastfeeding should be started as soon as possible after birth, so it is vital that staff at your unit are trained to help you initiate breastfeeding.

Units that wish to demonstrate their commitment to breastfeeding can apply for UNICEF breast accreditation, which requires that they undergo rigorous assessment in this area every two years. They can achieve full 'UNICEF baby friendly status' or part recognition with a 'certificate of commitment'. Sustaining breastfeeding requires continued support, and some maternity services run breastfeeding clinics as part of their postnatal care. You may also have access to breastfeeding counsellors who can visit you at home or a specialist breastfeeding helpline.

Breastfeeding

It is universally acknowledged that, except in a few very rare situations, the best food for newborn babies is their mother's breast milk. This is because:

- Breast milk contains the ideal balance of nutrients for the human baby, and is easily digested.
- The production of breast milk is tailored to the individual baby's needs. For example, in hot weather you will produce more of the dilute foremilk to give your baby extra fluid, so there is no need to give bottles of water between feeds.
- Neither breast milk nor your nipples need to be sterilised.

- Breast milk contains antibodies to protect your baby from infectious diseases, particularly gastroenteritis.
- Breast milk is always available 'on tap'. Going out even on a short journey with a small baby involves taking an amazing amount of baggage with you – if you breastfeed, you can dispense with bottles and bottle-warmers.
- Breastfeeding is cheaper than formula feeding, even taking into account the cost of nursing bras and the extra food you need to eat.
- It is thought that the action of suckling makes breastfed babies less likely to get ear infections following a cold.
- Breastfed babies do not become constipated, and the dirty nappies of a breastfed baby smell less unpleasant than those of a formula fed baby.
- For most women, breastfeeding is psychologically satisfying.

It sounds perfect. There must be drawbacks, or every mother would breastfeed.
In the 1960s, many health professionals involved with maternity care discouraged breastfeeding and advised women to give their babies formula feeds. It was thought that formula feeding was more hygienic, scientific, and convenient for the mother. It was certainly easier to fit formula feeding into the rigid feeding schedules which were considered appropriate for babies in those days. It took a very brave woman to resist the trend and breastfeed her baby.

As a result, the generation of women who are now becoming grandmothers are not in a position to offer their daughters practical advice and support with breastfeeding, and may even, with the best of intentions, try to pressurise them into formula feeding.
Although we now know that the experts of the 1960s were wrong, breastfeeding does have a few genuine disadvantages compared with formula feeding.
- It can only be done by the mother (unless she expresses milk, which some women find tough to do), so fathers and grandparents may feel excluded. Changing a nappy does not give quite the same satisfaction as feeding the baby.

Birth Story Marion Frost

In the early months of my pregnancy I decided that I would breastfeed my baby and simply assumed that because I wanted to, it would be easy. I'd heard the stories about women who tried to breastfeed and gave up, either because the baby couldn't do it or because they were simply too exhausted, but I dismissed these as feeble excuses. How wrong could I be?

I thought that babies were born knowing how to breastfeed, but while it is easy for a few, the vast majority of babies – and mothers – have to learn. The baby's head and body need to be in the right position and he needs to 'latch-on' correctly – that is, to have a large area of breast in his mouth and use his entire jaw to suck – otherwise he doesn't get any milk. He should also be hungry. My baby was born after a long and difficult labour and for the first 12 hours wasn't the slightest bit interested in food.

Nevertheless, during my time in hospital, breastfeeding seemed, if not easy, then at least a very real possibility, as there was always someone to show me how to hold him and to help him latch on. Once he got going he was ok, but even the midwives sometimes took 20 minutes to get him started. My birth hadn't gone to plan and it slowly began to dawn on me that breastfeeding wasn't going to be easy either. But it wasn't until we got home that the difficulties really started.

It seems ridiculous now, but it would take me up to an hour to get him to latch on. And every time he 'fell off' the breast – which he did frequently – it would take all that time to get him on again. After my labour, I felt more tired than I had ever been in my life and that first night his feed took six hours from midnight. By morning I was beginning to feel wildly hysterical and a complete failure. At seven o'clock I gave him a bottle.

But I was determined not to give up, and the community midwives who visited me at home were hugely encouraging. One in particular was amazingly supportive, visiting me every day for the first five days, which were by far the worst, lending me books and putting me in touch with local support groups. She told me that it could take up to six weeks to learn how to breastfeed and, very gently, that if it didn't work out, I wasn't a failure.

After two weeks it still took up to 2 hours for each feed, but this was at least manageable and it was becoming less and less each day. At the end of six weeks, it was completely sorted. Breastfeeding became the calm oasis of my day. I would sit down, put my feet up and just relax. It was wonderful. As he got older, the interaction became more intense. He would stare into my eyes or play with my clothes while attached firmly to my breast. I loved it.

I continued to breastfeed throughout his early months and let myself be guided by him. At six months old he was down to one feed a day. Then suddenly, around the ten-month mark, he lost interest, latching on and becoming instantly distracted, and so I stopped. My baby didn't miss breastfeeding in the slightest. I can't say the same for me.

- Breastfed babies tend to need a night feed for longer than formula fed babies.
- At the beginning, breastfeeding can be painful due to cracked nipples – which, whatever you may read in the baby books, can occur even if your baby's position at the breast is perfect. If you persevere, this does settle down.

Will I be offered help to start breastfeeding?

Yes. The World Health Organisation Baby Friendly Hospital Initiative has been widely adopted by British hospitals, and includes the following ten points:
- There should be a written breastfeeding policy of which all healthcare staff should routinely be made aware.
- All healthcare staff should be trained in the skills necessary to implement this policy.
- Every pregnant woman should be given information about the benefits and management of breastfeeding.
- Mothers should be helped to start breastfeeding within 30 minutes of giving birth (it is now also known that breastfeeding is more likely to succeed if the mother, rather than the midwife, puts the baby to the breast).
- Mothers should be shown how to breastfeed, and how to maintain their milk supply, even if they are separated from their babies.
- Babies should not be given any food or drink apart from breast milk, unless there is a medical reason to do so.
- Mothers and babies should be allowed to stay together 24 hours a day.
- Breastfeeding on demand should be encouraged.
- Breastfeeding babies should not be given a dummy or pacifier.
- Breastfeeding support groups should be encouraged and recommended to mothers on discharge from hospital.
- You can contact UNICEF UK Baby Friendly Initiative on tel 020 7312 7652, www.babyfriendly.org.uk. Alternatively, the NCT has a breastfeeding helpline on 0870 444 8708, 8am – 10pm, 7 days a week.

What if I don't seem to be producing any milk after my baby is born?

Don't worry, it is normal to produce nothing apart from a clear yellowish fluid called colostrum for the first 48 hours or so after your baby is born. Colostrum is rich in protein and antibodies against infection. A full term baby has sufficient reserves to need nothing else, and it is important to resist the temptation to give your baby a drink of water or formula milk during this time unless his blood sugar drops so low that he develops symptoms of hypoglycaemia. Do allow your baby to suckle regularly – this will help your milk supply.

Are there any situations in which I shouldn't breastfeed?

If you are HIV positive, or are on chemotherapy for cancer, drugs for an overactive thyroid gland, or an antidepressant called lithium, you will be advised not to breastfeed.

If your baby is very premature, they may need a special high-energy formula feed. However, you will be encouraged to try to express breast milk so that he can benefit from it and to keep your milk supply going so that you can breastfeed him when he is ready.

Will breastfeeding stop me from getting pregnant again?

Breastfeeding a baby is an effective form of contraception provided the following conditions apply:

- Your baby is less than six months old.
- You are not giving your baby any food apart from breast milk.
- Your periods have not returned.
- As soon as you start to introduce even a small amount of formula milk or weaning food, you should start to use alternative contraception unless you plan to become pregnant again quickly.

What forms of contraception can I use when I am breastfeeding?

The only form of contraception which you should avoid is the combined pill, which may reduce your milk supply. All other forms are safe to use. If the pill is your preferred form of contraception, a good compromise is to take the progestogen-only pill (the mini-pill) while you are breastfeeding, and go back on to the combined pill once your baby is weaned.

Can I continue to breastfeed even if I do become pregnant again?

Yes, although you may find that your milk supply starts to diminish.

Are there any national organisations which offer help and support to breastfeeding mothers?

The National Childbirth Trust has a breastfeeding information line (0870 444 8708) which can give you contact details of breastfeeding counsellors in your area.

La Leche League is an international organisation which promotes breastfeeding, and it has branches in the UK and Ireland. They have a 24 hour advice line (020 7242 1278) which can give you contact details for breastfeeding counsellors in your area.

If I decide not to breastfeed, will I be pressurised to change my mind?

No. If you decide from the start that you do not want to breastfeed, you should be shown how to make up and give formula feeds. However, you should be fully counselled to ensure that you are making a truly informed decision.

Can I have medication to dry up my milk if I do not breastfeed?

There are drugs available which can stop your milk coming in, but they are expensive and have unpleasant side effects so they are not prescribed routinely. Wearing a firm support bra, taking painkillers such as aspirin or paracetamol, and resisting the temptation to relieve the pressure in your breasts by expressing some of the milk, will stop your milk production within a few days. Applying an ice pack, or a pack of frozen peas wrapped in a tea towel around your breasts helps to settle the swelling and discomfort.

There are so many formula milks. Which should I choose?

All of the leading brand first-stage milks are suitable for babies from birth, and there is little to choose between them. They have been heavily modified to give them a similar nutritional content to human breastmilk as possible. They all cost around the same amount. Always make formula milk up to the correct strength using the scoop provided and freshly boiled tap water, not bottled or chemically sterilised water.

Don't be tempted to try formula products which are advertised as being suitable for 'hungrier babies'. There is no evidence that they really do make a hungry baby less demanding, and the high casein (curd) content makes them quite different from human breastmilk and can make babies more likely to suffer from constipation and vomiting. Do not give your baby soy formula unless a paediatrician has made a definite diagnosis of intolerance to lactose or cow's milk protein. In these rare situations, your GP will prescribe soy formula or another special milk for your baby. There is no evidence that babies with colic, eczema or recurrent colds benefit from being put on soy formula.

Dried skimmed milk, tinned evaporated milk and ordinary pasteurised cow's, goat's or sheep's milk are not suitable for babies in the first year of life.

Wound Care

What will happen about my caesarean section wound?
The midwife will check it every day, and will clean the wound site and change the dressing if you have one. If there is any sign of infection, such as redness or increasing tenderness, you may be prescribed a course of antibiotics and some of your stitches or clips may be removed.

If you have clips or non-absorbable stitches, these will be taken out after 5-7 days. Absorbable stitches such as catgut or vicryl will dissolve by themselves within a week or two. Having regular baths or showers will speed up this process. Most caesarean section wounds fade to a very thin line similar in colour to your skin within a few months.

How should I look after my episiotomy site?

When you have had stitches in your perineum, especially if these were the result of a forceps delivery, the area around your vagina will be very sore for a few days. Avoid sitting, even on a rubber ring, for long periods – stay up and about, or lie on one side to rest. Applying an ice pack for no more than a few minutes at a time can be soothing.

Wash the stitched area after going to the toilet – a bidet is useful for this, but pouring a jug of water over your perineum while you sit on the toilet is equally effective. Dry gently with a clean towel.

If your perineum becomes very swollen and the stitches are cutting into the skin, your midwife may suggest taking them out. This is a good idea – you will have immediate relief from pain, and you will heal up just as quickly. Infection can occur, but this is surprisingly uncommon considering how close the perineum is to the anus.

What are afterpains?

Afterpains are contraction-type pains from the muscle of your womb which occur in the 24-48 hours after your baby is born. They can be quite severe, although rarely as bad as labour itself – more like a really bad period pain. Afterpains tend to get worse with successive babies. Painkillers such as paracetamol or ibuprofen can help, and are safe even if you are breastfeeding. Aspirin, however, should be avoided.

How long will I bleed after giving birth?

For the first few days, you may have quite heavy, fresh red blood loss with a few small clots. The bleeding then gives way to a pinkish-brown watery fluid called lochia which normally lasts for 2-3 weeks, but you may have a pinkish discharge for up to 5-6 weeks. If you are passing large clots and your blood loss cannot be contained by maternity pads, or if your lochia suddenly changes back to fresh red blood, tell your midwife – you may have a retained piece of placenta or have developed an infection of the womb.

How will I know if I have an infection of the womb?

Infection of the womb (puerperal sepsis, or endometritis) is rare after an uncomplicated normal delivery, but is more likely if you have had a very long labour with lots of internal examinations, a caesarean section, or if the placenta did not come away completely after the baby was born.

Infection of the womb typically develops 5-7 days after delivery, so it is unlikely to show up while you are still in hospital. It can present with the following symptoms:

- Fever, possibly with sweating and shivering.
- A fast pulse – this is one of the reasons why the midwife measures your pulse rate at every postnatal check.
- Instead of being well contracted, your womb becomes soft and tender and may rise above your umbilicus.
- Sudden increase in blood loss, or a smelly vaginal discharge.
- Vomiting, headache and a general feeling of exhaustion.
- If diagnosed early, infections of the womb can be treated very effectively with antibiotic tablets unless a large piece of placenta has been left behind. If this is suspected, you will be sent back into hospital for a scan and, if necessary, a small internal operation to remove the retained placenta.

If I have my baby in hospital, how long will I stay in afterwards?

This can range from a few hours to five days, depending on the type of delivery you had, whether or not you had any complications such as haemorrhage or retained placenta, and how much support you have at home. It is no longer considered medically necessary for women to stay in hospital for a long time after delivery. Getting mobile early reduces the risk of venous thrombosis (blood clots in the legs or lungs), and you are at much lower risk of infection in your own home than in the postnatal ward.

If you have a caesarean section, you can expect to stay in hospital for around 5 days, although some units allow you to go home after three days if you are well enough. If you have a forceps delivery, you will be able to stay in for 2-3 days.

Birth Story Sue Morris

As my due date approached, my baby suddenly stopped moving around. I immediately checked into the Hospital, and was soon rigged up to a monitor which showed my baby's heart beating, safe and sound. Although I had attended antenatal classes with midwives and at a yoga clinic, no one had told me that this is a regular occurrence prior to the onset of labour – the baby shuts up as it gets ready for the big plunge.

I was advised to stay in overnight so that the hospital could monitor me, but, although my contractions had now begun, they were barely noticeable, so I went home. I slept pretty well, and then went for a walk in the park the next day. The contractions were now getting stronger, and I had to stop every ten minutes or so, bent over double against a tree or bench. By midnight I was crawling on the floor in agony. I rang the hospital. 'It sounds as if you are ready', was the calm reply.

I actually walked into the foyer and even climbed the stairs to the maternity unit, where, happily, a midwife from my practice was on duty. She examined me in a delivery suite – I was already 5cm dilated. 'You are a star!' she said, and repeated it regularly over the next painful 6 hours. She broke my waters there and then and put me on a monitor for the first 20 minutes, which was agony, as I had to remain totally still. At last I was allowed to move around – on the bed, off the bed, crouched on all fours on a mat on the floor – all the time taking deep draughts of the magical gas and air.

The second stage was agony, and I begged for an epidural – 'Sorry, it's too late'! I just remember screaming

'I can't do it, I can't do it', 'you can, you can' said the midwife. I pushed with all my force. The crowning was excruciating, the delivery of the head and body amazingly quick and light. A second midwife appeared, plunged a big needle into my thigh and then disappeared as quickly as she had come. This was the Syntometrin – a drug given as a matter of course to speed up the delivery of the placenta from a natural half hour to 7 minutes. To extract the (giant) placenta in just a few minutes must be tricky. I coughed, as directed, and the midwife drew it out and carried it back-stage.

Back at home four days later, the visiting midwife was examining an alarming piece of blackened flesh hanging from between my legs, 'Oh dear, you will have to go into hospital for this one' she said. I heard her talking calmly on the phone to the maternity ward nurse, 'I think we have a prolapsed vagina here'. I had to go back to hospital and was terrified, and pretty weepy, but once there the registrar rapidly identified the real problem. It wasn't a prolapse, which, by the way, is extremely rare, especially in women in their 30s. However, a piece of placenta as big as a lamb's liver had been left behind after delivery. Apparently I got away lightly, as this can cause a fever and really bad infection, or necessitate a DNC for some women. But in my case, once the placenta was removed, a course of antibiotics soon sorted the problem.

What can I do if I feel I'm being sent home too early?

Tell the ward manager, or the midwife who is looking after you. If you are not well enough to go home, or do not have the social support you need, they can usually let you stay a little longer.

How do I know that my baby is well enough to go home?

The midwife will check your baby regularly while you are on the postnatal ward, and before you take your baby home he or she will be examined thoroughly by a paediatrician (usually a senior house officer). If the senior house officer thinks there may be a problem, they will either arrange for a more senior paediatrician to see your baby before you go home, or make an appointment for you to bring your baby to the outpatient clinic. In some units, your baby will be checked by a specially trained midwife instead of a paediatrician.

Who will I see when I go home from hospital?

Your community midwife – probably the same midwife who looked after you during your pregnancy – will visit you for up to 28 days. Most community midwives will visit when needed rather than routinely visiting every day. Some GPs routinely visit every woman who has had a baby, while others only visit if the midwife asks them to do so because there is a problem.

What will the community midwife do when she visits me?

She will ask how you are feeling and how well your baby is feeding, sleeping, and filling its nappies. She will examine the following:

- **Your abdomen,** to check that your womb is shrinking properly and that your caesarean section scar, if you have one, is healing.
- **Your perineum,** if you have tears or stitches.
- **Your maternity pad,** to make sure your lochia is normal.
- **Your breasts,** to check for engorgement, mastitis, or cracked nipples.
- **Your temperature, pulse and blood pressure.**

She will be able to advise you on how to manage some of the discomforts of the postnatal period, such as constipation and sore breasts and she will examine and weigh your baby.

Why did the community midwife take blood from my baby?
There are two likely reasons. First, if your baby is jaundiced (yellow), the midwife may take a blood sample to the hospital to make sure that this is not severe enough to need treatment. Second, at the age of 5-7 days, all babies have a blood test called a Guthrie test to check for an underactive thyroid gland and phenylketonuria – both serious, though rare, conditions which respond well to being treated promptly. More recently, the Guthrie test has been extended to include cystic fibrosis and sickle cell disease.

What will happen after the midwife has stopped visiting me?
When your baby is about ten days old, your health visitor will contact you to arrange a convenient time to visit you at home, tell you about the care she offers, and give you a personal child health record ('red book') in which all of your baby's routine health care will be recorded.

What will happen at my postnatal check?
When your baby is about six weeks old, you should be invited to attend your GP's surgery for a postnatal check. The purpose of this is:
- To make sure that you have recovered, physically and mentally, from your pregnancy and delivery.
- To check that your perineum has healed up sufficiently to allow you to have sex.
- To check, if you are bottlefeeding, that you have had a period.
- To make sure you are confident in looking after your baby, and to discuss feeding.
- To check for postnatal depression.
- To take a cervical smear test, if you have not had a normal one within the past 3 years.
- To discuss contraception.
- To offer you advice about health related issues such as diet and smoking.

If the practice nurse does your postnatal check, she will refer you to the GP if you have problems such as a perineal wound which is slow to heal.

Postnatal Emotional Problems

The incidence of mental illness and suicide in women falls during pregnancy, but rises again after giving birth. The majority of women will suffer a brief attack of 'maternity blues' starting within a week of giving birth and lasting no more than a few days. However, at least one woman in ten develops postnatal depression, and in many cases the condition is not diagnosed. This is because either the woman does not realise that what she is experiencing is different to the normal process of adjustment of having a baby, or because health professionals do not think of it.

How will I know whether I have postnatal depression or just maternity blues?

Maternity blues usually occur around 3-5 days after delivery, and are often preceded by a day or two of feeling particularly positive and energetic. The symptoms are entirely mood-related, particularly tearfulness and irritability.

Postnatal depression typically starts later – between two weeks and three months after delivery, although occasionally it does not develop until the baby is six months old – and it may not be obvious at first that you are depressed. Although postnatal depression can cause tearfulness, anxiety and feelings of guilt, it can present instead with physical symptoms like tiredness and loss of appetite, or extreme anxiety about your baby's health. Mothers who are always consulting the GP or health visitor about their baby's feeding and sleeping pattern or minor disorders like snuffles and rashes are very often found to have postnatal depression.

What causes postnatal depression?

Some experts think it is caused by hormonal changes and others think it is a purely psychological illness caused by the major lifestyle changes involved in becoming a mother. There is evidence to support both views, which suggests that postnatal depression is either a group of symptoms which can develop for more than one reason, or a condition caused by a combination of physical and social factors.

Will any tests be done to see if I have postnatal depression?

In the first few weeks after your baby is born, your health visitor may ask you to do a test called the Edinburgh Postnatal Depression Score. This asks you to choose a response to each of ten questions, each of which has a score. If your total score is more than 13 it is likely that you are suffering from postnatal depression. The test may be repeated later if you request it, or if your health visitor, practice nurse or GP suspect that you may be developing postnatal depression.

My GP diagnosed postnatal depression without doing any tests.

Sometimes the signs and symptoms of depression are so obvious that there is no need to do the Edinburgh Postnatal Depression Score. Other tests, such as blood tests and brain scans, do not help with the diagnosis of postnatal depression, although they may occasionally be needed to rule out physical causes for your symptoms such as anaemia or an underactive thyroid gland.

What treatment will I be given?

For mild postnatal depression, antidepressant medication and counselling are equally effective and you should be able to choose the one with which you feel most comfortable. You will be able to remain in your own home and continue to look after your baby. As you may feel physically tired and lack confidence, this will be easier if you have a supportive partner or someone else to whom you can turn for practical help and emotional support. If you have more severe postnatal depression, you may need to be looked after by the home treatment team, or be admitted to hospital – usually to a mother and baby unit. In most areas, every effort will be made to support you in your own home.

What is a mother and baby unit?

This is a psychiatric unit with inpatient beds, daycare and outpatient facilities for women who have postnatal mental illness, including severe postnatal depression. The unit is designed and staffed to allow women to keep their babies with them, as it is important to maintain the bond between mother and baby and help the mother to gain confidence in her ability to look after her baby.

What is puerperal psychosis?

This is a relatively rare condition, occurring after about one delivery in 500. It starts within four weeks of delivery, and the woman rapidly becomes severely depressed (although a few become overactive). She also suffers from confusion, hallucinations and paranoid ideas. Puerperal psychosis is most common after the first baby, but in some women it recurs after every pregnancy.

How is puerperal psychosis treated?

By admission to hospital – usually a mother and baby unit – and treatment with drugs.

Will I be able to continue to breastfeed while I am having treatment for postnatal depression or puerperal psychosis?

Yes. If you are breastfeeding, you will be strongly encouraged to continue, and medication which is safe for use while breastfeeding will be selected for you.

Where can I find out more information?

For advice, and to be put in contact with other mothers who have suffered postnatal depression, contact The Association for Postnatal Illness (APNI), Helpline 0207 386 0868, www.apni.org.

Your New Baby

The first days and weeks at home with a new baby can be a daunting experience. Having sole responsibility (even if you have a partner or a whole extended family sharing the job with you) is terrifying at first, and you can be certain that your baby will do something that the parentcraft classes and baby books did not prepare you for.

When your baby is ten days old, the health visitor will arrange to come and see you at home. If your area has parent-held records for children, she will bring you a set and help you to fill in the background details. During the first year of your child's life, expect to see the health visitor regularly. She will weigh and measure your baby, perform developmental checks, and discuss matters such as feeding and sleeping. She is also in the best position to identify whether you have postnatal depression. As your child approaches school age, the health visitor will become less involved with their care unless there are problems.

Who is the health visitor, and what does she do?
The health visitor is a nurse who has done a special training course in health visiting. She may also be qualified as a midwife or a children's nurse. She will normally be based at a community clinic or at your GP's surgery. You may even meet your health visitor in the antenatal clinic before your baby is born. As well as being an expert in normal child development and behaviour, the health visitor is well placed to liaise with other agencies such as your GP, the community paediatrician, or social services. She will also know about local sources of support and funding for families with special needs.

What precautions should I take when I put my baby in his cot at night?
Make sure your baby is not overwrapped and the room is not overheated – as a rough guide, if you are comfortable in a nightshirt, your baby needs no more than a cotton vest, a sleepsuit, and perhaps a thin cardigan. If your baby is too cold, he will let you know by crying, but he may not alert you if he is too hot.
- Put your baby on his back to sleep.
- Don't use duvets, cot bumpers or a pillow for your baby.
- Put his feet at the bottom of the cot, and make sure his head cannot go under the bedclothes.
- Ensure that his clothes and toys have no dangling lengths of cloth or loose pieces on which he could choke.

What causes cot death?
Cot death, or sudden infant death syndrome, is the unexplained death of a baby aged under one year. About one baby in 500 will die in this way, most of them before the age of six months. Nobody knows for certain what causes it. In previous centuries, it was

attributed to parents rolling over and suffocating their babies. Over the years, theories have included viruses, chemicals in cot mattresses, air travel, and infanticide. We do know, however, that certain babies are at increased risk of cot death. These include:

- Boys, and babies born in the winter.
- Babies of very young mothers.
- Babies who were born prematurely.
- Babies who were small for gestational age.
- Twins.
- Babies who had an episode of stopping breathing while in the maternity unit.
- Babies born into a family where another baby died in a cot death.
- Babies whose parents smoke.

Should I buy a breathing monitor?

There is no evidence that these help prevent cot death – false alarms due to normal changes in the baby's breathing pattern are common, and there have been cases of babies dying while the breathing monitor was being used without the alarm being triggered. The false reassurance they give can be dangerous.

If you have had a previous cot death and have been lent an oxygen saturation monitor by the hospital, you should certainly use it. These monitors measure the concentration of oxygen in the baby's blood through the skin, and are highly reliable.

In what situations should I call an ambulance?

This is very rarely necessary. Most worries about babies can be resolved by a visit to the GP or a chat with the health visitor. However, there are a few situations in which you should seek attention immediately:

- **If your baby suddenly becomes very breathless or wheezy.**
- **If your baby has severe diarrhoea with vomiting and is refusing to feed.** Small babies quickly become dehydrated in these conditions. Diarrhoea alone in an alert baby who is taking feeds and has vomited only once or twice does not need hospital attention.

- **If your baby is floppy and lethargic** with or without a high temperature.
- **If your baby is irritable** – if he appears to be in pain, dislikes being handled and cannot be distracted from his misery by a feed or by your voice.
- **If he screams inconsolably at a high pitch.**
- **If he develops a speckled or blotchy purplish rash which does not disappear when you press a glass on it.**
- **If he appears to be choking.**
- **If he has a convulsion (fit).**
- **If he is dropped from a height or on to a hard surface.**

How do I find a GP for my child?

You must register your baby's birth at the Register Office before they are six weeks old. When you do this, as well as a birth certificate, you will be given a form which confirms that your baby is entitled to NHS treatment. The form should be signed by someone with parental responsibility and handed in to the practice at which you wish to register your baby. A few weeks later, you will receive a medical card – but you do not have to wait for this to arrive before you can consult the GP about your baby.

Do GPs know anything about child health?

The vast majority of child health problems are managed entirely by the GP and other members of the primary health care team. Most GPs have spent at least six months working in the children's ward of a hospital, and can offer a full range of child health services, including developmental checks, immunisation, routine consultations, fast-track surgery consultations for sick children, and referrals for tests or specialist opinions.

What about home visits?

You should only ask your GP to visit your child at home if they have a medical problem which would be made worse by being taken to the surgery. If your child is seriously ill call an ambulance rather than wait for your GP to visit.

In practice, a GP is obliged to put themselves in a position to assess the patient's condition and act appropriately, so if the GP thinks that your child needs to be examined, and you refuse to take them to the surgery or A&E, they will do a house call.

Do I have to register my child with my own GP?
No. In theory, you could choose any GP. However, GPs are, above all, family doctors, and it makes sense for your baby to be under the care of the same GP as you are. If you feel strongly that you do not trust your GP to provide adequate care for your baby, register at a different practice.

For the first fourteen days after your baby is born, your GP has to provide medical care for your child provided you are living within the practice area.

When Things go Wrong

I'm not happy with the care my baby and I received in hospital. What can I do?

Try to arrange a meeting with your consultant and, if appropriate, the midwifery manager for a full and open discussion. Remember that you are entitled to read your medical records and those of your baby.

What if I'm still not satisfied?

Write to the trust manager, outlining your concerns. The trust manager may arrange a further meeting after investigating your complaint, and will give you a full written reply within 28 days.

And if that is still not adequate?

Within 28 days of receiving your written reply, you can write back to the trust manager requesting an independent review. A convenor from outside the trust will decide whether or not this is appropriate.

What about the health service ombudsman?

If a complaint cannot be resolved at local level, the health service ombudsman may be able to help. You can submit your complaint to the ombudsman in a letter or using a special form. There is no charge for doing this and you do not need to use a solicitor. Contact the health service ombudsman on tel: 020 7217 4051 or www.ombudsman.org.uk.

What if I want to claim compensation for medical negligence?

The hospital trust, and the health service ombudsman, cannot award compensation. You will need to take legal advice. At present, you are only likely to be awarded compensation if negligence on the part of those responsible for your care during pregnancy and delivery can be proved. You should seek the advice of a legal firm with particular expertise in medical negligence. They will be able to advise you whether or not you have a case worth pursuing.

Section 4:
Maternity Unit Profiles

Comparing maternity units

In the following pages there are descriptions of nearly every maternity unit in the UK along with key facts and figures about each. They are designed to help you think about the following issues:

Type of unit Midwife units can provide an environment conducive to natural childbirth. Many larger consultant hospitals try to create a similar atmosphere in parts of the labour ward and you can have midwife-led care in most large midwife and consultant hospitals.

Size of unit Smaller units sometimes have better continuity of care but may not have all the facilities of a larger unit. We tell you the number of beds in the unit (including delivery beds) and, for midwife units, the number of births that took place in the unit (ie excluding home births) as well as the number WTE* midwives working at the unit.

Continuity of care Women prefer it if they are looked after by one midwife or a small number of midwives through their pregnancy. In many large hospitals the first time you ever see the midwife who delivers you is when you arrive at the unit in labour. Many hospitals now operate systems such as caseload midwifery, group practice and team midwifery which are all designed to improve continuity of care. The domino system is different but can have the same effect. (see page 25).The key measure of success is how many women were delivered by a midwife they know. The figures range from less than one per cent to 100 per cent.

* WTE is whole time equivalalantes. A unit with 3 midwives, two of whom work half time, would have two whole time equivalent midwives.

Staffing A maternity service providing antenatal, delivery and postnatal care can sensibly cope with 35 births per year according to academic studies. At many hospitals, particularly in the South East and London, the workload on midwives is higher. This can make it harder to provide personal attention such as one-to-one care in labour. One-to-one care in labour, where there is a midwife on the labour ward dedicated to looking after you, can greatly improve women's experience of childbirth but is something that many hospitals are unable to provide.

Crowding The number of deliveries per day per delivery bed in a unit can range from less than 0.5 to over 1.5. This gives an indication of which units are more crowded than others. Some are well prepared for this and may have additional facilities that can be quickly put to use. Others will find that their units can become overcrowded.

Home births Studies show that one in five women is interested in having their baby at home. But across the county less than one in fifty actually has a home birth. But home birth rates vary. In Torquay, ten per cent of women now have their babies at home. In contrast some other large hospitals deliver less than 0.1 per cent of babies at home. Hospitals with higher home birth rates are likely to give you good support if you decide you would like a home birth. (See page 82).

Antenatal scans and tests Many women want to know as early as possible if there are any problems with their pregnancy. But not all units offer or make available the full range of screening services. The tables tell you which units routinely offer triple testing for Down's syndrome (see page29) and which can arrange nuchal fold scans although this may require referral to another unit. Note that if a unit does not offer nuchal fold scans they may still help to arrange a private scan for you.

Pain relief Attitudes to pain vary. Some units may discourage women from epidural pain relief in labour on the grounds that it can slow labour. Other units may encourage it. Some may have better availability of anaesthetists than others. We tell you the percentage of women who had epidurals in each hospital which can vary from as little as 15 per cent to as much as 60 per cent. This figure includes epidurals given in labour and epidurals given for caesareans. In a few cases the figure is high because of epidurals used for caesareans rather than pain relief in labour. We have usually identified this in the text. In the tables we tell you about different pain relief methods including mobile epidurals, water and entonox (see page73). Other options are often described in the text.

Medical support Most large hospitals will have a paediatrician and an obstetrician on site 24 hours a day. Having doctors close to hand can be important in an emergency. If doctors are not on site, there may be doctors on call who can come into the hospital at short notice.

Water birth We identify units that have a full service – a water birth pool and midwives trained in water births on duty at all times. In the text we identify some units that have a more limited service, for example home water birth services where you have to hire your own pool.

Caesarean deliveries Some hospitals are twice as likely to perform a caesarean as others – an issue both if you are someone who would like to avoid a caesarean or someone who believes this would be the best way to deliver your baby. At most hospitals, caesareans are done most often as emergencies – usually after an attempted natural delivery has run into difficulties. There are a minority of hospitals where the majority of caesareans are elective suggesting a greater willingness at these hospitals to book operations. We give you the figures for both types. (See page 109)

Instrumental deliveries and episiotomies Around one in ten deliveries is by forceps or ventouse. For some women, a caesarean would be preferable to a difficult instrumental delivery. For others a vaginal birth is better, even if assisted. There are hospitals that have much lower rates of instrumental deliveries – sometimes in conjunction with higher caesarean rates. Others have much higher rates. Also hospitals differ in the instruments the use. A minority use forceps more often than the ventouse. Episiotomy rates also vary greatly. (See page 102-106)

Adjusted and crude figures For English units only we have adjusted the key intervention rates – caesarean, ventouse, forceps and epidurals – to take account of the types of women using the unit. Adjusted rates take account of average maternal age and average social deprivation of the mothers who use the unit. The purpose of this is to iron out some of the differences that arise because of the different types of patients treated in hospitals and makes the figures a more useful for comparison. Figures for Northern Ireland, Scotland and Wales are not adjusted.

The East

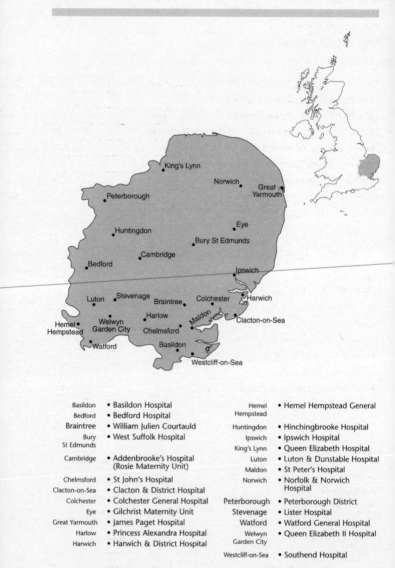

Basildon	• Basildon Hospital	Hemel Hempstead	• Hemel Hempstead General
Bedford	• Bedford Hospital		
Braintree	• William Julien Courtauld	Huntingdon	• Hinchingbrooke Hospital
Bury St Edmunds	• West Suffolk Hospital	Ipswich	• Ipswich Hospital
		King's Lynn	• Queen Elizabeth Hospital
Cambridge	• Addenbrooke's Hospital (Rosie Maternity Unit)	Luton	• Luton & Dunstable Hospital
		Maldon	• St Peter's Hospital
Chelmsford	• St John's Hospital	Norwich	• Norfolk & Norwich Hospital
Clacton-on-Sea	• Clacton & District Hospital		
Colchester	• Colchester General Hospital	Peterborough	• Peterborough District
Eye	• Gilchrist Maternity Unit	Stevenage	• Lister Hospital
Great Yarmouth	• James Paget Hospital	Watford	• Watford General Hospital
Harlow	• Princess Alexandra Hospital	Welwyn Garden City	• Queen Elizabeth II Hospital
Harwich	• Harwich & District Hospital		
		Westcliff-on-Sea	• Southend Hospital

Basildon · **Basildon Hospital**

Nethermayne, Basildon
Essex, SS16 5NL
Phone: 01268 533 911
Fax: 01268 593 757

Trust: Basildon and Thurrock General
Hospitals NHS Trust

The maternity unit at Basildon hospital offers shared care between consultants and midwives. Epidurals are available 24hrs a day and there are two obstetric theatres if you need a caesarean. The maternity unit is above the Hospital's children unit, which has a specialist neonatal intensive care unit, for the care of very small, premature or ill babies. There is also a day assessment unit. The unit has a water birth pool, which many women use for relaxation and pain relief during labour. As well as preparation for childbirth and parentcraft classes for pregnant women and their partners, there are physiotherapist-run relaxation sessions twice a week and a monthly class for grandmothers, designed to bring them up to date with current practice.

Consultant and Midwife Unit

Number of beds	55
Births per midwife	35
Births per bed	0.73
Home births	1%
Amenity Rooms, Price	£35

Obstetrician 24 hours	Yes
Paediatrician 24 hours	Yes
Full Water Birth Service	Yes

Tests

Routine Triple Testing	No
Nuchal Fold Scan	Yes
Fetal Assessment Unit	Yes

Pain Relief

24 hour epidural	Yes
Mobile epidural	No
Pethidine injections	Yes
Water (eg bath)	Yes

Intervention Rates	%	regional average %	national average %
Epidural	36	31	33
Elective Caesarean	9	8	8
Emergency Caesarean	12	13	12
Induction	21	20	20
Forceps	4	4	4
Ventouse	9	8	7
Episiotomy	27	17	14

Bedford · **Bedford Hospital**

Kempston Road
Bedford, MK42 9DJ
Phone: 01234 355122
Fax: 01234 218106

Trust: Bedford Hospital
NHS Trust

The Cygnet Wing at Bedford Hospital was opened in 1996 and combines maternity, paediatric and gynaecological services. There are 8 delivery rooms, a maternity operating theatre and 14 neonatal cots. Care is shared between consultants and midwives. If your pregnancy is low-risk you will be cared for by midwives in both the hospital and the community. The unit is able to offer antenatal classes during the daytime, evenings and weekend. You will be offered a range of antenatal screening tests and can be referred to London for nuchal fold scans. Intervention rates at the hospital are around the national average. The unit has full water birth facilities and midwives trained in water births are available 24 hrs a day.

Consultant and Midwife Unit

Number of beds	40
Births per midwife	31
Births per bed	0.91
Home births	3%
Amenity Rooms, Price	£47

Obstetrician 24 hours	Yes
Paediatrician 24 hours	Yes
Full Water Birth Service	Yes

Tests

Routine Triple Testing	Yes
Nuchal Fold Scan	Yes
Fetal Assessment Unit	Yes

Pain Relief

24 hour epidural	Yes
Mobile epidural	No
Pethidine injections	Yes
Water (eg bath)	Yes

Intervention Rates

	%	regional average %	national average %
Epidural	37	31	33
Elective Caesarean	7	8	8
Emergency Caesarean	12	13	12
Induction	17	20	20
Forceps	4	4	4
Ventouse	10	8	7
Episiotomy	27	17	14

Braintree · **William Julien Courtauld Hospital**

London Road, Braintree
Essex CM7 2LJ
Phone: 01376 551 221
Fax: 01376 553 241

Trust: Mid-Essex Hospital Services NHS Trust

This is a small midwife-led unit that offers low-tech care with minimal intervention for low-risk births. Women who choose to deliver at the local consultant-led unit, however, can receive antenatal and postnatal care from midwives at William Julian Courtauld. Continuity of care is high at the unit since with two teams of midwives, each team looking after an allocated group of women. Three-quarters of women who give birth there know the midwife who delivers them. The unit runs a regular consultant clinic and has scanning facilities and a blood-testing services as well as clinic facilities for local GPs, enabling women to access all their care in one place. Classes include one-to-one groups for special needs and teenage mothers.

Midwife Unit

Number of beds	11
Births	123
Midwives	10
Home births	-
Amenity Rooms, Price	-
Obstetrician 24 hours	No
Paediatrician 24 hours	No
Full Water Birth Service	No

Tests

Routine Triple Testing	Yes
Nuchal Fold Scan	No
Fetal Assessment Unit	No

Pain Relief

24 Hour epidural	No
Mobile epidural	No
Pethidine injections	Yes
Water (eg Bath)	Yes

Midwife-led units are adequately equipped to care for women whose pregnancy is progressing normally without complications. As a result, intervention tends to be low in these units. Basic pain relief will be offered, but any woman requesting an epidural during the delivery will need to be transferred to the nearest consultant-led unit. A woman will also be transferred to the obstetric unit if any complications develop during the delivery.

Bury St Edmunds · **West Suffolk Hospital**

Hardwick Lane, Bury St Edmunds
Suffolk, IP33 2QZ
Phone: 01284 713000
Fax: 01284 701992

Trust: West Suffolk Hospitals
NHS Trust

The maternity unit covers all aspects of care from high-risk obstetric cases to low-risk midwifery-led cases. The unit also has a network of community-based antenatal clinics. Although not all midwifery services are integrated, the majority of women who give birth here are looked after in labour by a midwife they know. The caesarean rate and in particular the emergency caesarean rate is higher than at most hospitals. Forceps however are used very rarely – the hospital has one of the lowest forceps rates in the country. A 24hr epidural service is led by dedicated obstetric anaesthetists. The central delivery suite offers a range of other facilities including a birthing pool, aromatherapy and reflexology.

Consultant and Midwife Unit

Number of beds	41
Births per midwife	32
Births per bed	0.65
Home births	3%
Amenity Rooms, Price	£50

Obstetrician 24 hours	Yes
Paediatrician 24 hours	Yes
Full Water Birth Service	Yes

Tests

Routine Triple Testing	Yes
Nuchal Fold Scan	No
Fetal Assessment Unit	Yes

Pain Relief

24 hour epidural	Yes
Mobile epidural	No
Pethidine injections	Yes
Water (eg bath)	Yes

Intervention Rates	%	regional average %	national average %
Epidural	32	31	33
Elective Caesarean	9	8	8
Emergency Caesarean	16	13	12
Induction	22	20	20
Forceps	0	4	4
Ventouse	7	8	7
Episiotomy	13	17	14

Cambridge · **Addenbrooke's Hospital**

Hills Road, Cambridge
Cambridgeshire, CB2 2QQ
Phone: 01223 245151
Fax: 01223 216520

Trust: Addenbrooke's
  NHS Trust

The Rosie maternity unit based on the Addenbrooke's site is a referral centre for women and their babies with complex medical problems as well as providing services to its local population. Intervention rates are above average with a higher number of emergency caesarean deliveries and more frequent use of forceps.

    Facilities include a dedicated ultrasound scanning department, an emergency and day assessment unit, a central delivery suite and adjacent obstetric theatres and inpatient wards. Water births can be supervised if done at home. Home birth services are offered and the home birth rate is in line with the national average. A wide range of antenatal tests are offered and the hospital is now introducing nuchal fold scans.

Consultant and Midwife Unit

Number of beds	76
Births per midwife	37
Births per bed	0.79
Home births	2%
Amenity Rooms, Price	£100

Obstetrician 24 hours	Yes
Paediatrician 24 hours	Yes
Full Water Birth Service	No

Tests

Routine Triple Testing	Yes
Nuchal Fold Scan	No
Fetal Assessment Unit	Yes

Pain Relief	
24 hour epidural	Yes
Mobile epidural	No
Pethidine injections	Yes
Water (eg bath)	Yes

Intervention Rates

	%	regional average %	national average %
Epidural	27	31	33
Elective Caesarean	8	8	8
Emergency Caesarean	15	13	12
Induction	21	20	20
Forceps	6	4	4
Ventouse	8	8	7
Episiotomy	18	17	14

Chelmsford · **St John's Hospital**

Wood Street, Chelmsford
Essex, CM1 9BG
Phone: 01245 491 149
Fax: 01245 513 671

Trust: Mid-Essex Hospital Services NHS
Trust

There are two teams of midwives which provide care though pregnancy, labour and postnatally. Separate teams of community midwives look after home births or provide domino deliveries. However, the work load for midwives is high with over 40 births per year per midwife. The unit is also the referral centre for the two midwife-led units at Braintree and Maldon.

The caesarean rate here is very high – one of the highest in the country – with above average rates of both elective and emergency caeasareans. The antenatal ward of the unit has a 3-bed postnatal area for mothers whose babies are in the Neonatal Unit which is adjacent to the antenatal ward.

Consultant and Midwife Unit

Number of beds	40
Births per midwife	44
Births per bed	0.69
Home births	-
Amenity Rooms, Price	£33

Obstetrician 24 hours	Yes
Paediatrician 24 hours	Yes
Full Water Birth Service	No

Tests

Routine Triple Testing	Yes
Nuchal Fold Scan	No
Fetal Assessment Unit	No

Pain Relief

24 hour epidural	Yes
Mobile epidural	No
Pethidine injections	Yes
Water (eg bath)	Yes

Intervention Rates	%	regional average %	national average %
Epidural	16	31	33
Elective Caesarean	13	8	8
Emergency Caesarean	15	13	12
Induction	18	20	20
Forceps	4	4	4
Ventouse	4	8	7
Episiotomy	15	17	14

Clacton-on-Sea · **Clacton Hospital**

Tower Road, Clacton
Essex, CO15 1LH
Phone: 01255 201 717
Fax: 01255 201 550

Trust: Essex Rivers Healthcare NHS
Trust

Clacton Maternity unit is a shared GP and midwife unit designed to provide a complete maternity service to low-risk women. The unit has 8 postnatal beds and 2 delivery rooms. Consultant clinics are held here and the unit is manned 24hrs a day with one midwife and one nursing auxiliary. Although medical intervention is relatively low, there are a small number of forceps deliveries and episiotomies. Emergency cases are transferred by ambulance to the main consultant unit in Colchester. The unit provides a full range of antenatal screening tests: the triple test is offered to all women and nuchal translucency scanning is offered to high-risk groups. Antenatal classes are only held on weekday evenings.

Midwife Unit

Number of beds	10
Births	147
Midwives	11
Home births	13%
Amenity Rooms, Price	-

Obstetrician 24 hours	No
Paediatrician 24 hours	No
Full Water Birth Service	No

Tests

Routine Triple Testing	Yes
Nuchal Fold Scan	No
Fetal Assessment Unit	No

Pain Relief

24 Hour epidural	No
Mobile epidural	No
Pethidine injections	Yes
Water (eg Bath)	No

Midwife-led units are adequately equipped to care for women whose pregnancy is progressing normally without complications. As a result, intervention tends to be low in these units. Basic pain relief will be offered, but any woman requesting an epidural during the delivery will need to be transferred to the nearest consultant-led unit. A woman will also be transferred to the obstetric unit if any complications develop during the delivery.

Colchester · **Colchester General Hospital**

Turner Road, Colchester
Essex, CO4 5JL
Phone: 01206 747 474
Fax: 01206 742 324

Trust: Essex Rivers Healthcare NHS
Trust

The maternity unit at Colchester General Hospital offers the option of GP-led care as well as midwife or consultant led care.

You will usually be put under the care of a team of midwives based on where you live. Continuity of care is reasonable but lower than at some hospitals with one in five chance of being delivered by a midwife they know. The unit has a slightly higher than average epidural rate overall, but many of these are for caesarean deliveries. The rate of use of epidurals for pain relief in labour is slightly lower than average. Consultants at the unit do practice ECV for breech babies but this is done selectively.

Consultant and Midwife Unit

Number of beds	64
Births per midwife	33
Births per bed	1
Home births	3%
Amenity Rooms, Price	£42

Obstetrician 24 hours	Yes
Paediatrician 24 hours	Yes
Full Water Birth Service	Yes

Tests

Routine Triple Testing	Yes
Nuchal Fold Scan	No
Fetal Assessment Unit	No

Pain Relief

24 hour epidural	Yes
Mobile epidural	No
Pethidine injections	Yes
Water (eg bath)	Yes

Intervention Rates	%	regional average %	national average %
Epidural	39	31	33
Elective Caesarean	8	8	8
Emergency Caesarean	11	13	12
Induction	19	20	20
Forceps	2	4	4
Ventouse	9	8	7
Episiotomy	16	17	14

Eye · **The Gilchrist Maternity Unit**

Castleton Way, Eye
Suffolk, IP23 7BH
Phone: 01379 870600

Trust: Salisbury District NHS Trust

Midwives provide care for women with low-risk pregnancies at The Gilchrist Birthing Unit.

However you will be offered a full range of scans and tests through consultant-led outreach clinics.

Almost half of the women who are cared for at the unit end up having their babies at home. Most women who deliver at the unit are back at home within six hours, with a midwife in attendance.

The unit is small and as a result most women are cared for during labour by a midwife they know. In keeping with the low-tech environment, epidurals are not available. However, should you want a water birth, there is a birthing pool at the unit.

Midwife Unit

Number of beds	2
Births	34
Midwives	6
Home births	31%
Amenity Rooms, Price	-
Obstetrician 24 hours	No
Paediatrician 24 hours	No
Full Water Birth Service	Yes

Tests

Routine Triple Testing	Yes
Nuchal Fold Scan	No
Fetal Assessment Unit	No

Pain Relief

24 Hour epidural	No
Mobile epidural	No
Pethidine injections	Yes
Water (eg bath)	Yes

Midwife-led units are adequately equipped to care for women whose pregnancy is progressing normally without complications. As a result, intervention tends to be low in these units. Basic pain relief will be offered, but any woman requesting an epidural during the delivery will need to be transferred to the nearest consultant-led unit. A woman will also be transferred to the obstetric unit if any complications develop during the delivery.

Great Yarmouth · **James Paget Hospital**

Lowestoft Road, Gorleston
Great Yarmouth, Norfolk, NR31 6LA
Phone: 01493 452452
Fax: 01493 452078

Trust: James Paget Healthcare NHS Trust

The midwives at this unit are divided into five teams, with midwives rotating between community and hospital placements. As a result, you may have continuity of midwife care pre- and post-natally, but it is unlikely that you will know the midwife caring for you in labour.

Home births are offered and the home birth rate is higher than at most hospitals.

There is a full range of options for pain relief, including patient-controlled systems which allow a woman in labour to directly manage the level of anaesthetic delivered. However, mobile epidurals are not available.

Overall, the take-up of epidurals for pain relief in the unit is average, as are the levels of medical intervention in birth.

Consultant and Midwife Unit

Number of beds	35
Births per midwife	35
Births per bed	0.67
Home births	3%
Amenity Rooms, Price	£35

Obstetrician 24 hours	Yes
Paediatrician 24 hours	Yes
Full Water Birth Service	No

Tests

Routine Triple Testing	Yes
Nuchal Fold Scan	No
Fetal Assessment Unit	No

Pain Relief

24 hour epidural	Yes
Mobile epidural	No
Pethidine injections	Yes
Water (eg bath)	Yes

Intervention Rates	%	regional average %	national average %
Epidural	33	31	33
Elective Caesarean	11	8	8
Emergency Caesarean	12	13	12
Induction	21	20	20
Forceps	3	4	4
Ventouse	8	8	7
Episiotomy	10	17	14

Harlow · **The Princess Alexandra Hospital**

Hamstel Road, Harlow
Essex, CM20 1QX
Phone: 01279 444 455
Fax: 01279 429 371

Trust: The Princess Alexandra Hospital
NHS Trust

The hospital operates a system of low and high-risk care. The majority of women are judged to be low-risk, and will be cared for in the community by a team of midwives and a GP. High-risk women will be given additional support by an obstetrician. Outpatient services are available on site as well as at St Margaret's Hospital in Epping and the Herts and Essex Hospital in Bishops Stortford. About half of women giving birth here know the midwife delivering them, and the unit hopes to increase this figure to 80 per cent.

For pain relief there is an epidural service and a slightly above average rate of epidurals. Alternative methods of pain management are also offered such as TENS and aromatherapy.

Consultant and Midwife Unit

Number of beds	35
Births per midwife	35
Births per bed	0.87
Home births	3%
Amenity Rooms, Price	£60

Obstetrician 24 hours	Yes
Paediatrician 24 hours	Yes
Full Water Birth Service	Yes

Tests

Routine Triple Testing	Yes
Nuchal Fold Scan	Yes
Fetal Assessment Unit	No

Pain Relief

24 hour epidural	Yes
Mobile epidural	Yes
Pethidine injections	Yes
Water (eg bath)	Yes

Intervention Rates	%	regional average %	national average %
Epidural	35	31	33
Elective Caesarean	10	8	8
Emergency Caesarean	14	13	12
Induction	20	20	20
Forceps	2	4	4
Ventouse	7	8	7
Episiotomy	14	17	14

Harwich · **Harwich & District Hospital**

419 Main Road, Dovercourt
Harwich, Essex, CO12 4EX
Phone: 01255 201 200
Fax: 01255 552 335

Trust: Essex Rivers Healthcare NHS
Trust

The small unit at Harwich maternity hospital provides GP-led care with GPs often assisting the midwives with deliveries. The unit is small and friendly and most women are cared for in labour by a midwife they know. Ultrasound scanning and antenatal screening is carried out in the clinic. Epidurals are not available for pain management, but full water birth facilities are offered and midwives trained in water delivery are available around the clock. Should you experience difficulties during labour, GPs are on call, or you will be transferred to the nearest consultant unit at Colchester which is 16 miles away.

Midwife Unit

Number of beds	8
Births	131
Midwives	9
Home births	1%
Amenity Rooms, Price	£42

Obstetrician 24 hours	No
Paediatrician 24 hours	No
Full Water Birth Service	Yes

Tests

Routine Triple Testing	Yes
Nuchal Fold Scan	No
Fetal Assessment Unit	No

Pain Relief

24 Hour epidural	No
Mobile epidural	No
Pethidine injections	Yes
Water (eg Bath)	Yes

Midwife-led units are adequately equipped to care for women whose pregnancy is progressing normally without complications. As a result, intervention tends to be low in these units. Basic pain relief will be offered, but any woman requesting an epidural during the delivery will need to be transferred to the nearest consultant-led unit. A woman will also be transferred to the obstetric unit if any complications develop during the delivery.

Huntingdon · **Hinchingbrooke Hospital**

Hinchingbrooke Park, Huntingdon
Cambridgeshire, PE29 6NT
Phone: 01480 416416
Fax: 01480 416561

Trust: Hinchingbrooke Healthcare
NHS Trust

This large maternity unit shares care between midwives and consultants. Water birth is offered, with trained midwives available 24 hours a day. Home births are not undertaken as frequently as in many large hospitals. The unit also offers domino deliveries. Continuity of care is lower than in many smaller hospitals with about a fifth of women being cared for in labour by a midwife they know.

The unit gives comprehensive antenatal testing to all women who need it. Intervention rates here are higher than average however over half of women giving birth here last year did so without any intervention.

You can consult a range of support services here, including antenatal and postnatal support lines and counsellors.

Consultant and Midwife Unit

Number of beds	30
Births per midwife	40
Births per bed	0.62
Home births	1%
Amenity Rooms, Price	-

Obstetrician 24 hours	No
Paediatrician 24 hours	Yes
Full Water Birth Service	Yes

Tests

Routine Triple Testing	Yes
Nuchal Fold Scan	Yes
Fetal Assessment Unit	Yes

Pain Relief

24 hour epidural	Yes
Mobile epidural	No
Pethidine injections	Yes
Water (eg bath)	Yes

Intervention Rates	%	regional average %	national average %
Epidural	19	31	33
Elective Caesarean	9	8	8
Emergency Caesarean	14	13	12
Induction	22	20	20
Forceps	5	4	4
Ventouse	4	8	7
Episiotomy	12	17	14

Ipswich · **The Ipswich Hospital**

Heath Road, Ipswich
Suffolk, IP4 5PD
Phone: 01473 712233
Fax: 01473 703400

Trust: Ipswich Hospital NHS Trust

This unit has six obstetric consultants and offers consultant-led, midwife-led and GP-led care.

Women are offered the choice of giving birth either in the hospital, the Gilchrist birthing unit, or at home. For a large unit Ipswich has more home births than many hospitals. The hospital has no central delivery suite, but has three multifunctional wards each offering antenatal, intrapartum and postnatal care.

As well as the usual antenatal education classes, the unit offers classes on breastfeeding and postnatal exercise. Aromatherapy during labour is offered and there is a full water birth service with midwives on hand all day to supervise.

Consultant and Midwife Unit

Number of beds	55
Births per midwife	31
Births per bed	1.3
Home births	3%
Amenity Rooms, Price	£35

Obstetrician 24 hours	Yes
Paediatrician 24 hours	Yes
Full Water Birth Service	Yes

Tests

Routine Triple Testing	Yes
Nuchal Fold Scan	No
Fetal Assessment Unit	Yes

Pain Relief

24 Hour epidural	Yes
Mobile epidural	No
Pethidine injections	Yes
Water (eg Bath)	Yes

Intervention Rates

	%	regional average %	national average %
Epidural	-	31	33
Elective Caesarean	8	8	8
Emergency Caesarean	12	13	12
Induction	18	20	20
Forceps	4	4	4
Ventouse	6	8	7
Episiotomy	5	17	14

King's Lynn · **The Queen Elizabeth Hospital**

Gayton Road, King's Lynn
Norfolk, PE30 4ET
Phone: 01553 613613
Fax: 01553 613700

Trust: King's Lynn and Wisbech
Hospitals NHS Trust

This unit offers a full range of maternity services for women with normal and complicated pregnancies. You can choose whether to be under midwife or consultant led care and there is a smooth transition between community and hospital-based care if your needs change. You will have a named midwife responsible for continuity of care and about a third of women are cared for in labour by a midwife they know – more than for most large hospitals. The unit has a high caesarean rate including a high elective caesarean rate which partly reflects women chosing caesareans. Inductions however are relatively rare and forceps are used much less frequently than in similar hospitals.

Consultant and Midwife Unit

Number of beds	31
Births per midwife	35
Births per bed	0.38
Home births	2%
Amenity Rooms, Price	£40

Obstetrician 24 hours	Yes
Paediatrician 24 hours	Yes
Full Water Birth Service	Yes

Tests

Routine Triple Testing	Yes
Nuchal Fold Scan	Yes
Fetal Assessment Unit	Yes

Pain Relief

24 hour epidural	Yes
Mobile epidural	No
Pethidine injections	Yes
Water (eg bath)	Yes

Intervention Rates	%	regional average %	national average %
Epidural	45	31	33
Elective Caesarean	14	8	8
Emergency Caesarean	15	13	12
Induction	10	20	20
Forceps	2	4	4
Ventouse	9	8	7
Episiotomy	10	17	14

Luton · **The Luton & Dunstable Hospital**

Lewsey Road, Luton
Bedfordshire, LU4 0DZ
Phone: 01582 491122
Fax: 01582 492130

Trust: The Luton and Dunstable
NHS Trust

The unit has two maternity wards, including transitional care cots, but most women will be transferred home after delivery. An early pregnancy assessment clinic runs every weekday morning. The delivery suite includes a birthing pool and bereavement suite.

Obstetric and gynaecological inpatients and day patients at the hospital are integrated into one unit, known as the Women's Health Unit, one of the busiest of its kind in the Eastern Region. A genetic clinic is held every month.

Antenatal classes run throughout the week and at weekends; the unit also runs sessions for ethnic minorities, teenage pregnancies and water births.

Consultant and Midwife Unit

Number of beds	59
Births per midwife	36.3
Births per bed	0.79
Home births	3%
Amenity Rooms, Price	£95

Obstetrician 24 hours	Yes
Paediatrician 24 hours	Yes
Full Water Birth Service	Yes

Tests

Routine Triple Testing	Yes
Nuchal Fold Scan	No
Fetal Assessment Unit	Yes

Pain Relief

24 hour epidural	Yes
Mobile epidural	Yes
Pethidine injections	Yes
Water (eg bath)	Yes

Intervention Rates	%	regional average %	national average %
Epidural	39	31	33
Elective Caesarean	6	8	8
Emergency Caesarean	16	13	12
Induction	21	20	20
Forceps	4	4	4
Ventouse	7	8	7
Episiotomy	14	17	14

Maldon · **St Peter's Hospital**

32a Spital Road, Maldon
Essex, CM9 6EG
Phone: 01621 854 344
Fax: 01621 851 034

Trust: **Mid-Essex Hospital Services NHS Trust**

The Maple Ward is a small, low-tech GP and midwife-led maternity unit providing a range of midwifery care from initial antenatal booking to 28 days post-delivery. You can also come here for antenatal care and postnatal recovery if you plan to give birth in the main unit in Colchester.

The unit provides a consultant clinic, ultrasound scanning, blood-testing and midwife antenatal clinics, this ensures that you will have access, in one place, to all those involved in your care. There are also plans in place to install a birthing pool at St Peter's later this year.

Antenatal classes cater to teenagers and those with special needs on a one-to-one basis.

Midwife Unit

Number of beds	13
Births	157
Midwives	11
Home births	-
Amenity Rooms, Price	-
Obstetrician 24 hours	No
Paediatrician 24 hours	No
Full Water Birth Service	No

Tests

Routine Triple Testing	Yes
Nuchal Fold Scan	No
Fetal Assessment Unit	No

Pain Relief

24 Hour epidural	No
Mobile epidural	No
Pethidine injections	Yes
Water (eg bath)	Yes

Midwife-led units are adequately equipped to care for women whose pregnancy is progressing normally without complications. As a result, intervention tends to be low in these units. Basic pain relief will be offered, but any woman requesting an epidural during the delivery will need to be transferred to the nearest consultant-led unit. A woman will also be transferred to the obstetric unit if any complications develop during the delivery.

Norwich · **Norfolk & Norwich Hospital**

Brunswick Road, Norwich
Norfolk, NR1 3SR
Phone: 01603 286286
Fax: 01603 287211

Trust: Norfolk and Norwich University
Hospital NHS Trust

The facilities at the hospital include a bath and two pools to help with pain management. Water births are also offered.

Intervention rates are broadly in line with national averages. A full range of pain relief is available although use of epidurals is lower than at most hospitals. Home births are offered and the home birth rate at 2 per cent is in line with other hospitals.

Community midwives offer special education classes for teenagers.

There are also midwife-led late pregnancy assessment, and pre-op assessment clinics.

There is a breastfeeding clinic and support services include bereavement counselling.

Consultant and Midwife Unit

Number of beds	70
Births per midwife	38
Births per bed	0.94
Home births	2%
Amenity Rooms, Price	£50

Obstetrician 24 hours	Yes
Paediatrician 24 hours	Yes
Full Water Birth Service	Yes

Tests

Routine Triple Testing	Yes
Nuchal Fold Scan	Yes
Fetal Assessment Unit	No

Pain Relief

24 hour epidural	Yes
Mobile epidural	Yes
Pethidine injections	Yes
Water (eg bath)	Yes

Intervention Rates	%	regional average %	national average %
Epidural	21	31	33
Elective Caesarean	9	8	8
Emergency Caesarean	13	13	12
Induction	21	20	20
Forceps	3	4	4
Ventouse	9	8	7
Episiotomy	14	17	14

Peterborough · **Peterborough District Hospital**

Thorpe Road, Peterborough
Cambridgeshire, PE3 6DA
Phone: 01733 874000
Fax: 01733 874001

Trust: Peterborough Hospitals
NHS Trust

The maternity unit at Peterborough District Hospital is a shared midwife and consultant unit, with the majority of care and deliveries undertaken by midwives.

Home births are offered but are relatively rare and water births are not available. Intervention rates are similar to most large hospital units.

The unit runs active birth and breast feeding classes as well a debriefing sessions. As well as the full range of traditional forms of pain relief, complementary therapies are available to help with pain management during labour. Mobile epidurals which allow greater feeling and movement during labour are also available.

Consultant and Midwife Unit

Number of beds	60
Births per midwife	36
Births per bed	0.92
Home births	0.47%
Amenity Rooms, Price	£35

Obstetrician 24 hours	Yes
Paediatrician 24 hours	Yes
Full Water Birth Service	No

Tests

Routine Triple Testing	Yes
Nuchal Fold Scan	No
Fetal Assessment Unit	Yes

Pain Relief

24 hour epidural	Yes
Mobile epidural	Yes
Pethidine injections	Yes
Water (eg bath)	Yes

Intervention Rates	%	regional average %	national average %
Epidural	32	31	33
Elective Caesarean	7	8	8
Emergency Caesarean	14	13	12
Induction	17	20	20
Forceps	5	4	4
Ventouse	9	8	7
Episiotomy	18	17	14

Stevenage · **Lister Hospital**

Coreys Mill Lane, Stevenage
Hertfordshire, SG1 4AB
Phone: 01438 314333
Fax: 01438 781306

Trust: East and North Hertfordshire
NHS Trust

The unit has two wards and a central delivery suite with seven delivery rooms. There is also a neonatal intensive care unit with 13 cots. Antenatal care is given wherever possible outside the hospital in GP surgeries and local health centres. Community midwives are attached to GP surgeries and provide both domino and home deliveries. The home birth service is popular with a home birth rate more than double the national average. There is a 24 hour epidural service dependent on availability of anaesthetists. Pethedine, diamorphine and gas and air are also available for pain relief. The unit has Baby Friendly accreditation for encouraging breastfeeding. It also supports environmental friendly practices, for example the use of reusable cotton nappies.

Consultant and Midwife Unit

Number of beds	32
Births per midwife	32
Births per bed	0.98
Home births	5%
Amenity Rooms, Price	-

Obstetrician 24 hours	Yes
Paediatrician 24 hours	Yes
Full Water Birth Service	Yes

Tests

Routine Triple Testing	No
Nuchal Fold Scan	Yes
Fetal Assessment Unit	No

Pain Relief

24 hour epidural	Yes
Mobile epidural	Yes
Pethidine injections	Yes
Water (eg bath)	Yes

Intervention Rates

	%	regional average %	national average %
Epidural	29%	31%	33%
Elective Caesarean	6%	8%	8%
Emergency Caesarean	11%	13%	12%
Induction	21%	20%	20%
Forceps	4%	4%	4%
Ventouse	4%	8%	7%
Episiotomy	16%	17%	14%

Watford · **Watford General Hospital**

Vicarage Road, Watford
Hertfordshire, WD1 80HB
Phone: 01923 244 366
Fax: 01923 217 824

Trust: West Hertfordshire Hospitals
  NHS Trust

This is a busy unit with midwives coping with 42 births per year – more than at most hospitals. However contintuity of care is good with 42 per cent of women looked after in labour by a midwife they know, which is high for this type of hospital.

There are a variety of options for care, including low-risk midwife-led care, high-risk shared care and a domino scheme. Home births are offered but not well used with very few women chosing this option. The unit has full facilities for water birth, with midwives trained in this procedure available around the clock.

A full range of tests are available, including the triple test for Down's syndrome. Women needing nuchal fold scans are referred to King's College Hospital.

Consultant and Midwife Unit

Number of beds	66
Births per midwife	42
Births per bed	0.81
Home births	0.13%
Amenity Rooms, Price	-

Obstetrician 24 hours	Yes
Paediatrician 24 hours	Yes
Full Water Birth Service	Yes

Tests

Routine Triple Testing	Yes
Nuchal Fold Scan	Yes
Fetal Assessment Unit	Yes

Pain Relief

24 hour epidural	Yes
Mobile epidural	No
Pethidine injections	Yes
Water (eg bath)	Yes

Intervention Rates	%	regional average %	national average %
Epidural	20%	31%	33%
Elective Caesarean	9%	8%	8%
Emergency Caesarean	12%	13%	12%
Induction	23%	20%	20%
Forceps	3%	4%	4%
Ventouse	10%	8%	7%
Episiotomy	18%	17%	14%

Welwyn Garden City · **Queen Elizabeth II Hospital**

Howlands, Welwyn Garden City
Hertfordshire, AL7 4HQ
Phone: 01707 328 111
Fax: 01707 373 359

Trust: East and North Hertfordshire
NHS Trust

Provision of midwifery care is organised around seven integrated midwifery teams providing the full range of care.

The majority of antenatal care is provided in the community. There are a number of 'drop-in' clinics for women seeking care without appointment and the unit also offers counselling services for women requiring support whilst undergoing fetal and maternal screening and diagnostic procedures.

Antenatal classes run during the day, evenings and weekends, and there are special teenage mother groups. Epidural and induction rates are relatively high. Other intervention rates are in line with national averages.

Consultant and Midwife Unit

Number of beds	46
Births per midwife	31.25
Births per bed	0.87
Home births	2%
Amenity Rooms, Price	-

Obstetrician 24 hours	Yes
Paediatrician 24 hours	Yes
Full Water Birth Service	No

Tests

Routine Triple Testing	Yes
Nuchal Fold Scan	Yes
Fetal Assessment Unit	Yes

Pain Relief

24 hour epidural	Yes
Mobile epidural	No
Pethidine injections	Yes
Water (eg bath)	Yes

Intervention Rates	%	regional average %	national average %
Epidural	41	31	33
Elective Caesarean	8	8	8
Emergency Caesarean	13	13	12
Induction	26	20	20
Forceps	3	4	4
Ventouse	8	8	7
Episiotomy	15	17	14

Westcliff-on-Sea · **Southend Hospital**

Prittlewell Chase, Westcliff-on-Sea
Essex, SS0 0RT
Phone: 01702 435 555
Fax: 01702 221 300

Trust: Southend Hospital
NHS Trust

Southend Maternity unit is a large shared-care facility, which has a high number of home births, and also offers women the choice of having a domino midwife. Water births are also offered and the unit can provide a pool for home births in addition to the pool in the unit. The midwifery teams aim to achieve a high level of familiarity between women and midwives with up to three-quarters of women being cared for in labour by a midwife they know from their antenatal care. Use of epidurals for pain relief in labour is more frequent than at most hospitals. Full water birth facilities are on offer, and the unit also offers bereavement counselling and a debriefing service after delivery.

Consultant and Midwife Unit

Number of beds	66
Births per midwife	31.4
Births per bed	0.89
Home births	4%
Amenity Rooms, Price	£50

Obstetrician 24 hours	Yes
Paediatrician 24 hours	Yes
Full Water Birth Service	Yes

Tests

Routine Triple Testing	No
Nuchal Fold Scan	Yes
Fetal Assessment Unit	Yes

Pain Relief

24 hour epidural	Yes
Mobile epidural	No
Pethidine injections	Yes
Water (eg bath)	Yes

Intervention Rates	%	regional average %	national average %
Epidural	43	31	33
Elective Caesarean	8	8	8
Emergency Caesarean	15	13	12
Induction	21	20	20
Forceps	4	4	4
Ventouse	4	8	7
Episiotomy	13	17	14

London

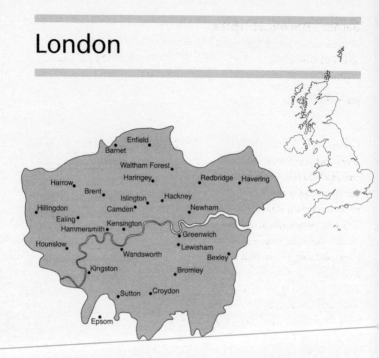

Barnet	• Barnet Hospital	Islington	• Whittington Hospital
	• Edgware Birth Centre	Kensington	• Chelsea & Westminster Hospital
Bexley	• Queen Mary's Hospital		
Brent	• Central Middlesex Hospital	Kingston upon Thames	• Kingston Hospital
Bromley	• Farnborough Hospital	Lewisham	• King's College Hospital
Camden	• Elizabeth Garrett Anderson and Obstetric Hospital		• University Hospital Lewisham
		Newham	• Newham General Hospital
	• Royal Free Hospital		• Newham General
Croydon	• Mayday Hospital		• Hospital (Midwife-led Unit)
Ealing	• Ealing Hospital	Redbridge	• King George Hospital
Enfield	• Chase Farm Hospital	St John's Wood	• Hospital of St John and St Elizabeth
Epsom	• Epsom General Hospital		
Greenwich	• Queen Elizabeth Hospital	Southwark	• Guy's Hospital
Hackney	• Homerton Hospital	Sutton	• St Helier Hospital
Hammersmith	• Queen Charlotte's & Chelsea	Tooting	• The Birth Centre
		Tower Hamlets	• Royal London Hospital
Haringey	• North Middlesex Hospital	Waltham Forest	• Whipps Cross Hospital
Harrow	• Northwick Park Hospital		• Whipps Cross Hospital (Midwife-led Unit)
Havering	• Harold Wood Hospital		
Hillingdon	• Hillingdon Hospital	Wandsworth	• St George's Hospital
Hounslow	• West Middlesex Hospital		• St Mary's Hospital
			• The Portland Hospital

Barnet · **Barnet Hospital**

Wellhouse Lane, Barnet
Hertfordshire, EN5 3DJ
Phone: 020 8216 4000
Fax: 020 8216 5426

Trust: Barnet and Chase Farm Hospitals
NHS Trust

Women at this maternity unit can choose between midwife-led care, consultant-led care, and integrated caseload midwifery (with two midwives working in tandem). Midwives are also able to offer the domino system for those who want it. Home births are not common but water births are offered: the unit has its own pool and midwives trained in water births are available around the clock. Antenatal classes include groups for couples and multiple births. There is also a weekly rolling programme of walk-in sessions.

The unit has an above average rate of epidurals and below average use of inductions. Other interventions are broadly in line with average.

Consultant and Midwife Unit

Number of beds	32
Births per midwife	33
Births per bed	0.86
Home births	1%
Amenity Rooms, Price	-

Obstetrician 24 hours	Yes
Paediatrician 24 hours	Yes
Full Water Birth Service	Yes

Tests

Routine Triple Testing	Yes
Nuchal Fold Scan	Yes
Fetal Assessment Unit	Yes

Pain Relief

24 hour epidural	Yes
Mobile epidural	Yes
Pethidine injections	Yes
Water (eg bath)	Yes

Intervention Rates	%	regional average %	national average %
Epidural	40	33	33
Elective Caesarean	7	8	8
Emergency Caesarean	12	12	12
Induction	17	20	20
Forceps	4	3	4
Ventouse	8	8	7
Episiotomy	14	15	14

Barnet · **Edgware Community Hospital**

Burnt Oak Broadway, Edgware
Middlesex, HA8 0AD
Phone: 020 8732 6777
Fax: 020 8732 6773

Trust: Barnet and Chase Farm Hospitals
NHS Trust

The centre is an innovative midwife-led unit, run as a 'home-from-home', for women experiencing a normal pregnancy who might have considered a home birth.

The midwives at the birth centre aim to facilitate informed choice and foster a non-intrusive, non-interventionist approach to birth.

Three quarters of women are cared for by a midwife known to them. Any interventions involve a transfer to Barnet or Chase Farm Hospitals.

The centre offers two water pools, and over many women deliver in water.

Bean bags, a Dutch birth stool and birth balls are all available.

Support services include antenatal and postnatal helplines, along with a breast feeding helpline and counsellors. Facilities for partners to stay are available.

Midwife Unit

Number of beds	5
Births	266
Midwives	8
Home births	0%
Amenity Rooms, Price	-
Obstetrician 24 hours	No
Paediatrician 24 hours	No
Full Water Birth Service	Yes

Tests

Routine Triple Testing	No
Nuchal Fold Scan	No
Fetal Assessment Unit	No

Pain Relief

24 Hour epidural	No
Mobile epidural	No
Pethidine injections	Yes
Water (eg bath)	Yes

Midwife-led units are adequately equipped to care for women whose pregnancy is progressing normally without complications. As a result, intervention tends to be low in these units. Basic pain relief will be offered, but any woman requesting an epidural during the delivery will need to be transferred to the nearest consultant-led unit. A woman will also be transferred to the obstetric unit if any complications develop during the delivery.

Bexley · **Queen Mary's Hospital**

Frognal Avenue, Sidcup
Kent, DA14 6LT
Phone: 020 8302 2678
Fax: 020 8308 3052

Trust: Queen Mary's Sidcup
NHS Trust

This is a large maternity unit which cares for a significant number of mothers from outside the area. Intervention rates are low – the caesarean rate is well below the national average. Also, although there is a 24 hour epidural service, relatively few women have these. As well as providing a full range of orthodox pain relief, including mobile epidurals, the unit offers complementary therapies, such as aromatherapy. Parent education sessions are run at available weekends and evenings. These include groups for teenagers, those with learning disabilities and those with physical disabilities.

Water birth is offered and midwives trained in such deliveries are available 24 hours a day, although women must bring their own pool.

Consultant and Midwife Unit

Number of beds	51
Births per midwife	37
Births per bed	0.71
Home births	1%
Amenity Rooms, Price	£27

Obstetrician 24 hours	Yes
Paediatrician 24 hours	Yes
Full Water Birth Service	No

Tests

Routine Triple Testing	No
Nuchal Fold Scan	Yes
Fetal Assessment Unit	Yes

Pain Relief

24 hour epidural	Yes
Mobile epidural	Yes
Pethidine injections	Yes
Water (eg bath)	Yes

Intervention Rates	%	regional average %	national average %
Epidural	16	33	33
Elective Caesarean	6	8	8
Emergency Caesarean	10	12	12
Induction	-	20	20
Forceps	-	3	4
Ventouse	-	8	7
Episiotomy	16	15	14

Brent · **Central Middlesex Hospital**

Acton Lane, Park Royal
London, NW10 7NS
Phone: 020 8965 5733
Fax: 020 8453 2069

Trust: North West London Hospitals
Trust

Care at this unit is shared between midwives and consultants and the domino system is offered.

Intervention rates are fairly low with few inductions and infrequent use of forceps. Elective caesareans are also done less often than in most hospitals although the emergency caesarean rate is above average. Although midwives trained in water birth are not available 24 hours a day, water birth is offered and the unit does have its own pool, so the midwives will try to accommodate your wishes.

Parent education sessions and antenatal classes are available during the evenings and during the daytime. Support services include an antenatal support line, postnatal support line and a breastfeeding helpline.

Consultant and Midwife Unit

Number of beds	37
Births per midwife	31
Births per bed	0.83
Home births	1%
Amenity Rooms, Price	£50

Obstetrician 24 hours	Yes
Paediatrician 24 hours	Yes
Full Water Birth Service	No

Tests

Routine Triple Testing	No
Nuchal Fold Scan	Yes
Fetal Assessment Unit	No

Pain Relief

24 hour epidural	Yes
Mobile epidural	No
Pethidine injections	Yes
Water (eg bath)	Yes

Intervention Rates	%	regional average %	national average %
Epidural	21	33	33
Elective Caesarean	6	8	8
Emergency Caesarean	15	12	12
Induction	13	20	20
Forceps	2	3	4
Ventouse	7	8	7
Episiotomy	14	15	14

Bromley · **Farnborough Hospital**

Farnborough Common, Orpington
Kent, BR6 8ND
Phone: 01689 814 000
Fax: 01689 814 127

Trust: Bromley Hospitals
   NHS Trust

The main maternity unit of Bromley Hospitals NHS Trust is situated here but there is a satellite clinic at Beckenham Hospital. Care is provided by a team of obstetricians and midwives, supported by medical staff and GPs in the community.

Antenatal sessions are organised for fathers and grandparents, and one-to-one sessions are offered as required. Home births are catered for and the home birth rate is higher than average. The caesarean rate is higher than average – both for elective and emergency operations.

Fathers are not usually allowed to stay with you if you on the antenatal or postnatal wards.

Consultant and Midwife Unit

Number of beds	48
Births per midwife	36
Births per bed	0.91
Home births	3%
Amenity Rooms, Price	£35
Obstetrician 24 hours	Yes
Paediatrician 24 hours	Yes
Full Water Birth Service	No

Tests

Routine Triple Testing	Yes
Nuchal Fold Scan	Yes
Fetal Assessment Unit	No

Pain Relief

24 hour epidural	Yes
Mobile epidural	No
Pethidine injections	Yes
Water (eg bath)	Yes

Intervention Rates	%	regional average %	national average %
Epidural	36	33	33
Elective Caesarean	10	8	8
Emergency Caesarean	15	12	12
Induction	22	20	20
Forceps	3	3	4
Ventouse	7	8	7
Episiotomy	19	15	14

Camden · **The Elizabeth Garrett Anderson Hospital**

Huntley St
London, WC1E 6AU
Phone: 0207 387 9300
Fax: 0207 380 9917

Trust: University College London
Hospitals NHS Trust

Care is shared between consultants and midwives at this unit and interventions are above average with close to one in four babies delivered by caesarean section. Elective caesareans are performed as often as emergency procedures which is unusual. Epidurals are available and are widely used for pain relief although alternatives are also available including a TENS machine and acupuncture. Midwife staffing levels are good for a London hospital although only a minimal number of women end up being delivered by one of the midwifes they know.

Parent education sessions and antenatal classes are available in the evenings and during the daytime, with special sessions organised for Chinese speaking women. The unit also runs a breastfeeding clinic.

Consultant and Midwife Unit

Number of beds	40
Births per midwife	35
Births per bed	0.62
Home births	1%
Amenity Rooms, Price	£80

Obstetrician 24 hours	Yes
Paediatrician 24 hours	Yes
Full Water Birth Service	Yes

Tests

Routine Triple Testing	No
Nuchal Fold Scan	Yes
Fetal Assessment Unit	Yes

Pain Relief

24 hour epidural	Yes
Mobile epidural	Yes
Pethidine injections	Yes
Water (eg bath)	Yes

Intervention Rates	%	regional average %	national average %
Epidural	29	33	33
Elective Caesarean	12	8	8
Emergency Caesarean	12	12	12
Induction	21	20	20
Forceps	3	3	4
Ventouse	9	8	7
Episiotomy	15	15	14

Camden · **Royal Free Hospital**

Pond Street, Hampstead
London, NW3 2QG
Phone: 020 7794 0500
Fax: 020 7830 2602

Trust: Royal Free Hampstead
NHS Trust

The Royal Free Hospital maternity service is situated within a major London teaching hospital with multi-disciplinary support and academic resources. Because of this, the hospital cares for a large number of women with high-risk pregnancies and medical conditions. However intervention rates, after some adjustment to allow for this, are no higher than at other large hospitals. If your pregnancy is normal you can choose to be under the care of a midwife rather than a doctor. Midwife staffing levels are better than at many inner London hospitals. Use of epidurals for pain relief is more common than at most hospitals. Home births are offered but are relatively infrequent. Antenatal classes are run at weekends as well as evenings.

Consultant and Midwife Unit

Number of beds	54
Births per midwife	34
Births per bed	0.75
Home births	1%
Amenity Rooms, Price	£90

Obstetrician 24 hours	Yes
Paediatrician 24 hours	Yes
Full Water Birth Service	No

Tests

Routine Triple Testing	No
Nuchal Fold Scan	Yes
Fetal Assessment Unit	Yes

Pain Relief

24 hour epidural	Yes
Mobile epidural	Yes
Pethidine injections	Yes
Water (eg bath)	Yes

Intervention Rates	%	regional average %	national average %
Epidural	34	33	33
Elective Caesarean	9	8	8
Emergency Caesarean	13	12	12
Induction	19	20	20
Forceps	3	3	4
Ventouse	6	8	7
Episiotomy	13	15	14

Croydon · **Mayday Hospital**

London Road, Thorton Heath
Croydon, CR7 7YE
Phone: 0208 401 3000
Fax: 0208 401 3681

Trust: Mayday Healthcare
NHS Trust

Staffing levels here are reasonable for the area and about one third of women are delivered by a midwife they know, something that many larger hospitals – particularly in London – find difficult to achieve. Antenatal and parent education classes are available for teenage mothers and non-English speaking women. There is a birthing pool which can be used for pain relief and may also be used for water births although the unit does guarantee to always have a midwife experienced in water births available.

The unit has a low caesarean rate for a large consultant unit, especially one in the London. There is a breastfeeding clinic, a drop in clinic for women with alcohol and drug problems and a psychiatric clinic for women with mental health problems.

Consultant and Midwife Unit

Number of beds	60
Births per midwife	37
Births per bed	0.96
Home births	2%
Amenity Rooms, Price	£40

Obstetrician 24 hours	Yes
Paediatrician 24 hours	Yes
Full Water Birth Service	No

Tests

Routine Triple Testing	No
Nuchal Fold Scan	Yes
Fetal Assessment Unit	Yes

Pain Relief

24 hour epidural	Yes
Mobile epidural	No
Pethidine injections	Yes
Water (eg bath)	Yes

Intervention Rates	%	regional average %	national average %
Epidural	18	33	33
Elective Caesarean	7	8	8
Emergency Caesarean	10	12	12
Induction	15	20	20
Forceps	2	3	4
Ventouse	9	8	7
Episiotomy	20	15	14

Ealing · **Ealing Hospital**

Uxbridge Road, Southall
Middlesex, UB1 3HW
Phone: 020 8967 5000
Fax: 020 8967 5636

Trust: Ealing Hospitals
NHS Trust

This maternity unit has its own fully equipped theatre and recovery room, as well as a Special Care Baby Unit. You may request a domino midwife, although normally new mothers go home when they wish to, providing they are medically fit. Water birth is available with midwives trained in this procedure available around the clock.

The unit offers a service for home birth, although home births may not be as frequently carried out here as in other district hospitals. The unit has good links for referral with tertiary centres in the event of high-risk pregnancies, particularly with the Fetal Medicine Unit at Hammersmith Hospitals NHS Trust.

Special antenatal classes include sessions for Somalian women, and a National Childbirth Trust counsellor is on hand for postnatal support.

Consultant and Midwife Unit

Number of beds	46
Births per midwife	37
Births per bed	0.64
Home births	1%
Amenity Rooms, Price	£45

Obstetrician 24 hours	Yes
Paediatrician 24 hours	Yes
Full Water Birth Service	Yes

Tests

Routine Triple Testing	Yes
Nuchal Fold Scan	No
Fetal Assessment Unit	No

Pain Relief

24 hour epidural	Yes
Mobile epidural	Yes
Pethidine injections	Yes
Water (eg bath)	Yes

Intervention Rates	%	regional average %	national average %
Epidural	27	33	33
Elective Caesarean	8	8	8
Emergency Caesarean	16	12	12
Induction	22	20	20
Forceps	4	3	4
Ventouse	4	8	7
Episiotomy	17	15	14

Enfield · **Chase Farm Hospital**

The Ridgeway, Enfield
Middlesex, EN2 8JL
Phone: 020 8366 6600
Fax: 020 8364 6331

Trust: Barnet and Chase Farm Hospitals
   NHS Trust

This consultant and midwife-led unit operates a caseload midwifery practice designed to ensure that where possible you will be looked after by the same midwife through pregnancy and labour. Around a third of women booked into this hospital will know the midwife who delivers their baby. This unit provides most scanning facilities, though you will need to be referred to University College Hospital for some tests. Epidural rates are high here and the anaesthetic service also offers mobile epidurals which allow greater feeling and movement.

Antenatal classes are organised at weekends as well as during the day and evenings. Women only groups are also offered.

Consultant and Midwife Unit

Number of beds	64
Births per midwife	32
Births per bed	0.68
Home births	23%
Amenity Rooms, Price	£80

Obstetrician 24 hours	Yes
Paediatrician 24 hours	Yes
Full Water Birth Service	No

Tests

Routine Triple Testing	Yes
Nuchal Fold Scan	Yes
Fetal Assessment Unit	Yes

Pain Relief

24 Hour epidural	Yes
Mobile epidural	Yes
Pethidine injections	Yes
Water (eg bath)	Yes

Intervention Rates	%	regional average %	national average %
Epidural	45	33	33
Elective Caesarean	8	8	8
Emergency Caesarean	12	12	12
Induction	20	20	20
Forceps	3	3	4
Ventouse	10	8	7
Episiotomy	19	15	14

Epsom · **Epsom General Hospital**

Dorking Road, Epsom
Surrey, KT18 7EG
Phone: 01372 735 735
Fax: 01372 735 159

Trust: Epsom and St Helier
NHS Trust

Both consultant obstetrician and midwife-led services are provided at this unit for women with high and low-risk pregnancies. As far as possible antenatal care is provided away from the hospital in the community at local surgeries or at your home.

Intervention rates are broadly in line with averages although inductions are rare. The epidural service offers mobile epidurals which allow for greater feeling and movement during labour. For antenatal screening, triple testing is not routinely offered but you can be referred to King's College Hospital for a nuchal fold scan. There is a special baby care unit on site.

Consultant and Midwife Unit

Number of beds	38
Births per midwife	38
Births per bed	0.87
Home births	1%
Amenity Rooms, Price	£110

Obstetrician 24 hours	Yes
Paediatrician 24 hours	Yes
Full Water Birth Service	No

Tests

Routine Triple Testing	No
Nuchal Fold Scan	Yes
Fetal Assessment Unit	No

Pain Relief

24 hour epidural	Yes
Mobile epidural	Yes
Pethidine injections	Yes
Water (eg bath)	Yes

Intervention Rates	%	regional average %	national average %
Epidural	36	33	33
Elective Caesarean	10	8	8
Emergency Caesarean	12	12	12
Induction	13	20	20
Forceps	4	3	4
Ventouse	7	8	7
Episiotomy	16	15	14

Greenwich · **Queen Elizabeth Hospital**

Stadium Road, Woolwich
London, SE18 4QH
Phone: 020 8858 8141
Fax: 020 8312 6205

Trust: Queen Elizabeth Hospital
NHS Trust

This brand new maternity unit has more comfortable facilities than many older hospitals. The delivery rooms have ensuite showers with special high seats to help tired mothers. They also have resuscitation units to provide instant help for a distressed baby within the delivery room.

Despite low midwife staffing levels – in common with much of London – the midwifery service is good, with women under the care of a named midwife and most women delivered by a midwife they know.

In addition to traditional pain management, acupuncture, aromatherapy and homoeopathy are all also offered. The unit has a high percentage of home births and is likely to support you if this is what you want.

Consultant and Midwife Unit

Number of beds	49
Births per midwife	40
Births per bed	0.68
Home births	5%
Amenity Rooms, Price	£50
Obstetrician 24 hours	Yes
Paediatrician 24 hours	Yes
Full Water Birth Service	Yes

Tests

Routine Triple Testing	No
Nuchal Fold Scan	Yes
Fetal Assessment Unit	Yes

Pain Relief

24 hour epidural	Yes
Mobile epidural	Yes
Pethidine injections	Yes
Water (eg bath)	Yes

Intervention Rates	%	regional average %	national average %
Epidural	31	33	33
Elective Caesarean	9	8	8
Emergency Caesarean	12	12	12
Induction	18	20	20
Forceps	3	3	4
Ventouse	7	8	7
Episiotomy	15	15	14

Hackney · **Homerton Hospital**

Homerton Row, Hackney
London, E9 6SR
Phone: 020 8510 5555
Fax: 020 8510 7608

Trust: Homerton Hospital
  NHS Trust

Homerton Hospital provides hospital and community based maternity care for the diverse local population. Continuity of care is reasonably good for a large hospital with around a third of women in labour cared for by a midwife they know.

The unit now has a full complement of 120 midwives so home birth is more readily available than it was in the past. Water birth is also offered, but the unit cannot always guarantee that midwives trained in this procedure will be available around the clock. Epidurals for pain relief are widely used so you should not have difficulty getting one. The unit runs yoga and relaxation classes, as well as classes for women expecting multiple births.

Consultant and Midwife Unit

Number of beds	70
Births per midwife	32
Births per bed	1.09
Home births	1%
Amenity Rooms, Price	£80
Obstetrician 24 hours	Yes
Paediatrician 24 hours	Yes
Full Water Birth Service	No

Tests

Routine Triple Testing	Yes
Nuchal Fold Scan	Yes
Fetal Assessment Unit	Yes

Pain Relief

24 hour epidural	Yes
Mobile epidural	No
Pethidine injections	Yes
Water (eg bath)	Yes

Intervention Rates	%	regional average %	national average %
Epidural	49	33	33
Elective Caesarean	8	8	8
Emergency Caesarean	13	12	12
Induction	22	20	20
Forceps	4	3	4
Ventouse	8	8	7
Episiotomy	13	15	14

Hammersmith · **Queen Charlotte's & Chelsea Hospital**

150 Du Cane Road, Hammersmith
London, W12 0HS
Phone: 020 8383 1111
Fax: 020 8383 3994

Trust: Hammersmith Hospitals
NHS Trust

Queen Charlotte's and Chelsea Hospital is a large teaching maternity hospital with a worldwide reputation. It offers a wide range of obstetric and midwifery services, from leading edge fetal medicine to the brand new, midwife-led Birthing Centre.

The delivery suite includes a section for women who are low-risk which allows them to stay in a room with ensuite facilities, where they deliver and then recover after birth for up to 12 hours. There is also a private wing.

The hospital has a reputation for performing a lot of caesareans but, after making some adjustment for the mix of patients, the emergency caesarean rate is lower than average but the unit has a greater tendency to book women in for elective caesareans.

Consultant and Midwife Unit

Number of beds	72
Births per midwife	34
Births per bed	0.66
Home births	1%
Amenity Rooms, Price	£100

Obstetrician 24 hours	Yes
Paediatrician 24 hours	Yes
Full Water Birth Service	No

Tests

Routine Triple Testing	Yes
Nuchal Fold Scan	Yes
Fetal Assessment Unit	Yes

Pain Relief

24 hour epidural	Yes
Mobile epidural	Yes
Pethidine injections	Yes
Water (eg bath)	Yes

Intervention Rates	%	regional average %	national average %
Epidural	-	33	33
Elective Caesarean	14	8	8
Emergency Caesarean	9	12	12
Induction	28	20	20
Forceps	4	3	4
Ventouse	7	8	7
Episiotomy	13	15	14

Haringey · **The North Middlesex Hospital**

Sterling Way, Edmonton
London, N18 1QX
Phone: 020 8887 2000
Fax: 020 8887 4219

Trust: The North Middlesex Hospital
NHS Trust

The North Middlesex hospital is unusual for a large hospital based maternity unit in the London region in that intervention rates are relatively low and the use of epidurals for pain relief is well below average. There are good midwife staffing levels, particularly for London, and staff are successful in helping more women to deliver naturally than in similar hospitals.

Water births are offered and the unit has a pool. However it cannot guarantee to have a midwife trained in water births available at all times. Home births are offered – with the number of home deliveries higher than average for this type of hospital. There are women-only antenatal classes as well as special classes for Turkish and Somali women.

Consultant and Midwife Unit

Number of beds	44
Births per midwife	32.6
Births per bed	0.54
Home births	3%
Amenity Rooms, Price	£33

Obstetrician 24 hours	Yes
Paediatrician 24 hours	Yes
Full Water Birth Service	No

Tests

Routine Triple Testing	No
Nuchal Fold Scan	Yes
Fetal Assessment Unit	Yes

Pain Relief

24 hour epidural	Yes
Mobile epidural	Yes
Pethidine injections	Yes
Water (eg bath)	Yes

Intervention Rates	%	regional average %	national average %
Epidural	13	33	33
Elective Caesarean	8	8	8
Emergency Caesarean	10	12	12
Induction	16	20	20
Forceps	2	3	4
Ventouse	4	8	7
Episiotomy	13	15	14

Harrow · **Northwick Park Hospital**

Watford Road, Harrow
Middlesex, HA1 3UJ
Phone: 020 8864 3232
Fax: 020 8869 2880

Trust: North West London Hospitals
Trust

This maternity unit is in the process of redeveloping its services and is waiting on funding for total refurbishment of the existing building.

Staff recruitment can be a problem here as in much of the South East and midwives are often under pressure. The unit has occasionally had to suspend services. Water births are offered but the unit does not guarantee that a midwife trained in water birth will be available at the time you want one.

A variety of pain relief is available, including mobile epidurals, and it is likely that you will be able to receive one when you want one. A TENS machine is also available.

Triple testing for Down's syndrome is offered, but nucal fold scan is not. Fetal assesment is provided at Queen Charlotte's & Chelsea Hospital.

Consultant and Midwife Unit

Number of beds	40
Births per midwife	42
Births per bed	0.82
Home births	0.5%
Amenity Rooms, Price	£75

Obstetrician 24 hours	Yes
Paediatrician 24 hours	Yes
Full Water Birth Service	No

Tests

Routine Triple Testing	Yes
Nuchal Fold Scan	No
Fetal Assessment Unit	Yes

Pain Relief

24 hour epidural	Yes
Mobile epidural	Yes
Pethidine injections	Yes
Water (eg bath)	Yes

Intervention Rates	%	regional average %	national average %
Epidural	30	33	33
Elective Caesarean	6	8	8
Emergency Caesarean	14	12	12
Induction	-	20	20
Forceps	2	3	4
Ventouse	9	8	7
Episiotomy	17	15	14

Havering · **Harold Wood Hospital**

Gubbins Lane, Harold Wood, Romford
Essex, RM3 0BE
Phone: 01708 345 533
Fax: 01708 376 717

Trust: Havering Hospitals
NHS Trust

This service is undergoing major change. A new philosophy and model of care will be implemented over the next two years. It is hoped that intervention rates, which are currently rather high overall, will decrease as midwife-led care for low-risk women is provided. The unit has a greater tendency than most hospitals to book women in for caesareans. This may in part contribute to its relatively low emergency caesarean rate.

Continuity of care is better than average for a large hospital with a third of women are cared for by a midwife known to them in labour. Home deliveries and domino deliveries are also offered although the home birth rate is below average.

Consultant and Midwife Unit

Number of beds	44
Births per midwife	35
Births per bed	0.86
Home births	1%
Amenity Rooms, Price	£25

Obstetrician 24 hours	Yes
Paediatrician 24 hours	Yes
Full Water Birth Service	No

Tests

Routine Triple Testing	Yes
Nuchal Fold Scan	Yes
Fetal Assessment Unit	Yes

Pain Relief

24 hour epidural	Yes
Mobile epidural	No
Pethidine injections	Yes
Water (eg bath)	Yes

Intervention Rates	%	regional average %	national average %
Epidural	38	33	33
Elective Caesarean	12	8	8
Emergency Caesarean	8	12	12
Induction	24	20	20
Forceps	4	3	4
Ventouse	10	8	7
Episiotomy	20	15	14

Hillingdon · **The Hillingdon Hospital**

Pield Heath Road, Uxbridge
Middlesex, UB8 3NN
Phone: 01895 238 282
Fax: 01895 811 687

Trust: Hillingdon Hospital
NHS Trust

As is typical of a district general hospital on the outskirts of London, staffing levels are a little stretched but the midwives manage to ensure that nearly a third of women are cared for in labour by a midwife they know.

Intervention rates are average and there is a full range of pain relief available. However the unit also encourages other approaches to pain management including massage, breathing techniques and music.

Water birth and home birth are offered and are supported by midwives experienced in these areas. The unit also runs a monthly drop-in breastfeeding session that mothers can attend both before and after the birth. As with most large hospitals, if you have to go into the antenatal ward before labour starts you partner will probably not be able to stay with you.

Consultant and Midwife Unit

Number of beds	63
Births per midwife	38
Births per bed	0.73
Home births	2%
Amenity Rooms, Price	£50

Obstetrician 24 hours	Yes
Paediatrician 24 hours	Yes
Full Water Birth Service	Yes

Tests

Routine Triple Testing	Yes
Nuchal Fold Scan	No
Fetal Assessment Unit	No

Pain Relief

24 hour epidural	Yes
Mobile epidural	Yes
Pethidine injections	Yes
Water (eg bath)	Yes

Intervention Rates

	%	regional average %	national average %
Epidural	34	33	33
Elective Caesarean	9	8	8
Emergency Caesarean	10	12	12
Induction	17	20	20
Forceps	3	3	4
Ventouse	5	8	7
Episiotomy	18	15	14

Twickenham Road, Isleworth
Middlesex, TW7 6AF
Phone: 020 8560 2121
Fax: 020 8565 2522

Trust: West Middlesex University
Hospital NHS Trust

The West Middlesex has a surprisingly low caesarean rate for a large hospital-based maternity unit. Only 6 per cent of women had a planned caesareans last year – less than half the number in some other units – and relatively few had emergency caesareans. At the same time there is a full pain relief service and above average use of epidurals. Interestingly, the unit runs special antenatal clinics for women who are particularly worried about pain relief.

Midwife staffing levels are good and the unit is relatively good at ensuring women are cared for in labour by a midwife they know. Parenting information sessions are also offered in Hindi.

Consultant and Midwife Unit

Number of beds	46
Births per midwife	37
Births per bed	0.91
Home births	3%
Amenity Rooms, Price	£50

Obstetrician 24 hours	Yes
Paediatrician 24 hours	Yes
Full Water Birth Service	No

Tests

Routine Triple Testing	Yes
Nuchal Fold Scan	Yes
Fetal Assessment Unit	No

Pain Relief

24 hour epidural	Yes
Mobile epidural	Yes
Pethidine injections	Yes
Water (eg bath)	Yes

Intervention Rates	%	regional average %	national average %
Epidural	37	33	33
Elective Caesarean	6	8	8
Emergency Caesarean	10	12	12
Induction	19	20	20
Forceps	4	3	4
Ventouse	8	8	7
Episiotomy	15	15	14

Islington · **The Whittington Hospital**

Highgate Hill, Archway
London, N19 5NF
Phone: 020 7272 3070
Fax: 020 7288 3390

Trust: Whittington Hospital
NHS Trust

The Whittington Hospital is well staffed for a London hospital but the facilities are at full capacity with over one birth per day for every labour bed in the unit. Women are sent home as soon as possible after delivery assuming they are well enough.

The unit has six transitional care rooms for mothers of small but well babies, and a neonatal intensive care unit is located alongside the maternity unit. There are four amenity rooms available for hire.

Elective caesareans are performed relatively infrequently here however the emergency caesarean rate is above average. Inductions are also more common than at other units, while epidural pain relief is not widely used.

Consultant and Midwife Unit

Number of beds	47
Births per midwife	32.5
Births per bed	1.21
Home births	3%
Amenity Rooms, Price	£70

Obstetrician 24 hours	Yes
Paediatrician 24 hours	Yes
Full Water Birth Service	Yes

Tests

Routine Triple Testing	No
Nuchal Fold Scan	Yes
Fetal Assessment Unit	No

Pain Relief

24 hour epidural	Yes
Mobile epidural	Yes
Pethidine injections	Yes
Water (eg bath)	Yes

Intervention Rates

	%	regional average %	national average %
Epidural	13	33	33
Elective Caesarean	6	8	8
Emergency Caesarean	14	12	12
Induction	24	20	20
Forceps	6	3	4
Ventouse	8	8	7
Episiotomy	19	15	14

Kensington · **Chelsea and Westminster Hospital**

369 Fulham Road
London, SW10 9NH
Phone: 020 8746 8000
Fax: 020 8846 6539

Trust: Chelsea and Westminster
Healthcare NHS Trust

This large maternity unit has fourteen midwifery teams, providing an integrated community and hospital midwifery service. Seven of the teams are community-based, caring for 2000 births a year. Home births and domino births are encouraged and supported by the community-based teams, and 8 out of 10 women know their midwife in labour .

A development project is underway to create extra birthing rooms, an operating theatre, more postnatal beds and a private wing.
The percentage of emergency caesareans and epidurals is high.

The unit's facilities include two birthing pools and other equipment, such as bean bags, floor mats and birthing stools to encourage and facilitate natural childbirth.

Consultant and Midwife Unit

Number of beds	51
Births per midwife	35
Births per bed	1.01
Home births	1%
Amenity Rooms, Price	-
Obstetrician 24 hours	Yes
Paediatrician 24 hours	Yes
Full Water Birth Service	Yes

Tests

Routine Triple Testing	Yes
Nuchal Fold Scan	Yes
Fetal Assessment Unit	Yes

Pain Relief

24 hour epidural	Yes
Mobile epidural	Yes
Pethidine injections	Yes
Water (eg bath)	Yes

Intervention Rates	%	regional average %	national average %
Epidural	48	33	33
Elective Caesarean	8	8	8
Emergency Caesarean	14	12	12
Induction	20	20	20
Forceps	4	3	4
Ventouse	6	8	7
Episiotomy	13	15	14

Kingston upon Thames · **Kingston Hospital**

Galsworthy Road, Kingston upon Thames
Surrey, KT2 7QB
Phone: 020 8546 7711
Fax: 020 8546 3295

Trust: Kingston Hospital NHS Trust

Kingston Hospital's new maternity unit and neonatal unit has comfortable modern accommodation, with single en suite rooms together with a five bedded bay and three two bedded rooms. Staff vacancies have put midwives under pressure recently but the unit runs a midwife-led service which is designed to ensure that the midwife who delivers you is someone you know. However, Kingston cannot guarantee this yet and most women who deliver at the unit do not know their midwife.

There is a full medical service at the unit: intervention rates are a little higher than average. Unusually, nuchal fold scans are offered to all. A counsellor is available for women suffering an early fetal loss.

Consultant and Midwife Unit

Number of beds	58
Births per midwife	43
Births per bed	1.55
Home births	1%
Amenity Rooms, Price	-
Obstetrician 24 hours	Yes
Paediatrician 24 hours	Yes
Full Water Birth Service	No

Tests

Routine Triple Testing	No
Nuchal Fold Scan	Yes
Fetal Assessment Unit	Yes

Pain Relief

24 hour epidural	Yes
Mobile epidural	No
Pethidine injections	Yes
Water (eg bath)	No

Intervention Rates	%	regional average %	national average %
Epidural	28	33	33
Elective Caesarean	9	8	8
Emergency Caesarean	11	12	12
Induction	21	20	20
Forceps	4	3	4
Ventouse	8	8	7
Episiotomy	-	15	14

Lewisham · **King's College Hospital**

Denmark Hill, Camberwell
London, SE5 9RS
Phone: 0207 737 4000
Fax: 0207 346 4815

Trust: King's College Hospital
NHS Trust

The hospital promotes works closely with local GPs and aims to provide care tailored to your needs. A drive to improve continuity of care has helped mean that now around 40 per cent of women in labour know their midwife. – higher than for most large hospitals. King's home birth rate of 7 per cent is one of the highest in the country for this type of unit.

Water births are offered and midwives trained in water births are available round the clock. The unit does not routinely offer triple testing, but it does offer nuchal fold scanning. Kings also has a feotal assessment and medicine centre, which offers specialised care. The maternity and neonatal services will be moving into new accomodation in 2002.

Consultant and Midwife Unit

Number of beds	65
Births per midwife	35
Births per bed	0.92
Home births	7%
Amenity Rooms, Price	-
Obstetrician 24 hours	Yes
Paediatrician 24 hours	Yes
Full Water Birth Service	Yes

Tests

Routine Triple Testing	No
Nuchal Fold Scan	Yes
Fetal Assessment Unit	Yes

Pain Relief

24 hour epidural	Yes
Mobile epidural	No
Pethidine injections	Yes
Water (eg bath)	Yes

Intervention Rates	%	regional average %	national average %
Epidural	30	33	33
Elective Caesarean	8	8	8
Emergency Caesarean	14	12	12
Induction	15	20	20
Forceps	3	3	4
Ventouse	5	8	7
Episiotomy	11	15	14

Lewisham · **University Hospital Lewisham**

University Hospital Lewisham
High street
London, SE13 6LH
Phone: 020 8333 3000
Fax: 0208 690 7540

Trust: The Lewisham Hospital
NHS Trust

The unit moved into a purpose built women and children's wing in 1996. Home births and domino deliveries have long been available at this unit and the home birth rate is in line with the national average.

Water births are not offered, but you can bring your own water pool and use it for pain relief during labour. The unit has a relatively low induction rate, which suggests that there is a policy of letting your labour progress naturally. Antenatal classes are held in the daytime and evening, and the unit runs group sessions for fathers and teenage mothers. Partners are not allowed to stay on the ward except in exceptional circumstances. The unit does not offer triple testing, but it does offer nuchal fold scanning.

Consultant and Midwife Unit

Number of beds	42
Births per midwife	39
Births per bed	0.89
Home births	2%
Amenity Rooms, Price	£35

Obstetrician 24 hours	Yes
Paediatrician 24 hours	Yes
Full Water Birth Service	No

Tests

Routine Triple Testing	No
Nuchal Fold Scan	Yes
Fetal Assessment Unit	Yes

Pain Relief

24 hour epidural	Yes
Mobile epidural	No
Pethidine injections	Yes
Water (eg bath)	Yes

Intervention Rates	%	regional average %	national average %
Epidural	-	33	33
Elective Caesarean	8	8	8
Emergency Caesarean	15	12	12
Induction	14	20	20
Forceps	-	3	4
Ventouse	-	8	7
Episiotomy	13	15	14

Newham · **Newham General Hospital**

Glen Road, Plaistow
London, E13 8SL
Phone: 020 7476 4000
Fax: 020 7363 8363

Trust: Newham Healthcare
  NHS Trust

The large shared midwife and consultant unit at Newham General Hospital is one of the busiest in the country, and the 11-bedded labour suite is likely to be close to capacity most of the time. Single rooms are available for hire, but the charge for this is one of the highest in the country. Despite relatively low staffing levels, continuity of care is better than average with about a third of women cared for in labour by a midwife they know. Home birth is an option but it is not often done at this unit. The domino system is also available.

Intervention rates at the unit are about average, but the number of forceps deliveries is low.

Consultant and Midwife Unit

Number of beds	79
Births per midwife	47
Births per bed	1.03
Home births	0.3%
Amenity Rooms, Price	£165
Obstetrician 24 hours	Yes
Paediatrician 24 hours	Yes
Full Water Birth Service	Yes

Tests

Routine Triple Testing	Yes
Nuchal Fold Scan	Yes
Fetal Assessment Unit	Yes

Pain Relief

24 hour epidural	Yes
Mobile epidural	No
Pethidine injections	Yes
Water (eg bath)	Yes

Intervention Rates	%	regional average %	national average %
Epidural	24	33	33
Elective Caesarean	8	8	8
Emergency Caesarean	10	12	12
Induction	22	20	20
Forceps	3	3	4
Ventouse	8	8	7
Episiotomy	14	15	14

Newham · **Newham General Hospital**

Glen Road, Plaistow
London, E13 8SL
Phone: 020 7476 4000
Fax: 020 7363 8102

Trust: Newham Healthcare NHS Trust

This unit is attached to the main unit (see previous page) and is staffed by a small team of midwives. The unit provides a separate environment for women with uncomplicated pregnancies who want to give birth naturally without epidural pain relief or doctors present.

However should any complications arise you are only seconds away from the main consultant unit. Water birth is offered with midwives trained in this procedure available around the clock.

A TENS machine is available for pain relief. Support services include giving up smoking, bereavement and HIV counselling.

Midwife Unit

Number of beds	8
Births	213
Midwives	0
Home births	0%
Amenity Rooms, Price	-
Obstetrician 24 hours	Yes
Paediatrician 24 hours	Yes
Full Water Birth Service	Yes

Tests

Routine Triple Testing	Yes
Nuchal Fold Scan	Yes
Fetal Assessment Unit	Yes

Pain Relief

24 Hour epidural	No
Mobile epidural	No
Pethidine injections	Yes
Water (eg bath)	Yes

Midwife-led units are adequately equipped to care for women whose pregnancy is progressing normally without complications. As a result, intervention tends to be low in these units. Basic pain relief will be offered, but any woman requesting an epidural during the delivery will need to be transferred to the nearest consultant-led unit. A woman will also be transferred to the obstetric unit if any complications develop during the delivery.

Redbridge · **King George Hospital**

Barley Lane, Goodmayes, Ilford
Essex, IG3 8YB
Phone: 020 8983 8000
Fax: 020 8970 8001

Trust: Redbridge Healthcare
NHS Trust

The unit attempts to provide women with continuity of care so that they can establish a good relationship with their midwife. The service aims to be flexible with antenatal classes at the weekends as well as evenings.
A home birth service is available, although the number of women delivered at home is below the national average. Water births are also on offer. The unit has its own pool, but there may not always be a midwife trained in water birth available.

Intervention rates are in line with national averages for a large maternity unit, although inductions are more common than average.

Consultant and Midwife Unit

Number of beds	61
Births per midwife	45
Births per bed	1.06
Home births	1%
Amenity Rooms, Price	£45

Obstetrician 24 hours	Yes
Paediatrician 24 hours	Yes
Full Water Birth Service	No

Tests

Routine Triple Testing	No
Nuchal Fold Scan	Yes
Fetal Assessment Unit	Yes

Pain Relief

24 hour epidural	Yes
Mobile epidural	No
Pethidine injections	Yes
Water (eg bath)	Yes

Intervention Rates	%	regional average %	national average %
Epidural	28	33	33
Elective Caesarean	7	8	8
Emergency Caesarean	13	12	12
Induction	31	20	20
Forceps	3	3	4
Ventouse	8	8	7
Episiotomy	19	15	14

St John's Wood · **Hospital of St John and St Elizabeth**

60 Grove End Rd, St John's Wood
London, NW8 9NH
Tel: 020 7286 5126
Fax: 020 7266 4813

Private Hospital

The Birth Unit is a private maternity unit offering consultant and midwife led care – the latter accounting for 70 per cent of cases.

As you would expect of a private service, staffing levels are good and you would always have one midwife looking only after you in labour. The unit's accommodation consists of individual rooms with double beds. If you had to go into hospital early, your partner would be encouraged to stay with you.

Pain relief in labour is readily available, and around half of the women giving birth at the unit have an epidural. Complementary methods of pain management are also offered. Options include a full water birth service, massage, aromatherapy, homeopathy, baby massage, visualisation, and yoga.

Consultant and Midwife Unit

Number of beds	8
Births per midwife	-
Births per bed	0.51
Home births	0%
Amenity Rooms, Price	-

Obstetrician 24 hours	No
Paediatrician 24 hours	No
Full Water Birth Service	Yes

Tests

Routine Triple Testing	Yes
Nuchal Fold Scan	Yes
Fetal Assessment Unit	No

Pain Relief

24 hour epidural	Yes
Mobile epidural	Yes
Pethidine injections	No
Water (eg bath)	Yes

Intervention Rates	%	regional average %	national average %
Epidural	50	33	33
Elective Caesarean	11	8	8
Emergency Caesarean	10	12	12
Induction	12	20	20
Forceps	4	3	4
Ventouse	3	8	7
Episiotomy	5	15	14

Southwark · **Guy's Hospital**

St Thomas Street, Waterloo
London, SE1 9RT
Phone: 020 7955 5000
Fax: 020 7955 8803

Trust: Guy's and St Thomas' Hospital
NHS Trust

In March 2002, Guy's maternity services will move to a new unit currently being built on the St Thomas' Hospital site.

Midwifery caseload, where midwives work in pairs, is the usual model of care here. The pattern of interventions is unusual, with very few elective caesareans. Overall the caesarean rate is below average which is unusual for a large inner London hospital. The ventouse rate however is above average. Early ultrasound tests and blood screening tests are not routinely offered to all women but if you do need antenatal screening the unit provides nuchal fold translucency scans. There is a private service here which for a fee of £525 will give you a private room and a range of other benefits.

Consultant and Midwife Unit

Number of beds	107
Births per midwife	29
Births per bed	1.03
Home births	2%
Amenity Rooms, Price	£525

Obstetrician 24 hours	Yes
Paediatrician 24 hours	Yes
Full Water Birth Service	Yes

Tests

Routine Triple Testing	No
Nuchal Fold Scan	Yes
Fetal Assessment Unit	Yes

Pain Relief

24 Hour epidural	Yes
Mobile epidural	No
Pethidine injections	No
Water (eg bath)	Yes

Intervention Rates	%	regional average %	national average %
Epidural	46	33	33
Elective Caesarean	4	8	8
Emergency Caesarean	14	12	12
Induction	22	20	20
Forceps	3	3	4
Ventouse	10	8	7
Episiotomy	6	15	14

Sutton · **St Helier Hospital**

Wrythe Lane, Carshalton
Surrey, SM5 1AA
Phone: 020 8296 2000
Fax: 020 8641 9391

Trust: Epsom and St Helier
NHS Trust

This unit offers a wide range of services catering for both high- and low-risk care, including early pregnancy assessment, a fetal assessment day unit and an obstetric medicine clinic. Midwives working in the community provide antenatal care to women with normal or low-risk pregnancies, and the domino system of care is an option.

The unit does not routinely offer triple testing to all women, but nuchal fold scanning can be arranged. Obstetricians are experienced in breech delivery and external cephalic version.

A full range of pain relief is offered, including mobile epidurals, and a water birth service is available 24 hours a day.

Consultant and Midwife Unit

Number of beds	58
Births per midwife	34
Births per bed	0.76
Home births	2%
Amenity Rooms, Price	-
Obstetrician 24 hours	Yes
Paediatrician 24 hours	Yes
Full Water Birth Service	Yes

Tests

Routine Triple Testing	No
Nuchal Fold Scan	Yes
Fetal Assessment Unit	Yes

Pain Relief

24 hour epidural	Yes
Mobile epidural	Yes
Pethidine injections	Yes
Water (eg bath)	Yes

Intervention Rates

	%	regional average %	national average %
Epidural	31	33	33
Elective Caesarean	5	8	8
Emergency Caesarean	11	12	12
Induction	18	20	20
Forceps	5	3	4
Ventouse	12	8	7
Episiotomy	17	15	14

Tooting · **The Birth Centre**

37 Coverton Road
London, SW17 0QW
Phone: 0208 767 8294
Fax: 0207 498 0698

Private Hospital

The Birth Centre is a private maternity unit based next door to the high tech obstetric and paediatric units at St George's Hospital in South London. Care at the unit is midwife led, but if complications arise, you can be transferred to the consultant unit where a full range of medical interventions are performed.

The unit's rate for emergency caesarean sections is slightly above average, but rates for instrumental deliveries, episiotomies and epidurals are low.

The unit consists of three birth rooms, all equipped with double beds and ensuite facilities. There are also two consulting rooms where you may stay before or after the birth. Because all rooms are single, partners are allowed to stay. Midwives at the unit attend a large number of home deliveries.

Midwife Unit

Number of beds	5
Births	59
Midwives	3
Home births	49%
Amenity Rooms, Price	-
Obstetrician 24 hours	No
Paediatrician 24 hours	No
Full Water Birth Service	Yes

Tests

Routine Triple Testing	No
Nuchal Fold Scan	Yes
Fetal Assessment Unit	Yes

Pain Relief

24 hour epidural	Yes
Mobile epidural	Yes
Pethidine injections	Yes
Water (eg bath)	Yes

Midwife-led units are adequately equipped to care for women whose pregnancy is progressing normally without complications. As a result, intervention tends to be low in these units. Basic pain relief will be offered, but any woman requesting an epidural during the delivery will need to be transferred to the nearest consultant-led unit. A woman will also be transferred to the obstetric unit if any complications develop during the delivery.

Tower Hamlets · **The Royal London Hospital**

Whitechapel
London, E1 1BB
Phone: 020 7377 7000
Fax: 020 7377 7666

Trust: Barts and The London
 NHS Trust

The Royal London is currently undergoing a major refurbishment which will be completed by March 2002. An obstetric operating theatre has just opened.

The unit is the main referral centre in East London for sick and/or premature neonates, neonatal surgery and for major medical conditions affecting women in pregnancy. Traditionally, the unit has low intervention rates compared with the national averages. The number of inductions, forceps deliveries, and elective caesareans are below the national average. The service has recently introduced a revised model of midwifery care, which is improving continuity of care throughout the pregnancy and labour. The unit offers a full range of pain relief, including mobile epidurals, and water births are available.

Consultant and Midwife Unit

Number of beds	56
Births per midwife	34
Births per bed	0.87
Home births	1.5%
Amenity Rooms, Price	-

Obstetrician 24 hours	Yes
Paediatrician 24 hours	Yes
Full Water Birth Service	Yes

Tests

Routine Triple Testing	Yes
Nuchal Fold Scan	Yes
Fetal Assessment Unit	Yes

Pain Relief

24 hour epidural	Yes
Mobile epidural	Yes
Pethidine injections	Yes
Water (eg bath)	Yes

Intervention Rates	%	regional average %	national average %
Epidural	33	33	33
Elective Caesarean	7	8	8
Emergency Caesarean	12	12	12
Induction	17	20	20
Forceps	4	3	4
Ventouse	7	8	7
Episiotomy	14	15	14

Waltham Forest · **Whipps Cross Hospital**

Whipps Cross Road, Leytonstone
London, E11 1NR
Phone: 020 8539 5522
Fax: 020 8558 8115

Trust: Whipps Cross University
NHS Trust

This unit is well staffed, intervention rates are average and there is a full pain relief service, although epidurals are used much more rarely than in other hospitals.

Although an early ultrasound scans are not done routinely a 24hr assessment unit means you can drop in at any time to be assessed by a midwife and treatment can be undertaken if necessary.

There is also a 24hr help line and antenatal clinics between 8.30am and 5.00pm on weekdays in addition to normal antenatal visits.

Although we do not have a breakdown of caesarean rates, the overall caesarean rate is 20%, slightly below average.

Consultant and Midwife Unit

Number of beds	67
Births per midwife	36
Births per bed	0.67
Home births	1%
Amenity Rooms, Price	£40
Obstetrician 24 hours	Yes
Paediatrician 24 hours	Yes
Full Water Birth Service	Yes

Tests

Routine Triple Testing	Yes
Nuchal Fold Scan	Yes
Fetal Assessment Unit	Yes

Pain Relief

24 hour epidural	Yes
Mobile epidural	Yes
Pethidine injections	Yes
Water (eg bath)	Yes

Intervention Rates	%	regional average %	national average %
Epidural	16	33	33
Elective Caesarean	-	8	8
Emergency Caesarean	-	12	12
Induction	15	20	20
Forceps	2	3	4
Ventouse	5	8	7
Episiotomy	7	15	14

Waltham Forest · **Whipps Cross Hospital**

Whipps Cross Road, Leytonstone
London, E11 1NR
Phone: 020 8539 5522
Fax: 020 8558 8115

Trust: Whipps Cross University NHS
Trust

The midwife-led unit at Whipps Cross Hospital provides care for low-risk women who wish to deliver with a minimum of intervention.

The unit is situated in Whipps Cross Hospital (see previous page) where there is also a full medical maternity unit offering epidural pain relief and obstetricians able to intervene should problems occur during labour.

The domino system is offered.

Water births are offered, but only if a midwife trained in water birth is available at the time. For pain relief there is water, gas and air plus a TENS machine.

Midwives encourage women to use different positions to help manage pain.

Midwife Unit

Number of beds	8
Births	271
Midwives	8
Home births	-
Amenity Rooms, Price	£75

Obstetrician 24 hours	Yes
Paediatrician 24 hours	Yes
Full Water Birth Service	No

Tests

Routine Triple Testing	Yes
Nuchal Fold Scan	Yes
Fetal Assessment Unit	Yes

Pain Relief

24 Hour epidural	No
Mobile epidural	No
Pethidine injections	Yes
Water (eg bath)	Yes

Midwife-led units are adequately equipped to care for women whose pregnancy is progressing normally without complications. As a result, intervention tends to be low in these units. Basic pain relief will be offered, but any woman requesting an epidural during the delivery will need to be transferred to the nearest consultant-led unit. A woman will also be transferred to the obstetric unit if any complications develop during the delivery.

Wandsworth · St George's Hospital

Blackshaw Road
London, SW17 0QT
Phone: 020 8672 1255
Fax: 0208 672 5304

**Trust: St George's Healthcare
NHS Trust**

Care at this unit is shared between midwives and consultants. Continuity of care is less good than in most hospitals with only one in ten women being delivered by a midwife they know. However domino deliveries are available as an option.

The unit offers several methods of pain relief during labour, including epidurals which are more widely used here than at most hospitals. Intervention in labour is, overall, no higher than for most large hospitals, although forceps are used much more frequently than in similar units.

The unit also offers women-only antenatal groups, a general counselling service and support services for teenagers and for women with HIV.

Consultant and Midwife Unit

Number of beds	52
Births per midwife	35
Births per bed	0.82
Home births	2%
Amenity Rooms, Price	£75
Obstetrician 24 hours	Yes
Paediatrician 24 hours	Yes
Full Water Birth Service	Yes

Tests

Routine Triple Testing	No
Nuchal Fold Scan	Yes
Fetal Assessment Unit	Yes

Pain Relief

24 hour epidural	Yes
Mobile epidural	Yes
Pethidine injections	Yes
Water (eg bath)	Yes

Intervention Rates

	%	regional average %	national average %
Epidural	37	33	33
Elective Caesarean	8	8	8
Emergency Caesarean	13	12	12
Induction	19	20	20
Forceps	6	3	4
Ventouse	9	8	7
Episiotomy	16	15	14

Westminster · **St Mary's Hospital**

Praed Street
London, W2 1NY
Phone: 020 7886 6666
Fax: 020 7886 6200

Trust: St Mary's
NHS Trust

St Mary's is a major London teaching hospital. Home birth, water birth and domino birth facilities are available for women with low-risk pregnancies. A midwife-led unit is currently being built within the main labour ward as well as dedicated water birth room. Both are due for completion in May 2002. Those women with high-risk pregnancies benefit from the specialist obstetric services such as a recurrent miscarriage clinic, specialist medical teams, a fetal medicine unit and a Maternity Day Care facility. It is also a regional referral centre for neonatal and paediatric services.

Intervention rates are much in line with national averages, apart from caesarean rates, which are higher than average.

Consultant and Midwife Unit

Number of beds	52
Births per midwife	35
Births per bed	0.76
Home births	2%
Amenity Rooms, Price	-
Obstetrician 24 hours	Yes
Paediatrician 24 hours	Yes
Full Water Birth Service	Yes

Tests

Routine Triple Testing	Yes
Nuchal Fold Scan	Yes
Fetal Assessment Unit	Yes

Pain Relief

24 hour epidural	Yes
Mobile epidural	No
Pethidine injections	Yes
Water (eg bath)	Yes

Intervention Rates

	%	regional average %	national average %
Epidural	33	33	33
Elective Caesarean	10	8	8
Emergency Caesarean	14	12	12
Induction	18	20	20
Forceps	3	3	4
Ventouse	7	8	7
Episiotomy	14	15	14

Westminster · **The Portland Hospital**

205-209 Great Portland Street
London, W1W 5AH
Phone: 0207 5804400
Fax: 0207 3908012

Private Hospital

The Portland is the largest private maternity unit in the UK, with 2165 deliveries last year.

There are 32 antenatal/postnatal bedrooms all with ensuite bathrooms. The unit is predominantly obstetric-led and can care for mothers with high-risk pregnancies, although a small proportion of care is also midwife-led.

Intervention rates are high: of all the non-caesarean births last year, 89 per cent of women had an epidural. Planned caesareans are very common here, with 26 per cent of women last year giving birth this way.

The unit offers a full range of pain relief options, including TENS machines.

The unit does not offer the triple test to all women, however, nuchal fold scans are available to those in risk groups.

Consultant and Midwife Unit

Number of beds	37
Births per midwife	-
Births per bed	1.19
Home births	0%
Amenity Rooms, Price	-
Obstetrician 24 hours	Yes
Paediatrician 24 hours	Yes
Full Water Birth Service	No

Tests

Routine Triple Testing	No
Nuchal Fold Scan	Yes
Fetal Assessment Unit	Yes

Pain Relief

24 hour epidural	Yes
Mobile epidural	Yes
Pethidine injections	Yes
Water (eg bath)	Yes

Intervention Rates	%	regional average %	national average %
Epidural	92	33	33
Elective Caesarean	26	8	8
Emergency Caesarean	18	12	12
Induction	-	20	20
Forceps	7	3	4
Ventouse	7	8	7
Episiotomy	20	15	14

The Northwest

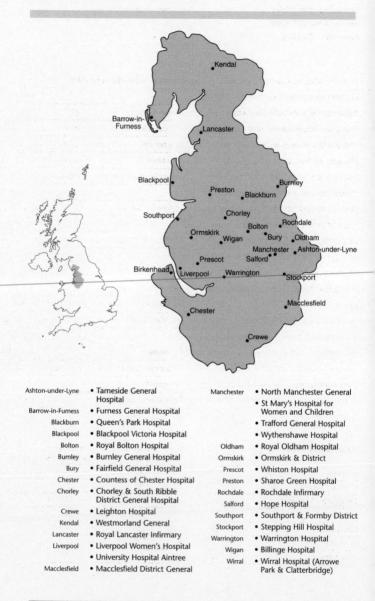

Ashton-under-Lyne	• Tameside General Hospital	Manchester	• North Manchester General
Barrow-in-Furness	• Furness General Hospital		• St Mary's Hospital for Women and Children
Blackburn	• Queen's Park Hospital		• Trafford General Hospital
Blackpool	• Blackpool Victoria Hospital		• Wythenshawe Hospital
Bolton	• Royal Bolton Hospital	Oldham	• Royal Oldham Hospital
Burnley	• Burnley General Hospital	Ormskirk	• Ormskirk & District
Bury	• Fairfield General Hospital	Prescot	• Whiston Hospital
Chester	• Countess of Chester Hospital	Preston	• Sharoe Green Hospital
Chorley	• Chorley & South Ribble District General Hospital	Rochdale	• Rochdale Infirmary
		Salford	• Hope Hospital
Crewe	• Leighton Hospital	Southport	• Southport & Formby District
Kendal	• Westmorland General	Stockport	• Stepping Hill Hospital
Lancaster	• Royal Lancaster Infirmary	Warrington	• Warrington Hospital
Liverpool	• Liverpool Women's Hospital	Wigan	• Billinge Hospital
	• University Hospital Aintree	Wirral	• Wirral Hospital (Arrowe Park & Clatterbridge)
Macclesfield	• Macclesfield District General		

Ashton-under-Lyne · **Tameside General Hospital**

Fountain Street, Ashton-Under-Lyne
Lancashire, OL6 9RW
Phone: 0161 331 6000
Fax: 0161 331 6074

Trust: Tameside & Glossop Acute
Sevices NHS Trust

The service is well staffed but few women here have their babies delivered by a midwife they know. There are also relatively few homebirths. However, the unit has plans to address this and improve both figures. Caseload midwifery was introduced last year – under which you are looked after by one named midwife and a second backup throughout your pregnancy and labour. Intervention rates are low, with very few planned caesareans. Epidurals are available but used less widely for pain relief in labour than at other hospitals. Aquanatal classes are arranged and there is a weekly support group for breastfeeding. For antenatal screening double testing is used rather than triple testing. Women needing a nuchal fold scan are referred to a nearby hospital.

Consultant and Midwife Unit

Number of beds	40
Births per midwife	24
Births per bed	1.28
Home births	0.5%
Amenity Rooms, Price	£25

Obstetrician 24 hours	Yes
Paediatrician 24 hours	Yes
Full Water Birth Service	No

Tests

Routine Triple Testing	No
Nuchal Fold Scan	Yes
Fetal Assessment Unit	Yes

Pain Relief

24 hour epidural	Yes
Mobile epidural	No
Pethidine injections	Yes
Water (eg bath)	Yes

Intervention Rates	%	regional average %	national average %
Epidural	25	29	33
Elective Caesarean	4	8	8
Emergency Caesarean	13	12	12
Induction	17	21	20
Forceps	1	3	4
Ventouse	7	7	7
Episiotomy	8	15	14

Barrow-in-Furness · **Furness General Hospital**

Dalton Lane, Barrow-in-Furness
Cumbria, LA14 4LF
Phone: 01229 870 870
Fax: 01229 491 270

Trust: Morecambe Bay Hospitals
NHS Trust

Furness General Hospital maternity provides care for women from the Furness Peninsula and parts of South Lakeland. Booking ultrasound scans are not usually carried out until 16-19 weeks unlike the more usual 12 weeks. Intervention rates are broadly average although you are more likely to be induced than at other hospitals. In contrast, instrumental deliveries are done less often than in most hospitals. Relatively few women have epidurals for pain relief in labour although it is available.

There is full medical cover and a special care baby unit on site to deal with more difficult deliveries. Home births and water births are both options. However home births are done very rarely. Breast feeding workshops are held every six weeks.

Consultant and Midwife Unit

Number of beds	39
Births per midwife	24
Births per bed	0.40
Home births	1%
Amenity Rooms, Price	£27

Obstetrician 24 hours	Yes
Paediatrician 24 hours	Yes
Full Water Birth Service	Yes

Tests

Routine Triple Testing	Yes
Nuchal Fold Scan	Yes
Fetal Assessment Unit	Yes

Pain Relief

24 hour epidural	Yes
Mobile epidural	No
Pethidine injections	Yes
Water (eg bath)	Yes

Intervention Rates	%	regional average %	national average %
Epidural	25	29	33
Elective Caesarean	10	8	8
Emergency Caesarean	11	12	12
Induction	25	21	20
Forceps	2	3	4
Ventouse	4	7	7
Episiotomy	14	15	14

Blackburn · **Queen's Park Hospital**

Haslingden Road, Blackburn
Lancashire, BB2 3HH
Phone: 01245 263 555
Fax: 01245 263 555

Trust: Blackburn, Hyndburn & Ribble
Valley Healthcare NHS Trust

Queens Park Hospital's maternity facilities are well-staffed and midwives operate a caseload system, where you are looked after by one named midwife with a second backup throughout your pregnancy and labour. Over half of women giving birth here last year knew their midwife. However, figures for home births are low. The triple test for Down's is not available and women needing a nuchal fold scan would be referred to the regional centre at St Mary's Hospital in Manchester. Epidurals are offered for pain relief, but are not commonly used. However, a mobile service is being introduced in the near future.

You are more likely to be induced here than at other hospitals. Obstetricians are experienced in breech delivery and practice external cephalic version.

Consultant and Midwife Unit

Number of beds	80
Births per midwife	27
Births per bed	0.70
Home births	0.3%
Amenity Rooms, Price	£64
Obstetrician 24 hours	Yes
Paediatrician 24 hours	Yes
Full Water Birth Service	Yes

Tests

Routine Triple Testing	No
Nuchal Fold Scan	Yes
Fetal Assessment Unit	Yes

Pain Relief

24 hour epidural	Yes
Mobile epidural	No
Pethidine injections	Yes
Water (eg bath)	Yes

Intervention Rates	%	regional average %	national average %
Epidural	23	29	33
Elective Caesarean	6	8	8
Emergency Caesarean	12	12	12
Induction	27	21	20
Forceps	1	3	4
Ventouse	8	7	7
Episiotomy	19	15	14

Blackpool · **Blackpool Victoria Hospital**

Whinney Heys Road
Blackpool, FY3 8NR
Phone: 01253 300 000
Fax: 01253 306 979

Trust: Blackpool Victoria Hospital
NHS Trust

Pain relief methods available during labour include a TENS machine and aromatherapy. There is a full epidural service, although epidurals may not always be available if there is an emergency. However, epidurals for pain relief in labour are very widely used with about a third of women having them. Antenatal testing is more limited than in many units. Early ultrasound scans are only offered to high-risk groups and nuchal fold scans for Down's syndrome are not available although high-risk groups will be offered triple testing.

Parentcraft classes are held both during the day and in the evenings to enable as many parents as possible to attend. There are also classes for women only and for women and their partners. The unit also offers a breastfeeding helpline.

Consultant and Midwife Unit

Number of beds	60
Births per midwife	31
Births per bed	0.79
Home births	1%
Amenity Rooms, Price	£45

Obstetrician 24 hours	Yes
Paediatrician 24 hours	Yes
Full Water Birth Service	Yes

Tests

Routine Triple Testing	No
Nuchal Fold Scan	No
Fetal Assessment Unit	Yes

Pain Relief

24 hour epidural	Yes
Mobile epidural	Yes
Pethidine injections	Yes
Water (eg bath)	Yes

Intervention Rates	%	regional average %	national average %
Epidural	43	29	33
Elective Caesarean	8	8	8
Emergency Caesarean	13	12	12
Induction	23	21	20
Forceps	4	3	4
Ventouse	6	7	7
Episiotomy	5	15	14

Bolton · **Royal Bolton Hospital**

Minerva Road, Farnworth
Bolton, BL4 0JR
Phone: 01204 390 390
Fax: 01204 390 794

Trust: Bolton Hospitals
   NHS Trust

This is a well-staffed service with team midwifery, where a team of midwives look after you through pregnancy, labour and the postnatal period. This approach has improved continuity of care and around three quarters of women are now looked after in labour by a midwife they know. The caesarean rate here is lower than at similar hospitals although other intervention rates are broadly in line with averages. Epidurals for pain relief are available but are not widely used. Mobile epidurals are being introduced. There are specific parentcraft classes for Asian women and there are also groups for teenagers, and for women with multiple pregnancies.

Consultant and Midwife Unit

Number of beds	99
Births per midwife	22
Births per bed	0.69
Home births	0.5%
Amenity Rooms, Price	£26
Obstetrician 24 hours	Yes
Paediatrician 24 hours	Yes
Full Water Birth Service	Yes

Tests

Routine Triple Testing	No
Nuchal Fold Scan	No
Fetal Assessment Unit	Yes

Pain Relief

24 hour epidural	Yes
Mobile epidural	No
Pethidine injections	Yes
Water (eg bath)	Yes

Intervention Rates	%	regional average %	national average %
Epidural	19	29	33
Elective Caesarean	7	8	8
Emergency Caesarean	10	12	12
Induction	24	21	20
Forceps	4	3	4
Ventouse	7	7	7
Episiotomy	15	15	14

Burnley · **Burnley General Hospital**

Casterton Avenue, Burnley
Lancashire, BB10 2PQ
Phone: 01282 425071
Fax: 01282 474444

Trust: Burnley Health Care
NHS Trust

Burnley General Hospital offers a choice of consultant led care or midwife led care. As with many units in the North West there are good midwife staffing levels and over a third of women are looked after in labour by a midwife they know. The unit also operates one-to-one midwife care in labour making sure there is a midwife on the labour ward for every woman in labour. The purpose-built unit is modern with well appointed rooms and accommodation for fathers. There are 15 en suite rooms for postnatal care. Epidurals are available although they are used relatively infrequently for pain relief in labour. Inductions are relatively rare. Other intervention rates are average. Triple testing is not done, but the unit does do double testing, which is similar although less definitive.

Consultant and Midwife Unit

Number of beds	35
Births per midwife	27
Births per bed	0.44
Home births	1%
Amenity Rooms, Price	-

Obstetrician 24 hours	Yes
Paediatrician 24 hours	Yes
Full Water Birth Service	Yes

Tests

Routine Triple Testing	No
Nuchal Fold Scan	No
Fetal Assessment Unit	Yes

Pain Relief

24 hour epidural	Yes
Mobile epidural	Yes
Pethidine injections	Yes
Water (eg bath)	Yes

Intervention Rates	%	regional average %	national average %
Epidural	28	29	33
Elective Caesarean	8	8	8
Emergency Caesarean	11	12	12
Induction	16	21	20
Forceps	3	3	4
Ventouse	8	7	7
Episiotomy	7	15	14

Bury · **Fairfield General Hospital**

Rochdale Old Road, Jericho, Bury
Lancashire, BL9 7TD
Phone: 0161 764 6081
Fax: 0161 705 3656

Trust: **Bury Health Care
NHS Trust**

The maternity service is provided by hospital and community based midwives along with four consultant obstetricians and four consultant paediatricians. Intervention rates are somewhat lower than average and forceps are only used in exceptional circumstances. There is a full range of pain relief options, although epidurals are used infrequently. There is also a TENS machine for pain relief. In July 2001, the unit relocated to a new purpose-built maternity unit which includes a new antenatal day assessment unit led by midwives and an early pregnancy unit. Staffing levels are good, although the facility is heavily used with nearly one birth per day for every delivery bed in the unit.

Home births are offered but occur in only one in a hundred births.

Consultant and Midwife Unit

Number of beds	31
Births per midwife	31
Births per bed	0.95
Home births	1%
Amenity Rooms, Price	£50
Obstetrician 24 hours	Yes
Paediatrician 24 hours	Yes
Full Water Birth Service	No

Tests

Routine Triple Testing	Yes
Nuchal Fold Scan	Yes
Fetal Assessment Unit	Yes

Pain Relief

24 hour epidural	Yes
Mobile epidural	No
Pethidine injections	Yes
Water (eg bath)	Yes

Intervention Rates	%	regional average %	national average %
Epidural	20	29	33
Elective Caesarean	8	8	8
Emergency Caesarean	12	12	12
Induction	14	21	20
Forceps	1	3	4
Ventouse	7	7	7
Episiotomy	13	15	14

Chester · **Countess of Chester Hospital**

Liverpool Road, Chester
Cheshire, CH2 1UL
Phone: 01244 365 000
Fax: 01244 365 292

Trust: Countess of Chester Hospital
NHS Trust

The Countess of Chester Hospital has good midwife staffing levels and tends to intervene in labour less often than many large hospitals. In particular elective caesareans are done less. There is full medical cover and a full range of pain relief options, including epidurals which are widely used. The domino system of midwife care is offered. Water births are available in a special water birthing suite. Home births are also offered, although they are done relatively infrequently. Early ultrasound scans are not offered unless considered necessary and nuchal fold scans are only done if you pay. The unit also has a transitional care unit so that if babies that need extra support with feeding or other requirements after birth can be kept near their mothers.

Consultant and Midwife Unit

Number of beds	57
Births per midwife	29.58
Births per bed	0.96
Home births	1%
Amenity Rooms, Price	£43

Obstetrician 24 hours	Yes
Paediatrician 24 hours	Yes
Full Water Birth Service	Yes

Tests

Routine Triple Testing	Yes
Nuchal Fold Scan	No
Fetal Assessment Unit	Yes

Pain Relief

24 hour epidural	Yes
Mobile epidural	Yes
Pethidine injections	Yes
Water (eg bath)	Yes

Intervention Rates

	%	regional average %	national average %
Epidural	36	29	33
Elective Caesarean	6	8	8
Emergency Caesarean	12	12	12
Induction	19	21	20
Forceps	4	3	4
Ventouse	6	7	7
Episiotomy	12	15	14

Preston Road, Chorley
Lancashire, PR7 1PP
Phone: 01257 261 222
Fax: 01257 245 117

Trust: Chorley and South Ribble NHS
 Trust

This is a newly established, midwife-led unit where you can give birth naturally if you have an uncomplicated pregnancy.

The unit aims to assign each woman her own midwife for the duration of her pregnancy. At the moment about one in four women get to be looked after in labour by a midwife they already know. The aim is that around 400 women a year should give birth here although currently the level is below that number. The good thing about this is that the unit is well staffed and not overcrowded.

There is a water birth service and the unit has its own pool. Midwives are trained in water birth deliveries and are available around the clock.

Other support services include a physiotherapist.

Mid-wife Care Led Unit

Number of beds	21
Births	214
Midwives	36
Home births	30
Amenity Rooms, Price	£30
Obstetrician 24 hours	No
Paediatrician 24 hours	No
Full Water Birth Service	Yes

Tests

Routine Triple Testing	No
Nuchal Fold Scan	Yes
Fetal Assessment Unit	No

Pain Relief

24 Hour epidural	No
Mobile epidural	No
Pethidine injections	Yes
Water (eg bath)	Yes

Midwife-led units are adequately equipped to care for women whose pregnancy is progressing normally without complications. As a result, intervention tends to be low in these units. Basic pain relief will be offered, but any woman requesting an epidural during the delivery will need to be transferred to the nearest consultant-led unit. A woman will also be transferred to the obstetric unit if any complications develop during the delivery.

Crewe · **Leighton Hospital**

Middlewich Road, Crewe
Cheshire, CW1 4QJ
Phone: 01270 255 141
Fax: 01270 587 696

Trust: Mid Cheshire Hospitals Trust

You will be looked after here by a team of midwives throughout your pregnancy and birth – the system is designed to ensure that you get to know the people who look afer you. In effect over half the women who give birth here have their baby delivered by a midwife they know which is better than most large hospitals. The unit is not quick to intervene in childbirth. Caesarean rates are lower than at similar units and epidurals for pain relief in labour are not widely used. However a full range of pain relief is available including a TENS machine. Antenatal classes are run in the evenings and sometimes at weekends, with special classes for grandparents also offered. The unit carries out double tests rather than triple tests for Down's, and also offers nuchal fold scans for a fee.

Consultant and Midwife Unit

Number of beds	51
Births per midwife	28
Births per bed	0.66
Home births	1%
Amenity Rooms, Price	£32

Obstetrician 24 hours	Yes
Paediatrician 24 hours	Yes
Full Water Birth Service	Yes

Tests

Routine Triple Testing	No
Nuchal Fold Scan	Yes
Fetal Assessment Unit	Yes

Pain Relief

24 hour epidural	Yes
Mobile epidural	No
Pethidine injections	Yes
Water (eg bath)	Yes

Intervention Rates

	%	regional average %	national average %
Epidural	22	29	33
Elective Caesarean	7	8	8
Emergency Caesarean	11	12	12
Induction	14	21	20
Forceps	3	3	4
Ventouse	10	7	7
Episiotomy	14	15	14

Kendal · **Westmorland General Hospital**

Burton Road, Kendal
Cumbria, LA9 7RG
Phone: 01539 732 288
Fax: 01539 740 991

Trust: Morecambe Bay Hospitals NHS
Trust

This unit has recently switched to being a pure midwife-led unit, providing a service for women with low-risk pregnancies who want to give birth naturally and without the aid of epidural pain relief.

Continuity of care is good, so you should get to know the midwives looking after you. The midwives will encourage you to remain upright and mobile during labour as a way of helping you to give birth naturally.

To help with pain management, you can use water, gas and air and a TENS machine. Midwives can also administer meptazinol injections. Screening for Down's syndrome is not routinely offered and nuchal fold scans are not available. If this is a concern for you, discuss this with a midwife at the unit.

Midwife Unit

Number of beds	14
Births	511
Midwives	18
Home births	3%
Amenity Rooms, Price	£45

Obstetrician 24 hours	No
Paediatrician 24 hours	No
Full Water Birth Service	Yes

Tests

Routine Triple Testing	No
Nuchal Fold Scan	No
Fetal Assessment Unit	No

Pain Relief

24 Hour epidural	No
Mobile epidural	No
Pethidine injections	Yes
Water (eg bath)	Yes

Midwife-led units are adequately equipped to care for women whose pregnancy is progressing normally without complications. As a result, intervention tends to be low in these units. Basic pain relief will be offered, but any woman requesting an epidural during the delivery will need to be transferred to the nearest consultant-led unit. A woman will also be transferred to the obstetric unit if any complications develop during the delivery.

Lancaster · **Royal Lancaster Infirmary**

Ashton Road
Lancaster, LA1 4RP
Phone: 01524 659 44
Fax: 01524 846 346

Trust: Morecambe Bay Hospitals
   NHS Trust

The Royal Lancaster Infirmary's maternity unit is undergoing major refurbishment which will continue until 2003. Despite this the unit remains a fully functional high-tech facility and a regional referral centre for complicated pregnancies. Intervention rates are above average for induction and emergency caesarean section. Epidurals are available for pain relief, but as with most hospitals in the North West, the use of epidurals relatively infrequent.

The unit does not routinely offer screening for Down's Syndrome or other chromosomal abnormalities. Nuchal fold scans are not offered but both Furness General Hospital and Blackpool Victoria Hospital, both around 20 miles away, do provide this service.

Consultant and Midwife Unit

Number of beds	31
Births per midwife	34
Births per bed	0.65
Home births	1%
Amenity Rooms, Price	£25

Obstetrician 24 hours	Yes
Paediatrician 24 hours	Yes
Full Water Birth Service	Yes

Tests

Routine Triple Testing	No
Nuchal Fold Scan	No
Fetal Assessment Unit	No

Pain Relief

24 hour epidural	Yes
Mobile epidural	Yes
Pethidine injections	Yes
Water (eg bath)	Yes

Intervention Rates

	%	regional average %	national average %
Epidural	31	29	33
Elective Caesarean	7	8	8
Emergency Caesarean	14	12	12
Induction	27	21	20
Forceps	5	3	4
Ventouse	9	7	7
Episiotomy	21	15	14

Liverpool · **Liverpool Women's Hospital**

Crown Street
Liverpool, L8 7SS
Phone: 0151 708 9988
Fax: 0151 702 4058

Trust: Liverpool Women's Hospital NHS
Trust

You can either be under consultant-led care or, for low-risk pregnancies, midwife led care here. The hospital contains a number of specialist units such as the Fetal Centre – a regional unit providing specialist care to women with high-risk pregnancies.

The centre takes referrals from other hospitals throughout the country and provides counselling and diagnosis for women with medical conditions such as diabetes, epilepsy, haemolytic antibodies, women who have had a previous baby with chromosomal or structural abnormality or whose baby has an abnormality diagnosed on ultrasound. A number of specialist clinics are also provided for ultrasound and prenatal diagnosis such as twins clinic, pre-pregnancy counselling, genetic clinic, miscarriage clinic and fetal cardiac clinic.

Consultant and Midwife Unit

Number of beds	115
Births per midwife	34
Births per bed	0.74
Home births	0.4%
Amenity Rooms, Price	-
Obstetrician 24 hours	Yes
Paediatrician 24 hours	Yes
Full Water Birth Service	No

Tests

Routine Triple Testing	Yes
Nuchal Fold Scan	Yes
Fetal Assessment Unit	Yes

Pain Relief

24 Hour epidural	Yes
Mobile epidural	No
Pethidine injections	Yes
Water (eg bath)	Yes

Intervention Rates	%	regional average %	national average %
Epidural	32	29	33
Elective Caesarean	9	8	8
Emergency Caesarean	12	12	12
Induction	26	21	20
Forceps	5	3	4
Ventouse	5	7	7
Episiotomy	13	15	14

Liverpool · **University Hospital Aintree**

Longmoor Lane, Liverpool
Merseyside, L9 7AL
Phone: **0151 525 5980**
Fax: **0151 525 6086**

Trust: Aintree Hospitals
    NHS Trust

Midwife care here is good. Group midwifery means you are assigned a named midwife who has a second as backup. This increases the likelihood that you will know the midwife who delivers your baby. Also, most women receive one to one care in labour – where one midwife is exclusively looking after you during your labour. The clinic provides a full range of antenatal services, and has a popular creche facility. The maternity ward has a mixture of four-bedded bays and single rooms. Caesarean rates – and in particular elective caesarean rates – are high. You are also much more likely to be induced here than at other hospitals. The delivery suite includes a pool room for water births. There is also a dedicated obstetric theatre situated within the delivery suite.

Consultant and Midwife Unit

Number of beds	46
Births per midwife	26
Births per bed	0.65
Home births	0%
Amenity Rooms, Price	-

Obstetrician 24 hours	Yes
Paediatrician 24 hours	Yes
Full Water Birth Service	Yes

Tests

Routine Triple Testing	Yes
Nuchal Fold Scan	No
Fetal Assessment Unit	Yes

Pain Relief

24 hour epidural	Yes
Mobile epidural	No
Pethidine injections	Yes
Water (eg bath)	Yes

Intervention Rates	%	regional average %	national average %
Epidural	35	29	33
Elective Caesarean	11	8	8
Emergency Caesarean	11	12	12
Induction	25	21	20
Forceps	3	3	4
Ventouse	6	7	7
Episiotomy	14.5	15	14

Macclesfield · **Macclesfield District General Hospital**

Victoria Road, Macclesfield
Cheshire, SK10 3BL
Phone: 01625 421 000
Fax: 01625 661 644

Trust: East Cheshire
   NHS Trust

Macclesfield Hospital maternity is a modern unit serving a wide area, with women coming in from the Peak District and North Staffordshire. Staffing levels are good and intervention rates are low.

There is a full service of epidural pain relief and although the overall epidural rate is low, epidurals in labour are used by about one in four women. The service is more family friendly than many with antenatal classes held in the evening and a policy of allowing your partner to stay in the hospital if you need to stay overnight before going into labour.

The triple test is not routinely available but nuchal scans are available should you need one.

Water birth is offered and the unit has midwives who are trained in water birth available around the clock.

Consultant and Midwife Unit

Number of beds	32
Births per midwife	20.79
Births per bed	0.93
Home births	2%
Amenity Rooms, Price	£40
Obstetrician 24 hours	Yes
Paediatrician 24 hours	Yes
Full Water Birth Service	Yes

Tests

Routine Triple Testing	No
Nuchal Fold Scan	Yes
Fetal Assessment Unit	Yes

Pain Relief

24 hour epidural	Yes
Mobile epidural	No
Pethidine injections	Yes
Water (eg bath)	Yes

Intervention Rates	%	regional average %	national average %
Epidural	19	29	33
Elective Caesarean	9	8	8
Emergency Caesarean	9	12	12
Induction	20	21	20
Forceps	1	3	4
Ventouse	8	7	7
Episiotomy	15	15	14

Manchester · **North Manchester General Hospital**

Crumpsall
Manchester, M8 5RB
Phone: 0161 795 4567
Fax: 0161 720 2676

Trust: North Manchester Healthcare
NHS Trust

North Manchester General Hospital is well staffed and has recently introduced caseload midwifery which means that you should get one midwife looking after you throughout your pregnancy and birth, with a second providing backup. Women tend to prefer having this consistency of care. Intervention rates are relatively low, with elective caesareans much less common than in many units. There is a full pain relief service including epidurals. Aromatherapy and reflexology are offered during the antenatal period. Water birth is also offered, with midwives available around the clock who can supervise your delivery.

A modernisation programme will see the building of facilities for fathers to stay on the delivery suite overnight.

Consultant and Midwife Unit

Number of beds	37
Births per midwife	25
Births per bed	0.85
Home births	1%
Amenity Rooms, Price	£23
Obstetrician 24 hours	Yes
Paediatrician 24 hours	Yes
Full Water Birth Service	Yes

Tests

Routine Triple Testing	No
Nuchal Fold Scan	Yes
Fetal Assessment Unit	Yes

Pain Relief

24 hour epidural	Yes
Mobile epidural	Yes
Pethidine injections	Yes
Water (eg bath)	Yes

Intervention Rates	%	regional average %	national average %
Epidural	35	29	33
Elective Caesarean	8	8	8
Emergency Caesarean	10	12	12
Induction	18	21	20
Forceps	4	3	4
Ventouse	7	7	7
Episiotomy	11	15	14

Manchester · St Mary's Hospital

Whitworth Park
Manchester, M13 0JH
Phone: 0161 276 1234
Fax: 0161 276 6107

Trust: Central Manchester &
    Manchester Childrens University
    Hospital NHS Trust

As a teaching hospital, St Mary's has three university chairs in obstetrics and gynaecology, child health and medical genetics. It carries out extensive research and provides a regional service for women with obstetric problems including women with complex fetal diseases and congenital abnormalities. The caesarean rate at the hospital is lower than would be expected and, in particular, emergency caesareans are relatively infrequent. Despite having good midwife staffing levels and offering domino system deliveries continuity is poor and very few women are cared for in labour by a midwife they know. Less than one per cent of women use the domino system. A drug liason midwife is employed to support women and their families who use illicit drugs or abuse alcohol.

Consultant and Midwife Unit

Number of beds	75
Births per midwife	26
Births per bed	0.77
Home births	1%
Amenity Rooms, Price	£25

Obstetrician 24 hours	Yes
Paediatrician 24 hours	Yes
Full Water Birth Service	Yes

Tests

Routine Triple Testing	No
Nuchal Fold Scan	No
Fetal Assessment Unit	Yes

Pain Relief

24 hour epidural	Yes
Mobile epidural	Yes
Pethidine injections	Yes
Water (eg bath)	Yes

Intervention Rates	%	regional average %	national average %
Epidural	40	29	33
Elective Caesarean	8	8	8
Emergency Caesarean	9	12	12
Induction	22	21	20
Forceps	3	3	4
Ventouse	7	7	7
Episiotomy	12	15	14

Manchester · **Trafford General Hospital**

Moorside Road, Davyhulme
Manchester, M41 5SL
Phone: 0161 748 4022
Fax: 0161 746 8556

Trust: Trafford Healthcare
NHS Trust

The unit is set up with small nursing bays and single rooms, all with en suite facilities and with separate areas for antenatal and postnatal patients. There is a large day/dining room with TV and video where meals are served. The five birth rooms have birthing chairs, TVs, ensuite bathrooms and tea and coffee making facilities. Medical care is led by four consultant obstetricians, two of whom are female. Unusually for the North West intervention levels are high with only a minority of births taking place naturally. The level of emergency caesareans is particularly high. Also epidurals are very widely used for pain relief in labour. A number of different models of care are available including shared care, GP care, midwifery-led care, domino and home births. There is also a special care baby unit.

Consultant and Midwife Unit

Number of beds	29
Births per midwife	27
Births per bed	0.81
Home births	1%
Amenity Rooms, Price	£52

Obstetrician 24 hours	Yes
Paediatrician 24 hours	Yes
Full Water Birth Service	No

Tests

Routine Triple Testing	No
Nuchal Fold Scan	Yes
Fetal Assessment Unit	Yes

Pain Relief

24 hour epidural	Yes
Mobile epidural	No
Pethidine injections	Yes
Water (eg bath)	Yes

Intervention Rates

	%	regional average %	national average %
Epidural	50	29	33
Elective Caesarean	8	8	8
Emergency Caesarean	18	12	12
Induction	28	21	20
Forceps	3	3	4
Ventouse	8	7	7
Episiotomy	7	15	14

Manchester · **Wythenshawe Hospital**

Southmoor Road, Wythenshawe
Manchester, M23 9LT
Phone: 0161 998 7070
Fax: 0161 291 2037

Trust: South Manchester University
Hospitals NHS Trust

You can decide with you GP or midwife whether to have consultant led care, midwife led care or a domino or home delivery, all of which are offered. Two beds are set aside for domino deliveries. There are parentcraft classes as well as exercise (including aquantal) and relaxation classes. There is a full range of pain relief options and epidurals are widely used. Intervention rates are average. Specialist midwifery support is provided to clients in vulnerable groups including pioneering work with homeless families.

Specialist midwifery support is also available for bereaved families and the unit has two dedicated self-contained suites well away from the main ward areas where families can grieve in private.

Consultant and Midwife Unit

Number of beds	39
Births per midwife	26.6
Births per bed	0.70
Home births	1%
Amenity Rooms, Price	£48
Obstetrician 24 hours	Yes
Paediatrician 24 hours	Yes
Full Water Birth Service	No

Tests

Routine Triple Testing	Yes
Nuchal Fold Scan	Yes
Fetal Assessment Unit	Yes

Pain Relief

25 hour epidural	Yes
Mobile epidural	Yes
Pethidine injections	Yes
Water (eg bath)	Yes

Intervention Rates	%	regional average %	national average %
Epidural	42	29	33
Elective Caesarean	10	8	8
Emergency Caesarean	14	12	12
Induction	18	21	20
Forceps	3	3	4
Ventouse	9	7	7
Episiotomy	-	15	14

Oldham · **The Royal Oldham Hospital**

Rochdale Road
Oldham, OL1 2JH
Phone: 0161 624 0420
Fax: 0161 627 8119

Trust: Oldham
   NHS Trust

The Marron maternity unit at the Royal Oldham Hospital has one of the best levels of midwife staffing which should help provide a high level of personal care and attention. The hospital conducts more home births than many other units in the North West. However, the delivery suite is likely to be close to capacity at times, as there is more than one birth per delivery bed per day.

Although the unit does not have a pool for water births, there are midwives trained to do this who will deliver you at home if you hire your own pool. There is a full epidural service, but relatively few women who give birth at the hospital use this form of pain relief. There is a health care worker to cater to the needs of ethnic minority women and an ethnic health team for interpretation.

Consultant and Midwife Unit

Number of beds	60
Births per midwife	20
Births per bed	1.02
Home births	2%
Amenity Rooms, Price	£28

Obstetrician 24 hours	Yes
Paediatrician 24 hours	Yes
Full Water Birth Service	No

Tests

Routine Triple Testing	Yes
Nuchal Fold Scan	Yes
Fetal Assessment Unit	Yes

Pain Relief

24 hour epidural	Yes
Mobile epidural	Yes
Pethidine injections	Yes
Water (eg bath)	Yes

Intervention Rates

	%	regional average %	national average %
Epidural	21	29	33
Elective Caesarean	9	8	8
Emergency Caesarean	11	12	12
Induction	24	21	20
Forceps	1	3	4
Ventouse	9	7	7
Episiotomy	14	15	14

Ormskirk · **Ormskirk and District General Hospital**

Wigan Road, Ormskirk
Lancashire, L39 2AZ
Phone: 01695 577 111
Fax: 01695 656 665

Trust: Southport & Ormskirk Hospital
NHS Trust

The maternity unit at Ormskirk and District General Hospital offers a full range of midwifery and consultant based care. An integrated midwifery service and domino service provides continuity of carer for mothers in both the hospital and the community, and midwife staffing is high.

Intervention rates for forceps, ventouse, elective and emergency caesareans, and episiotomies are well below the national averages. Water births are an option if your can hire your own pool, and trained midwives are available around the clock to assist you. Home birth is available, although it does not happen often.

The unit has recently developed an early pregnancy assessment unit to compliment their established pregnancy assessment unit.

Consultant and Midwife Unit

Number of beds	18
Births per midwife	19
Births per bed	0.45
Home births	1%
Amenity Rooms, Price	£22

Obstetrician 24 hours	Yes
Paediatrician 24 hours	Yes
Full Water Birth Service	No

Tests

Routine Triple Testing	No
Nuchal Fold Scan	Yes
Fetal Assessment Unit	Yes

Pain Relief

24 hour epidural	Yes
Mobile epidural	No
Pethidine injections	Yes
Water (eg bath)	Yes

Intervention Rates	%	regional average %	national average %
Epidural	25	29	33
Elective Caesarean	7	8	8
Emergency Caesarean	8	12	12
Induction	18	21	20
Forceps	2	3	4
Ventouse	6	7	7
Episiotomy	4	15	14

Prescot · **Whiston Hospital**

Whiston, Prescot
Merseyside, L35 5DR
Phone: 0151 426 1600
Fax: 0151 426 8478

Trust: St Helens and Knowsley
   Hospitals NHS Trust

This consultant and midwife led unit is well staffed and offers a full range of pain relief, with a high take up of epidurals as a means of pain management. However the unit does not do mobile epidurals. Domino system births are offered and the unit aims to provide as much antenatal care as possible outside the hospital either in your home or in local clinics. Water births are not offered but some midwives do have training in this area and could assist with a home water birth. On the other hand, home births are not done that often by the midwives at this hospital. The unit also offers support for women with HIV and drug problems as well as smoking cessation support.

Consultant and Midwife Unit

Number of beds	62
Births per midwife	28
Births per bed	0.2
Home births	0%
Amenity Rooms, Price	-

Obstetrician 24 hours	Yes
Paediatrician 24 hours	Yes
Full Water Birth Service	No

Tests

Routine Triple Testing	Yes
Nuchal Fold Scan	Yes
Fetal Assessment Unit	Yes

Pain Relief

24 hour epidural	Yes
Mobile epidural	No
Pethidine injections	Yes
Water (eg bath)	Yes

Intervention Rates	%	regional average %	national average %
Epidural	43	29	33
Elective Caesarean	10	8	8
Emergency Caesarean	13	12	12
Induction	21	21	20
Forceps	2	3	4
Ventouse	8	7	7
Episiotomy	10	15	14

Preston · **Sharoe Green Hospital**

Sharoe Green Lane South, Fulwood
Preston, PR2 9HT
Phone: 01772 716 565
Fax: 01772 710 333

Trust: Preston Acute Hospitals
NHS Trust

The maternity unit at Sharoe Green Hospital encourages women with low-risk pregnancies to have midwife-led care although consultant-led care is also available. The facility aims to assign each pregnant woman with her own midwife for the duration of her pregnancy to ensure good continuity of care. The result is that about one in five women have their baby delivered by a midwife they know. This is lower than for most large hospitals, but perhaps reflects the fact that the workload for midwives here is higher than at other units in the North West. There is a full pain relief service and epidurals are used frequently.

The unit works in close partnership with the midwifery led maternity unit at Chorley and South Ribble District General Hospital.

Consultant and Midwife Unit

Number of beds	72
Births per midwife	36
Births per bed	0.82
Home births	0.3%
Amenity Rooms, Price	£30

Obstetrician 24 hours	Yes
Paediatrician 24 hours	Yes
Full Water Birth Service	No

Tests

Routine Triple Testing	No
Nuchal Fold Scan	Yes
Fetal Assessment Unit	Yes

Pain Relief

24 hour epidural	Yes
Mobile epidural	No
Pethidine injections	Yes
Water (eg bath)	Yes

Intervention Rates	%	regional average %	national average %
Epidural	42	29	33
Elective Caesarean	10	8	8
Emergency Caesarean	12	12	12
Induction	21	21	20
Forceps	2	3	4
Ventouse	6	7	7
Episiotomy	13	15	14

Rochdale · **Rochdale Infirmary**

Whitehall Street, Rochdale
Lancashire, OL12 0NB
Phone: 01706 377 777
Fax: 01706 755 344

Trust: Rochdale Healthcare
NHS Trust

The maternity unit at Rochdale Infirmary was developed in January 2001 to provide a much improved, modern environment for maternity care. Midwives care for women across a wide geographical area, providing antenatal and postnatal care to around 1200 women a year who deliver in maternity units other than Rochdale. So the relatively low number of births per midwife disguises the fact that many other women are also cared for by the service. Intervention rates are a little above average although forceps are not much used. Nuchal fold scans and triple testing are offered to screen for Down's Syndrome – the triple test is routinely offered to women over 35.

Consultant and Midwife Unit

Number of beds	39
Births per midwife	29
Births per bed	0.67
Home births	0.41%
Amenity Rooms, Price	£24

Obstetrician 24 hours	Yes
Paediatrician 24 hours	Yes
Full Water Birth Service	No

Tests

Routine Triple Testing	No
Nuchal Fold Scan	Yes
Fetal Assessment Unit	Yes

Pain Relief

24 hour epidural	Yes
Mobile epidural	No
Pethidine injections	Yes
Water (eg bath)	Yes

Intervention Rates	%	regional average %	national average %
Epidural	24	29	33
Elective Caesarean	9	8	8
Emergency Caesarean	13	12	12
Induction	22	21	20
Forceps	2	3	4
Ventouse	6	7	7
Episiotomy	11	15	14

Salford · **Hope Hospital**

Stott Lane
Salford, M6 8WH
Phone: 0161 789 7373
Fax: 0161 787 5974

Trust: Salford Royal Hospitals
NHS Trust

The unit offers consultant-led care or, for lower risk pregnancies, a service where your birth is managed by midwives in a home-from-home environment. There is an epidural service but the unit actively encourages other forms of pain relief that do not use drugs.

Water birth is a new service at the unit and training is ongoing so trained midwifes are not yet available 24hrs a day. However, there is a pool on site. There is an antenatal day care facility and an early pregnancy assessment unit which you can drop in to if you have concerns during pregnancy. Local antenatal classes are provided outside the hospital and aquanatal classes are also on offer. The hospital offers a home birth service but relatively few births take place at home.

Consultant and Midwife Unit

Number of beds	60
Births per midwife	25.2
Births per bed	0.55
Home births	0.2%
Amenity Rooms, Price	£34

Obstetrician 24 hours	Yes
Paediatrician 24 hours	Yes
Full Water Birth Service	No

Tests

Routine Triple Testing	Yes
Nuchal Fold Scan	Yes
Fetal Assessment Unit	Yes

Pain Relief

24 hour epidural	Yes
Mobile epidural	Yes
Pethidine injections	Yes
Water (eg bath)	Yes

Intervention Rates	%	regional average %	national average %
Epidural	-	29	33
Elective Caesarean	10	8	8
Emergency Caesarean	13	12	12
Induction	21	21	20
Forceps	2	3	4
Ventouse	8	7	7
Episiotomy	10	15	14

Southport · **Southport & Formby District General**

Town Lane, Kew, Southport
Merseyside, PR8 6PN
Phone: 01704 547 471
Fax: 01704 548 229

Trust: Southport & Ormskirk Hospital
   NHS Trust

Midwives provide antenatal care at your home or in your GP clinic as well as in the hopsital. The Antenatal Clinic and Pregnancy Assessment Unit are based in the Outpatient Department. There is a good number of midwives to deal with the workload and domino deliveries are offered as well as home births, although home births are very rarely done.

Intervention rates are average, although, unusually, forceps are used more often than ventouse in instrumental deliveries.

There is no water birth service at the hospital, but midwives may be able to help you with a home water birth.

The unit does double testing rather than triple testing, and nuchal fold scans are also offered to screen for Down's.

Consultant and Midwife Unit

Number of beds	22
Births per midwife	21
Births per bed	0.70
Home births	1%
Amenity Rooms, Price	£22

Obstetrician 24 hours	No
Paediatrician 24 hours	Yes
Full Water Birth Service	No

Tests

Routine Triple Testing	No
Nuchal Fold Scan	Yes
Fetal Assessment Unit	Yes

Pain Relief

24 hour epidural	Yes
Mobile epidural	Yes
Pethidine injections	Yes
Water (eg bath)	Yes

Intervention Rates	%	regional average %	national average %
Epidural	35	29	33
Elective Caesarean	10	8	8
Emergency Caesarean	12	12	12
Induction	19	21	20
Forceps	5	3	4
Ventouse	2	7	7
Episiotomy	-	15	14

Stockport · **Stepping Hill Hospital**

Poplar Grove, Stockport
Cheshire, SK2 7JE
Phone: 0161 483 1010
Fax: 0161 419 5558

Trust: Stockport
NHS Trust

Stepping Hill maternity unit is located just outside Stockport, and has six consultant obstetricians and six paediatricians. Midwife staffing levels are good. The unit is implementing a team approach to midwifery care and plans to ensure that all women have one-to-one care in labour.

The caesarean rate is below average. Caesareans deliveries are carried out less often here than at other units.

There is a water birth service and the delivery unit has a pool room. All midwives are trained in water births and provide a 24hr service.

The neonatal unit has two intensive care cots, and two family rooms in which mothers can remain with infants after discharge from the neonatal unit. The unit also has an early pregnancy unit.

Consultant and Midwife Unit

Number of beds	56
Births per midwife	30.6
Births per bed	0.64
Home births	1%
Amenity Rooms, Price	£50

Obstetrician 24 hours	Yes
Paediatrician 24 hours	Yes
Full Water Birth Service	Yes

Tests

Routine Triple Testing	Yes
Nuchal Fold Scan	No
Fetal Assessment Unit	Yes

Pain Relief

24 hour epidural	Yes
Mobile epidural	No
Pethidine injections	Yes
Water (eg bath)	Yes

Intervention Rates	%	regional average %	national average %
Epidural	-	29	33
Elective Caesarean	7	8	8
Emergency Caesarean	11	12	12
Induction	-	21	20
Forceps	4	3	4
Ventouse	7	7	7
Episiotomy	16	15	14

Warrington · **Warrington Hospital**

Lovely Lane, Warrington
Cheshire, WA5 1QG
Phone: 01925 635 911
Fax: 01925 662 099

Trust: Warrington Hospital
NHS Trust

There are seven consultants and about 120 midwives providing care through pregnancy, birth and afterwards. Antenatal care is provided, as far as possible, in your home or in local GP surgeries or clinics. Some of the midwives specialise in high dependency care of women during labour and afterwards. Midwife staffing levels are average – although lower than many hospitals in the North West. But very few women are looked after in labour by someone they know. The caesarean rate is high with a particularly high rate of elective caesareans. There are midwives on staff with specialist skills in drugs, child protection and domestic violence. The hospital actively promotes breastfeeding.

Consultant and Midwife Unit

Number of beds	51
Births per midwife	35
Births per bed	0.76
Home births	0.3%
Amenity Rooms, Price	£43

Obstetrician 24 hours	Yes
Paediatrician 24 hours	Yes
Full Water Birth Service	Yes

Tests

Routine Triple Testing	Yes
Nuchal Fold Scan	No
Fetal Assessment Unit	No

Pain Relief

25 hour epidural	Yes
Mobile epidural	No
Pethidine injections	Yes
Water (eg bath)	Yes

Intervention Rates	%	regional average %	national average %
Epidural	32	29	33
Elective Caesarean	11	8	8
Emergency Caesarean	13	12	12
Induction	22	21	20
Forceps	3	3	4
Ventouse	7	7	7
Episiotomy	20	15	14

Wigan · **Billinge Hospital**

Upholland Road, Billinge, Wigan
Lancashire, WN5 7ET
Phone: 01942 244 000
Fax: 01695 626 523

Trust: Wigan and Leigh Health Services
NHS Trust

Midwife staffing levels are high at this hospital which should enable a better level of personal attention particularly during labour. The hospital has a good record on ensuring that women are looked after in labour by somebody they know and who knows their case. Intervention rates in labour are fairly average although you are more likely to have your labour induced here than at other similar units. A range of pain relief methods are available for use during birth, including water, gas and air, intramuscular opiate injection and epidurals.

There is a home birth service, but home births are extremely rare. Parent education sessions and antenatal classes run both during the daytime and in the evenings. The unit also runs specific women-only groups and groups for teenage parents.

Consultant and Midwife Unit

Number of beds	54
Births per midwife	28
Births per bed	0.82
Home births	0.5%
Amenity Rooms, Price	£20

Obstetrician 24 hours	Yes
Paediatrician 24 hours	Yes
Full Water Birth Service	Yes

Tests

Routine Triple Testing	Yes
Nuchal Fold Scan	No
Fetal Assessment Unit	No

Pain Relief

24 hour epidural	Yes
Mobile epidural	Yes
Pethidine injections	Yes
Water (eg bath)	Yes

Intervention Rates	%	regional average %	national average %
Epidural	30	29	33
Elective Caesarean	8	8	8
Emergency Caesarean	13	12	12
Induction	24	21	20
Forceps	4	3	4
Ventouse	8	7	7
Episiotomy	19	15	14

Arrowe Park Road, Upton
Wirral, Merseyside, CH49 5PE
Phone: 0151 604 7198

Trust: Wirral Hospital NHS Trust

The purpose-built Duchess of Westminster Wing at Arrowe Park Hospital has seven consultants including a specialist in fetal medicine. There is good level of midwife staffing with 17 midwife teams providing care throughout pregnancy and labour. The idea is that you should get to know your named midwife and others in the team. The system is working well with over two thirds of women looked after in labour by a midwife they know.

Although the unit does not offer water births, you can have a home water birth if you supply your own pool and the midwife will come out with a supervisor to handle the birth. Breech presentations tend to now be done by caesarean although there is a consultant who will attempt to turn the baby.

Consultant and Midwife Unit

Number of beds	69
Births per midwife	25
Births per bed	0.74
Home births	1%
Amenity Rooms, Price	£30

Obstetrician 24 hours	Yes
Paediatrician 24 hours	Yes
Full Water Birth Service	No

Tests

Routine Triple Testing	Yes
Nuchal Fold Scan	Yes
Fetal Assessment Unit	Yes

Pain Relief

25 hour epidural	Yes
Mobile epidural	No
Pethidine injections	Yes
Water (eg bath)	No

Intervention Rates	%	regional average %	national average %
Epidural	33	29	33
Elective Caesarean	8	8	8
Emergency Caesarean	9	12	12
Induction	-	21	20
Forceps	6	3	4
Ventouse	11	7	7
Episiotomy	30	15	14

The North

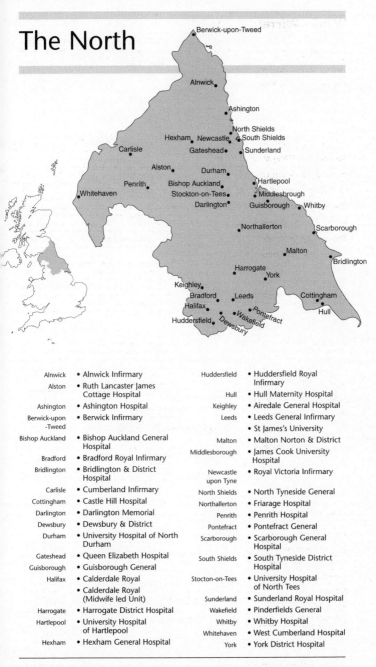

Berwick-upon-Tweed
Alnwick
Ashington
North Shields
Hexham Newcastle South Shields
Carlisle Gateshead Sunderland
Alston Durham
Penrith Bishop Auckland Hartlepool
Whitehaven Stockton-on-Tees Middlesbrough
Darlington Guisborough Whitby
Northallerton Scarborough
Malton
Bridlington
Harrogate
Keighley York
Bradford Leeds Cottingham
Halifax Pontefract Hull
Huddersfield Wakefield
Dewsbury

Alnwick	• Alnwick Infirmary
Alston	• Ruth Lancaster James Cottage Hospital
Ashington	• Ashington Hospital
Berwick-upon-Tweed	• Berwick Infirmary
Bishop Auckland	• Bishop Auckland General Hospital
Bradford	• Bradford Royal Infirmary
Bridlington	• Bridlington & District Hospital
Carlisle	• Cumberland Infirmary
Cottingham	• Castle Hill Hospital
Darlington	• Darlington Memorial
Dewsbury	• Dewsbury & District
Durham	• University Hospital of North Durham
Gateshead	• Queen Elizabeth Hospital
Guisborough	• Guisborough General
Halifax	• Calderdale Royal
	• Calderdale Royal (Midwife led Unit)
Harrogate	• Harrogate District Hospital
Hartlepool	• University Hospital of Hartlepool
Hexham	• Hexham General Hospital
Huddersfield	• Huddersfield Royal Infirmary
Hull	• Hull Maternity Hospital
Keighley	• Airedale General Hospital
Leeds	• Leeds General Infirmary
	• St James's University
Malton	• Malton Norton & District
Middlesborough	• James Cook University Hospital
Newcastle upon Tyne	• Royal Victoria Infirmary
North Shields	• North Tyneside General
Northallerton	• Friarage Hospital
Penrith	• Penrith Hospital
Pontefract	• Pontefract General
Scarborough	• Scarborough General Hospital
South Shields	• South Tyneside District Hospital
Stocton-on-Tees	• University Hospital of North Tees
Sunderland	• Sunderland Royal Hospital
Wakefield	• Pinderfields General
Whitby	• Whitby Hospital
Whitehaven	• West Cumberland Hospital
York	• York District Hospital

Alnwick · **Alnwick Infirmary**

Infirmary Drive, Alnwick
Northumberland, NE66 2NS
Phone: 01665 626700
Fax: 01665 626761

Trust: Northumbria Healthcare
    NHS Trust

The small maternity unit at Alnwick Infirmary has just one delivery bed. The unit used to operate shared care with GPs, however, it is now changing to a midwife-led service.

Alnwick has a small number of midwives who work as a team to care for all women booked with the service. This policy makes it likely that you will be familiar with the midwife who delivers you, though currently only around three-quarters of women fall into this category. Home birth is not available, nor is water birth.

The unit's low-tech approach extends to antenatal testing. Triple testing for Down's is not routinely offered to all women, and nuchal fold scans and chorionic villus sampling are not available.

Midwife Unit

Number of beds	8
Births	74
Midwives	11
Home births	0%
Amenity Rooms, Price	-
Obstetrician 24 hours	No
Paediatrician 24 hours	No
Full Water Birth Service	

Tests

Routine Triple Testing	No
Nuchal Fold Scan	No
Fetal Assessment Unit	No

Pain Relief

24 Hour epidural	No
Mobile epidural	No
Pethidine injections	Yes
Water (eg Bath)	Yes

Midwife-led units are adequately equipped to care for women whose pregnancy is progressing normally without complications. As a result, intervention tends to be low in these units. Basic pain relief will be offered, but any woman requesting an epidural during the delivery will need to be transferred to the nearest consultant-led unit. A woman will also be transferred to the obstetric unit if any complications develop during the delivery.

Alston · **Ruth Lancaster James Cottage Hospital**

Alston
Cumbria, CA9 3QX
Phone: 01434 381218
Fax: 01434 382134

Trust: North Cumbria Acute Hospitals NHS Trust

The maternity unit at Ruth Lancaster James Cottage Hospital has one labour bed and one other maternity bed used for antenatal and postnatal stays. Midwives and GPs share the care of women booked with the service, and strongly encourage home deliveries: in addition to the four babies born inthe unit a further eight were born at home. The triple test for Down's syndrome is available, but women must pay privately and travel to Newcastle for the more reliable nuchal fold scan. Routine scans are performed at Hexham, from where the unit receives input from consultants where necessary. As a small service offering a personalised care, antenatal education sessions can be arranged on an individual basis in the evenings or at weekends, though they are typically scheduled for the daytime.

Midwife Unit

Number of beds	1
Births	4
Midwives	1
Home births	66%
Amenity Rooms, Price	-

Obstetrician 24 hours	No
Paediatrician 24 hours	No
Full Water Birth Service	Yes

Tests

Routine Triple Testing	Yes
Nuchal Fold Scan	No
Fetal Assessment Unit	No

Pain Relief

24 Hour epidural	No
Mobile epidural	No
Pethidine injections	Yes
Water (eg Bath)	Yes

Midwife-led units are adequately equipped to care for women whose pregnancy is progressing normally without complications. As a result, intervention tends to be low in these units. Basic pain relief will be offered, but any woman requesting an epidural during the delivery will need to be transferred to the nearest consultant-led unit. A woman will also be transferred to the obstetric unit if any complications develop during the delivery.

Ashington · **Ashington Hospital**

West View, Ashington
Northumberland, NE63 0SA
Phone: 01670 521212
Fax: 01670 520034

Trust: Northumbria Healthcare
NHS Trust

This is a small unit with quite a high rate of induction although other forms of intervention are average.

The service does not offer the triple test as a screen for Down's, but nuchal fold scans, which are non-invasive, can be made available. If you need one of these you will be referred to the Royal Victoria Infirmary in Newcastle upon Tyne.

Home births are rare but there is a full water birth facility with midwives trained in this procedure available round the clock.

There is a Special Care Baby Unit, the only one of its type in the country, with 14 cots, two of which are high dependency cots. A team of neonatal nurse practitioners with support from other neonatal staff provide 24hr care, though a paediatrician will not necessarily be on site at all times.

Consultant and Midwife Unit

Number of beds	30
Births per midwife	38.3
Births per bed	0.63
Home births	0.4%
Amenity Rooms, Price	£37
Obstetrician 24 hours	Yes
Paediatrician 24 hours	No
Full Water Birth Service	Yes

Tests

Routine Triple Testing	No
Nuchal Fold Scan	Yes
Fetal Assessment Unit	Yes

Pain Relief

24 hour epidural	Yes
Mobile epidural	No
Pethidine injections	Yes
Water (eg bath)	Yes

Intervention Rates	%	regional average %	national average %
Epidural	35	33	33
Elective Caesarean	9	8	8
Emergency Caesarean	14	12	12
Induction	25	20	20
Forceps	4	4	4
Ventouse	8	6	7
Episiotomy	16	13	14

Berwick-upon-Tweed · **Berwick Infirmary**

Infirmary Square, Berwick on Tweed
Northumberland, TD15 1LT
Phone: 01289 307484
Fax: 01289 356667

Trust: Northumbria Healthcare
NHS Trust

This small unit operates shared care between midwives and GPs. Access to tests is limited: the triple test, nuchal fold scanning and chorionic villus sampling are not available.

High-risk patients are cared for at the consultant-led units at the Royal Victoria Hospital Newcastle, the Borders General Hospital, Melrose and Simpsons Memorial Hospital, Edinburgh. Because the unit is relatively well staffed for a small amount of births, 99 per cent of women know the midwife who delivers them. Antenatal classes are organised during the day or evening. There are women only groups as well as special groups for partners. Because six of the unit's eight beds are in single rooms, your partner is likely to be allowed to stay with you if you are going into labour overnight.

Midwife Unit

Number of beds	8
Births	47
Midwives	7
Home births	0%
Amenity Rooms, Price	-

Obstetrician 24 hours	No
Paediatrician 24 hours	No
Full Water Birth Service	

Tests

Routine Triple Testing	No
Nuchal Fold Scan	No
Fetal Assessment Unit	Yes

Pain Relief

24 hour epidural	No
Mobile epidural	No
Pethidine injections	Yes
Water (eg Bath)	Yes

Midwife-led units are adequately equipped to care for women whose pregnancy is progressing normally without complications. As a result, intervention tends to be low in these units. Basic pain relief will be offered, but any woman requesting an epidural during the delivery will need to be transferred to the nearest consultant-led unit. A woman will also be transferred to the obstetric unit if any complications develop during the delivery.

Cockton Hill Road, Bishop Auckland
Co Durham, DL14 6AD
Phone: 01388 454000
Fax: 01388 454127

Trust: South Durham Healthcare
  NHS Trust

This unit provides services to women in South Durham. The facility is well-staffed and a high proportion of women are cared for in labour by a midwife who also looked after them during their pregnancy.

The unit provides the domino system for births and home births, although its rate of home births is very low.

The unit is introducing double testing for Down's. Nuchal fold tests can be provided through the regional centre. Aquanatal classes, breastfeeding support and full water birth facilities are available, as well as facilities to accommodate partners. There is a 24-hour epidural service. Staff run breastfeeding support groups where mothers can get experience and support from midwives as well as benefiting from sharing their experiences with other mothers.

Consultant and Midwife Unit

Number of beds	27
Births per midwife	25
Births per bed	0.39
Home births	0.5%
Amenity Rooms, Price	£31

Obstetrician 24 hours	Yes
Paediatrician 24 hours	No
Full Water Birth Service	Yes

Tests

Routine Triple Testing	No
Nuchal Fold Scan	Yes
Fetal Assessment Unit	No

Pain Relief

24 hour epidural	Yes
Mobile epidural	No
Pethidine injections	Yes
Water (eg bath)	Yes

Intervention Rates	%	regional average %	national average %
Epidural	-	33	33
Elective Caesarean	8	8	8
Emergency Caesarean	12	12	12
Induction	23	20	20
Forceps	4	4	4
Ventouse	6	6	7
Episiotomy	10	13	14

Bradford · **Bradford Royal Infirmary**

Duckworth Lane, Bradford
West Yorkshire, BD9 6RJ
Phone: 01274 542 200
Fax: 01274 364 026

Trust: Bradford Hospitals
NHS Trust

Bradford Royal Infirmary is a large facility, delivering around 5000 babies a year. Its team of bilingual health support workers provide support to the high proportion of women from the Indian subcontinent, for whom English is not their first language. Women-only and evening antenatal classes are available.

Ultrasound and amniocentesis are offered, though the nearest facility offering triple testing and nuchal fold scanning is Leeds General Infirmary. Intervention rates are broadly in line with national averages for a unit of this type although the induction rate is low. Breastfeeding is deemed a priority within the unit and strongly encouraged.

Consultant and Midwife Unit

Number of beds	93
Births per midwife	32
Births per bed	0.82
Home births	0.4%
Amenity Rooms, Price	£31

Obstetrician 24 hours	No
Paediatrician 24 hours	Yes
Full Water Birth Service	No

Tests

Routine Triple Testing	No
Nuchal Fold Scan	No
Fetal Assessment Unit	Yes

Pain Relief

24 hour epidural	Yes
Mobile epidural	No
Pethidine injections	Yes
Water (eg bath)	Yes

Intervention Rates	%	regional average %	national average %
Epidural	39	33	33
Elective Caesarean	8	8	8
Emergency Caesarean	12	12	12
Induction	16	20	20
Forceps	4	4	4
Ventouse	5	6	7
Episiotomy	10	13	14

Bridlington · **Bridlington and District Hospital**

Bessingby Road, Bridlington
North Yorkshire
YO16 4QP
Tel: 01262 606 666
Fax: 01262 400 583

Trust: Scarborough & North East
Yorkshire Healthcare NHS Trust

Bridlington is a small midwifery led unit for low-risk women delivering about 120 births per year. Epidurals are not offered, but water, gas and air, intramuscular opiate injection are all used as methods of pain relief during labour.

If a woman needs medical assistance during labour, she will be transferred to Scarborough Hospital where there are obstetricians available.

Midwife Unit	
Number of beds	-
Births	-
Midwives	-
Home births	-
Amenity Rooms, Price	-
Obstetrician 24 hours	-
Paediatrician 24 hours	-
Full Water Birth Service	-

Tests	
Routine Triple Testing	-
Nuchal Fold Scan	-
Fetal Assessment Unit	-

Pain Relief	
24 hour epidural	-
Mobile epidural	-
Pethidine injections	-
Water (eg bath)	-

Midwife-led units are adequately equipped to care for women whose pregnancy is progressing normally without complications. As a result, intervention tends to be low in these units. Basic pain relief will be offered, but any woman requesting an epidural during the delivery will need to be transferred to the nearest consultant-led unit. A woman will also be transferred to the obstetric unit if any complications develop during the delivery.

Carlisle · **Cumberland Infirmary**

Newtown Road, Carlisle
Cumbria, CA2 7HY
Phone: 01228 523444
Fax: 01228 591889

Trust: Carlisle Hospitals
NHS Trust

This unit has a relaxed home-from-home environment; the rooms are en-suite and are equipped with reclining chairs and sofa beds. Water birth is also available although there is a charge for birthing pool hire. As with many other large consultant units, the first time you meet the midwife who delivers your baby will probably be when you arrive at the labour ward. However you could opt for a domino delivery which should ensure better continuity of care. Epidurals for pain relief in labour are not currenlty offered although the unit plans to introduce this service in the near future. Intervention rates are not high – forceps are rarely used and the induction rate is well below average.

Consultant and Midwife Unit

Number of beds	24
Births per midwife	35
Births per bed	0.38
Home births	1%
Amenity Rooms, Price	-

Obstetrician 24 hours	Yes
Paediatrician 24 hours	Yes
Full Water Birth Service	Yes

Tests

Routine Triple Testing	Yes
Nuchal Fold Scan	No
Fetal Assessment Unit	Yes

Pain Relief

24 hour epidural	No
Mobile epidural	No
Pethidine injections	Yes
Water (eg bath)	No

Intervention Rates	%	regional average %	national average %
Epidural	-	33	33
Elective Caesarean	8	8	8
Emergency Caesarean	10	12	12
Induction	16	20	20
Forceps	1	4	4
Ventouse	6	6	7
Episiotomy	14	13	14

Cottingham · **Castle Hill Hospital**

Castle Road, Cottingham
East Yorkshire, HU16 5JQ
Phone: 01482 875875
Fax: 01482 623209

Trust: Hull and East Yorkshire Hospitals
NHS Trust

Staffing levels are relatively good in this relatively large unit with 30 births to each midwife. There is an epidural service which is widely used. Other forms of pain relief are available such as opiate injections and TENS machines. The hospital has its own pool and water births are available. Induction rates are relatively high. But the caesarean rate is average. Forceps are rarely used. The unit is strong on antenatal testing with triple testing, booking scans and anomaly scans offered to all women. In addition, nuchal translucency scans, amniocentesis and chorionic villus sampling are available to women who need them.

Consultant and Midwife Unit

Number of beds	36
Births per midwife	30
Births per bed	0.66
Home births	1%
Amenity Rooms, Price	£30
Obstetrician 24 hours	Yes
Paediatrician 24 hours	No
Full Water Birth Service	Yes

Tests

Routine Triple Testing	Yes
Nuchal Fold Scan	Yes
Fetal Assessment Unit	Yes

Pain Relief

24 hour epidural	Yes
Mobile epidural	No
Pethidine injections	Yes
Water (eg bath)	Yes

Intervention Rates	%	regional average %	national average %
Epidural	55	33	33
Elective Caesarean	7	8	8
Emergency Caesarean	12	12	12
Induction	25	20	20
Forceps	2	4	4
Ventouse	11	6	7
Episiotomy	11	13	14

Darlington · **Darlington Memorial Hospital**

Hollyhurst Road, Darlington
Co Durham, DL3 6HW
Phone: 01325 380100
Fax: 01325 743622

Trust: South Durham Healthcare
NHS Trust

This medium sized unit is well staffed. Midwifes can be contacted by telephone for advice 24hrs a day. Staff run breastfeeding support groups where mothers can get experience and support from midwives as well as benefiting from sharing their experiences with other mothers.

The unit has its own birthing pool, if you want a water birth. The caesarean rate is higher than at similar hospitals but instrumental deliveries are less frequent. Antenatal sessions include physiotherapy and special classes for water births. The triple test for Down's syndrome is not routinely offered to all women, although the double test is. If you want a nuchal fold scan, you will be referred to the regional centre at Royal Victoria Hospital.

Consultant and Midwife Unit

Number of beds	41
Births per midwife	27
Births per bed	0.38
Home births	1%
Amenity Rooms, Price	£38

Obstetrician 24 hours	Yes
Paediatrician 24 hours	No
Full Water Birth Service	Yes

Tests

Routine Triple Testing	No
Nuchal Fold Scan	Yes
Fetal Assessment Unit	No

Pain Relief

24 hour epidural	Yes
Mobile epidural	Yes
Pethidine injections	Yes
Water (eg bath)	Yes

Intervention Rates	%	regional average %	national average %
Epidural	-	33	33
Elective Caesarean	9	8	8
Emergency Caesarean	15	12	12
Induction	-	20	20
Forceps	2	4	4
Ventouse	6	6	7
Episiotomy	11	13	14

Dewsbury · **Dewsbury and District Hospital**

Halifax Road, Dewsbury
West Yorkshire, WF13 4HS
Phone: 01924 512 000
Fax: 01924 816 081

Trust: Dewsbury District
   NHS Trust

This unit is currently moving towards midwife-led care, although at the moment care is shared between midwives and consultants. The unit offers 'ultra-early' discharges within six hour of giving birth – many women would prefer to get home as fast as possible to recuperate. Full pain relief facilities include a mobile epidural service. Water birth is also offered here and the unit has its own pool.

Scans and tests are performed selectively according to factors such as genetic family history and triple-testing is not always given to women without proven clinical necessity. Women needing a nuchal fold scan for Down's screening would be referred to a unit in Leeds. The induction rate is much higher than at similar units but other intervention rates are average.

Consultant and Midwife Unit

Number of beds	52
Births per midwife	38
Births per bed	0.52
Home births	1%
Amenity Rooms, Price	£25

Obstetrician 24 hours	Yes
Paediatrician 24 hours	Yes
Full Water Birth Service	Yes

Tests

Routine Triple Testing	No
Nuchal Fold Scan	Yes
Fetal Assessment Unit	Yes

Pain Relief

24 hour epidural	Yes
Mobile epidural	Yes
Pethidine injections	Yes
Water (eg bath)	Yes

Intervention Rates	%	regional average %	national average %
Epidural	31	33	33
Elective Caesarean	7	8	8
Emergency Caesarean	12	12	12
Induction	28	20	20
Forceps	5	4	4
Ventouse	6	6	7
Episiotomy	14	13	14

Durham · **University Hospital of North Durham**

North Road, Dryburn
Co Durham, DH1 5TW
Phone: 0191 333 2333
Fax: 0191 332 2699

Trust: North Durham Healthcare
NHS Trust

Instead of a traditional labour ward, this unit is based around 16 Labour, Delivery, Recovery, Postnatal (LDRP) rooms, all of which are equipped with ensuite baths for pain management. An LDRP room offers greater privacy and comfort in labour than a traditional bed. There is a 24 hour epidural service but epidurals for pain relief in labour are used infrequently. Other intervention rates are in line with national averages. The antenatal testing on offer is more limited than at some units. Neither the triple test nor alpha-feto protein testing are routinely offered to all women, though the unit intends to start offering the double test in the near future. If you wish to have a nuchal fold scan, this will need to be arranged privately.

Consultant and Midwife Unit

Number of beds	32
Births per midwife	28
Births per bed	0.37
Home births	2%
Amenity Rooms, Price	-
Obstetrician 24 hours	Yes
Paediatrician 24 hours	Yes
Full Water Birth Service	No

Tests

Routine Triple Testing	No
Nuchal Fold Scan	No
Fetal Assessment Unit	Yes

Pain Relief

24 hour epidural	Yes
Mobile epidural	No
Pethidine injections	Yes
Water (eg bath)	Yes

Intervention Rates	%	regional average %	national average %
Epidural	27	33	33
Elective Caesarean	8	8	8
Emergency Caesarean	11	12	12
Induction	20	20	20
Forceps	3	4	4
Ventouse	7	6	7
Episiotomy	9	13	14

Gateshead · **Queen Elizabeth Hospital**

Queen Elizabeth Avenue, Sheriff Hill
Gateshead, Tyne & Wear, NE9 6SX
Phone: 0191 482 0000
Fax: 0191 491 1823

Trust: Gateshead Health
** NHS Trust**

The maternity unit provides all aspects of maternity care including day care, fetal assessment and special care baby facilities. Intervention rates are typical of a unit of this type.

With regard to antenatal testing, anomaly ultrasound scans are offered to all women, but the double test is offered in preference to the triple test. The unit does not normally allow partners to stay with women going into labour on the antenatal ward overnight but you may be able to hire an amenity room. Antenatal classes are held in the evenings and on weekdays. A major modernisation is being planned for the unit for the coming year.

Consultant and Midwife Unit

Number of beds	29
Births per midwife	29
Births per bed	0.78
Home births	2%
Amenity Rooms, Price	£50

Obstetrician 24 hours	Yes
Paediatrician 24 hours	Yes
Full Water Birth Service	No

Tests

Routine Triple Testing	No
Nuchal Fold Scan	Yes
Fetal Assessment Unit	Yes

Pain Relief

24 hour epidural	Yes
Mobile epidural	No
Pethidine injections	Yes
Water (eg bath)	Yes

Intervention Rates	%	regional average %	national average %
Epidural	-	33	33
Elective Caesarean	9	8	8
Emergency Caesarean	13	12	12
Induction	18	20	20
Forceps	3	4	4
Ventouse	7	6	7
Episiotomy	11	13	14

Guisborough · **Guisborough General Hospital**

Northgate, Guisborough
Yorkshire, TS14 6HZ
Phone: 01287 284000
Fax: 01287 610 508

Trust: Tees and North East Yorkshire NHS Trust

This is a satellite facility run by the James Cook University Hospital 12 miles away. The unit is well staffed which should help enable the unit to give you a high level of personal attention. As is the case with most midwife-led units, few interventions are carried out, although episiotomies are performed. The service's role is under review and a wider range of interventions may be practised here in future. Pain management options include baths, gas and air, and opiate injections. A spa is also planned to be fitted this year for pain relief.

Security at the unit was upgraded in 1998. Alarmed cot matresses are now fitted to all cots, making here as safe as the main unit.

Midwife Unit

Number of beds	12
Births	145
Midwives	5
Home births	0%
Amenity Rooms, Price	-

Obstetrician 24 hours	No
Paediatrician 24 hours	No
Full Water Birth Service	

Tests

Routine Triple Testing	Yes
Nuchal Fold Scan	No
Fetal Assessment Unit	No

Pain Relief

24 Hour epidural	No
Mobile epidural	No
Pethidine injections	Yes
Water (eg Bath)	Yes

Midwife-led units are adequately equipped to care for women whose pregnancy is progressing normally without complications. As a result, intervention tends to be low in these units. Basic pain relief will be offered, but any woman requesting an epidural during the delivery will need to be transferred to the nearest consultant-led unit. A woman will also be transferred to the obstetric unit if any complications develop during the delivery.

Halifax · **The Calderdale Royal Hospital**

Salterhebble
Halifax, HX3 0PW
Phone: 01422 357 171
Fax: 01422 380 357

Trust: Calderdale Healthcare
NHS Trust

The consultant and midwife maternity unit at Calderdale Royal Hospital is newly built and abandons the traditional labour ward for ten Labour Delivery Recovery Postnatal (LDRP) rooms. These ensuite single rooms allow for a much higher level of privacy and comfort during your labour and afterwards. Additional single and shared rooms are available for antenatal care and for those who need to stay in hospital longer than 48 hours. An additional LDRP room equipped with a birthing pool is available for water birth.

There is an infant-feeding advisor in the hospital and all staff have received further training in supporting and enabling breastfeeding. Intervention rates are broadly in line with other large hospitals.

Consultant and Midwife Unit

Number of beds	33
Births per midwife	34
Births per bed	0.36
Home births	2%
Amenity Rooms, Price	-
Obstetrician 24 hours	Yes
Paediatrician 24 hours	Yes
Full Water Birth Service	Yes

Tests

Routine Triple Testing	Yes
Nuchal Fold Scan	No
Fetal Assessment Unit	Yes

Pain Relief

24 hour epidural	Yes
Mobile epidural	Yes
Pethidine injections	Yes
Water (eg bath)	Yes

Intervention Rates	%	regional average %	national average %
Epidural	37	33	33
Elective Caesarean	9	8	8
Emergency Caesarean	13	12	12
Induction	22	20	20
Forceps	5	4	4
Ventouse	5	6	7
Episiotomy	14	13	14

The Calderdale Royal Hospital (Midwife Unit)

Salterhebble
Halifax, HX3 0PW
Phone: 01422 357171
Fax: 01422 380357

Trust: Calderdale and Huddersfield NHS
Trust

Like the shared midwife and consultant unit at the same hospital, the Calderdale Royal Hospital midwife-led unit, which was completed in April 2001, is based around Ladour Delivery Recovery Postnatal (LDRP) single room accomodation. The LDRP rooms offer greater privacy and a more homely environment than a traditional labour ward. The unit aims to provide low-tech care to low-risk women, and its midwives also manage a siginficant number of home births. Because of this, you will not necessarily be offered antenatal tests such as a booking ultrasound scan.

Antenatal education sessions are held on weekdays, in the evenings and at weekends.

Midwife Unit

Number of beds	6
Births	128
Midwives	4
Home births	-
Amenity Rooms, Price	-

Obstetrician 24 hours	Yes
Paediatrician 24 hours	Yes
Full Water Birth Service	Yes

Tests

Routine Triple Testing	Yes
Nuchal Fold Scan	No
Fetal Assessment Unit	Yes

Pain Relief

24 Hour epidural	No
Mobile epidural	No
Pethidine injections	Yes
Water (eg Bath)	Yes

Midwife-led units are adequately equipped to care for women whose pregnancy is progressing normally without complications. As a result, intervention tends to be low in these units. Basic pain relief will be offered, but any woman requesting an epidural during the delivery will need to be transferred to the nearest consultant-led unit. A woman will also be transferred to the obstetric unit if any complications develop during the delivery.

Harrogate · **Harrogate District Hospital**

Lancaster Park Road
Harrogate, HG2 7SX
Phone: 01423 885 959
Fax: 01423 555 353

Trust: Harrogate Health Care
NHS Trust

The maternity unit at Harrogate General Hospital delivers about 1500 babies a year with shared midwife and consultant care. It has a greater tendency to intervene than many similar units with a high rate of caesarean delivery – particularly emergency caesareans – and an above average use of induction. There is an epidural service plus a range of other pain management options are including TENS machines and water. There is a full water birth service and home births are done, though not very often. Although the domino system is not available, rapid discharge after delivery can be arranged. Continuity of care is a little above average with one third of women are familiar with the midwife caring for them in labour.

Consultant and Midwife Unit

Number of beds	30
Births per midwife	34
Births per bed	0.61
Home births	1%
Amenity Rooms, Price	£35

Obstetrician 24 hours	Yes
Paediatrician 24 hours	Yes
Full Water Birth Service	Yes

Tests

Routine Triple Testing	No
Nuchal Fold Scan	Yes
Fetal Assessment Unit	No

Pain Relief

24 hour epidural	Yes
Mobile epidural	No
Pethidine injections	Yes
Water (eg bath)	Yes

Intervention Rates	%	regional average %	national average %
Epidural	36	33	33
Elective Caesarean	8	8	8
Emergency Caesarean	17	12	12
Induction	24	20	20
Forceps	6	4	4
Ventouse	5	6	7
Episiotomy	20	13	14

Hartlepool · **University Hospital of Hartlepool**

Holdforth Road
Hartlepool, TS24 9AH
Phone: 01429 266654
Fax: 01429 235389

Trust: North Tees and Hartlepool
NHS Trust

This unit has been developing antenatal care services for women with low-risk pregnancies based in the community, in preference to hospital based services. Intervention rates are in line with national averages except for the forceps rate which is unusually low. The relatively low total epidural disguises the fact that the rate for epidurals used for pain relief in labour is average.

Antenatal classes are typically offered on weekday evenings, but this is flexible – classes and even one-to-one sessions can be organised at weekends or during working hours. Continuity of care is better than many units with one in five women knowing the midwife who looks after them in labour. Domino deliveries are also available.

Consultant and Midwife Unit

Number of beds	26
Births per midwife	28
Births per bed	0.73
Home births	0.3%
Amenity Rooms, Price	£17

Obstetrician 24 hours	Yes
Paediatrician 24 hours	Yes
Full Water Birth Service	No

Tests

Routine Triple Testing	No
Nuchal Fold Scan	Yes
Fetal Assessment Unit	Yes

Pain Relief

24 hour epidural	Yes
Mobile epidural	No
Pethidine injections	Yes
Water (eg bath)	Yes

Intervention Rates

	%	regional average %	national average %
Epidural	35	33	33
Elective Caesarean	8	8	8
Emergency Caesarean	12	12	12
Induction	20	20	20
Forceps	2	4	4
Ventouse	5	6	7
Episiotomy	7	13	14

Hexham · **Hexham General Hospital**

Corbridge Road, Hexham
Northumberland, NE46 1QJ
Phone: 01434 655655
Fax: 01434 655613

Trust: Northumbria Healthcare
NHS Trust

The Hexham General Hospital maternity unit is small for a shared consultant and midwife facility. The pattern of intervention is unusual with elective caesareans taking place more often than emergency caesareans. The induction rate is above average. And forceps are used more frequently than the ventouse for instrumental deliveries. Staffing levels are good for a unit of this size as is continuity of care. Almost two thirds of women are cared for in labour by a midwife they know. Domino system deliveries are also an option. The 'triple test', early pregnancy ultrasound scans and anomaly ultrasound scans are offered to all women booked with the service, and risk groups can be referred to the Royal Victoria Infirmary for amniocentesis or chorionic villus sampling.

Consultant and Midwife Unit

Number of beds	16
Births per midwife	24
Births per bed	0.36
Home births	0.15%
Amenity Rooms, Price	£23

Obstetrician 24 hours	No
Paediatrician 24 hours	No
Full Water Birth Service	No

Tests

Routine Triple Testing	Yes
Nuchal Fold Scan	Yes
Fetal Assessment Unit	Yes

Pain Relief

24 hour epidural	Yes
Mobile epidural	No
Pethidine injections	Yes
Water (eg bath)	Yes

Intervention Rates	%	regional average %	national average %
Epidural	40	33	33
Elective Caesarean	11	8	8
Emergency Caesarean	10	12	12
Induction	23	20	20
Forceps	6	4	4
Ventouse	5	6	7
Episiotomy	11	13	14

Huddersfield · **Huddersfield Royal Infirmary**

Acre Street, Lindley, Huddersfield
Yorkshire, HD3 3EA
Phone: 01484 342000
Fax: 01484 482888

Trust: Huddersfield Healthcare Services
NHS Trust

The infirmary is a district general unit, where women can choose between consultant-led, shared community and hospital care, GP-led and midwifery-led care. The delivery suite has seven rooms including a home from home room and a birthing pool. There is a 24-hour obstetric theatre in the delivery suite. Community midwives are available for women who choose a home birth. Several midwives are qualified to give aromatherapy and massage to mothers and babies. Alternatively, epidurals are used very widely so there should be no problem getting this form of pain relief if you want it. Partners are welcome to stay if you have to go into the unit before labour has started. Support services are organised for for diabetic mothers, women subject to abuse and those suffering postnatal depression.

Consultant and Midwife Unit

Number of beds	31
Births per midwife	33.25
Births per bed	0.92
Home births	2%
Amenity Rooms, Price	£25

Obstetrician 24 hours	Yes
Paediatrician 24 hours	Yes
Full Water Birth Service	Yes

Tests

Routine Triple Testing	Yes
Nuchal Fold Scan	No
Fetal Assessment Unit	No

Pain Relief

24 hour epidural	Yes
Mobile epidural	No
Pethidine injections	Yes
Water (eg bath)	Yes

Intervention Rates	%	regional average %	national average %
Epidural	31	33	33
Elective Caesarean	8	8	8
Emergency Caesarean	11	12	12
Induction	14	20	20
Forceps	2	4	4
Ventouse	8	6	7
Episiotomy	-	13	14

Hull · **Hull Maternity Hospital**

Hedon Road, Hull
North Humberside, HU9 5LX
Phone: 01482 376215
Fax: 01482 374542

Trust: Hull and East Yorkshire Hospitals
NHS Trust

This large consultant and midwife-led unit has an unusually high use of epidurals for pain relief. Other options for pain management include gas and air, opiate injections, and TENS machines. There is no pool in the unit but water births can be done as home births if you hire your own pool. Also, amenity rooms in the unit can be made available but this is negotiated on an individual basis.

Antenatal tests are made available to everyone with routine ultrasound scans and triple testing. Nuchal fold scans can also be arranged as can amniocentesis and CVS.

The caesarean rate is broadly in line with the national average, although emergency caesareans are more frequent. Instrumental deliveries are relatively rare but unusually, forceps are used more often than ventouse.

Consultant and Midwife Unit

Number of beds	63
Births per midwife	27
Births per bed	0.44
Home births	1%
Amenity Rooms, Price	-
Obstetrician 24 hours	Yes
Paediatrician 24 hours	Yes
Full Water Birth Service	No

Tests

Routine Triple Testing	Yes
Nuchal Fold Scan	Yes
Fetal Assessment Unit	Yes

Pain Relief

24 hour epidural	Yes
Mobile epidural	No
Pethidine injections	Yes
Water (eg bath)	Yes

Intervention Rates	%	regional average %	national average %
Epidural	53	33	33
Elective Caesarean	8	8	8
Emergency Caesarean	14	12	12
Induction	15	20	20
Forceps	3	4	4
Ventouse	2	6	7
Episiotomy	13	13	14

Keighley · **Airedale General Hospital**

Skipton Road, Steeton, Keighley
West Yorkshire, BD20 6TD
Phone: 01535 652 511
Fax: 01535 655 129

Trust: Airedale
NHS Trust

The maternity unit at Airedale General Hospital has good midwife staffing levels with only twenty two births per midwife per year. Continuity of care, however, is not good, with only about one percent of women being looked after in labour by a midwife they know. Intervention rates are in line with national averages although elective caesareans take place a little more often than at most units of this type. The unit does not routinely offer either alpha feto protein testing or the 'triple test' to all women. However, nuchal fold translucency scans are available to those in risk groups. There is a water birth service, and staff are trained in delivering babies in water. However demand for this has not been great so midwives might need to refresh their skills.

Consultant and Midwife Unit

Number of beds	32
Births per midwife	22
Births per bed	0.78
Home births	1%
Amenity Rooms, Price	£40

Obstetrician 24 hours	Yes
Paediatrician 24 hours	No
Full Water Birth Service	Yes

Tests

Routine Triple Testing	No
Nuchal Fold Scan	Yes
Fetal Assessment Unit	Yes

Pain Relief

24 hour epidural	Yes
Mobile epidural	No
Pethidine injections	Yes
Water (eg bath)	Yes

Intervention Rates	%	regional average %	national average %
Epidural	34	33	33
Elective Caesarean	10	8	8
Emergency Caesarean	12	12	12
Induction	23	20	20
Forceps	3	4	4
Ventouse	4	6	7
Episiotomy	17	13	14

Leeds · **Leeds General Infirmary**

Great George Street, Leeds
West Yorkshire, LS1 3EX
Phone: 0113 243 2799
Fax: 0113 392 6336

Trust: Leeds Teaching Hospitals
NHS Trust

The unit aims to provide care, as much as possible, in the community so that no more than three hospital visits should be necessary throughout the course of each pregnancy unless complications arise. You may have midwife-led care if your pregnancy and labour is straightforward.

The unit is very busy with more than one birth per delivery bed per day. Furthermore, midwives will have their hands full, as there is only one midwife per forty births per year. The caesarean rate overall is average but elective operations happen more often than emergency procedures suggesting that the unit is more prepared than other units to book women in for the operation.

Consultant and Midwife Unit

Number of beds	54
Births per midwife	40
Births per bed	1.15
Home births	-
Amenity Rooms, Price	£60

Obstetrician 24 hours	Yes
Paediatrician 24 hours	Yes
Full Water Birth Service	Yes

Tests

Routine Triple Testing	No
Nuchal Fold Scan	Yes
Fetal Assessment Unit	Yes

Pain Relief

24 hour epidural	Yes
Mobile epidural	Yes
Pethidine injections	Yes
Water (eg bath)	Yes

Intervention Rates

	%	regional average %	national average %
Epidural	46	33	33
Elective Caesarean	11	8	8
Emergency Caesarean	9	12	12
Induction	18	20	20
Forceps	6	4	4
Ventouse	4	6	7
Episiotomy	10	13	14

Leeds · St James's University Hospital

Beckett Street, Leeds
West Yorkshire, LS9 7TF
Phone: 0113 243 3144
Fax: 0113 242 6496

Trust: Leeds Teaching Hospitals
 NHS Trust

The St James's University Hospital maternity service has rates for elective caesarean sections and epidural anaesthesia that are among the highest in the country. Almost half of the women who deliver at the unit do so under an epidural. However for women with uncomplicated pregnancies who wish to give birth naturally, midwife-led care is available including domino deliveries. Also alternative approaches to pain management are encouraged including beanbags, mats and cushions for alternative positions, baths, and TENS machines. Unusually for such a large unit, almost a third of women have met the midwife who looks after them through their labour during their pregnancy. Home births are managed by a separate service for the whole of Leeds.

Consultant and Midwife Unit

Number of beds	54
Births per midwife	35
Births per bed	0.83
Home births	-
Amenity Rooms, Price	£60

Obstetrician 24 hours	Yes
Paediatrician 24 hours	Yes
Full Water Birth Service	No

Tests

Routine Triple Testing	No
Nuchal Fold Scan	Yes
Fetal Assessment Unit	Yes

Pain Relief

24 hour epidural	Yes
Mobile epidural	Yes
Pethidine injections	Yes
Water (eg bath)	Yes

Intervention Rates	%	regional average %	national average %
Epidural	48	33	33
Elective Caesarean	13	8	8
Emergency Caesarean	10	12	12
Induction	20	20	20
Forceps	5	4	4
Ventouse	4	6	7
Episiotomy	15	13	14

Leeds · James Cook University Hospital

Marton Rd
Middlesbrough, TS4 3BW
Phone: 01642 850850

Trust: South Tees Hospitals
NHS Trust

This purpose-built maternity unit at James Cook University Hospital has been open for 12 years, and offers a combined consultant and midwife-led service. The elective caesarean rate is much higher than at most hospitals – but this may be one factor that has helped keep the emergency caesarean rate below average.

A full range of antenatal scans and tests is available, though patients requiring nuchal fold tests attend the Royal Victoria Infirmary. Pain management options include aromatherapy and a TENS machine as well as epidurals. More than half of women who deliver at the unit do so without intervention. Water birth facilities are offered and midwives who are trained in water birth deliveries are available around the clock.

Consultant and Midwife Unit

Number of beds	50
Births per midwife	25
Births per bed	1.02
Home births	-
Amenity Rooms, Price	£35
Obstetrician 24 hours	No
Paediatrician 24 hours	Yes
Full Water Birth Service	Yes

Tests

Routine Triple Testing	Yes
Nuchal Fold Scan	Yes
Fetal Assessment Unit	Yes

Pain Relief

24 hour epidural	Yes
Mobile epidural	Yes
Pethidine injections	Yes
Water (eg bath)	Yes

Intervention Rates

	%	regional average %	national average %
Epidural	42	33	33
Elective Caesarean	14	8	8
Emergency Caesarean	10	12	12
Induction	23	20	20
Forceps	3	4	4
Ventouse	9	6	7
Episiotomy	9	13	14

Malton · **Malton Norton & District Hospital**

Middlecave Road, Malton
North Yorkshire, YO17 7NG
Phone: 01653 693 041
Fax: 01653 600 589

Trust: Scarborough & North East
Yorkshire Healthcare NHS Trust

This relatively small, midwife-led unit delivered 98 births last year, and as with most low-tech units, intervention is kept to a minimum. The atmosphere is friendly and women can usually be accommodated without charge in the unit's side rooms.

The unit offers water births in their own pool and midwives trained in such deliveries are available 24 hours a day. Home births are popular here, and midwives also offer domino deliveries. Most scans can be done, although booking ultrasounds are not offered routinely. If you want a nuchal fold scan you will be referred to Leeds, where they will do this for a fee unless there is considered to be a clinical necessity.

Midwife Unit

Number of beds	8
Births	98
Midwives	10
Home births	3%
Amenity Rooms, Price	-

Obstetrician 24 hours	No
Paediatrician 24 hours	No
Full Water Birth Service	Yes

Tests

Routine Triple Testing	Yes
Nuchal Fold Scan	No
Fetal Assessment Unit	Yes

Pain Relief

24 Hour epidural	No
Mobile epidural	No
Pethidine injections	Yes
Water (eg Bath)	Yes

Midwife-led units are adequately equipped to care for women whose pregnancy is progressing normally without complications. As a result, intervention tends to be low in these units. Basic pain relief will be offered, but any woman requesting an epidural during the delivery will need to be transferred to the nearest consultant-led unit. A woman will also be transferred to the obstetric unit if any complications develop during the delivery.

Newcastle upon Tyne · **Royal Victoria Infirmary**

Queen Victoria Road
Newcastle Upon Tyne, NE1 4LP
Phone: 0191 232 5131
Fax: 0191 201 0155

Trust: The Newcastle upon Tyne
   Hospitals NHS Trust

As a regional referral centre for fetal medicine, the Royal Victoria Infirmary deals with many higher risk pregnancies. The hospital is a centre of excellence in performing amniocentesis and chorionic villus sampling, the most reliable diagnostic tests for a number of common developmental abnormalities. Maternal blood tests such as the 'triple test' are not routinely performed for all women, but nuchal fold scanning is available to those considered at risk.

The frequent use of instrumental deliveries- and in particular forceps which are used twice as often as in similar hospitals – is unusual. In contrast, the rate of caesarean deliveries is below average.

Consultant and Midwife Unit

Number of beds	85
Births per midwife	34
Births per bed	0.92
Home births	0.4%
Amenity Rooms, Price	£52

Obstetrician 24 hours	Yes
Paediatrician 24 hours	Yes
Full Water Birth Service	No

Tests

Routine Triple Testing	No
Nuchal Fold Scan	Yes
Fetal Assessment Unit	Yes

Pain Relief

24 hour epidural	Yes
Mobile epidural	No
Pethidine injections	Yes
Water (eg bath)	Yes

Intervention Rates	%	regional average %	national average %
Epidural	36	33	33
Elective Caesarean	7	8	8
Emergency Caesarean	11	12	12
Induction	-	20	20
Forceps	8	0	4
Ventouse	11	6	7
Episiotomy	20	13	14

North Shields · **North Tyneside General Hospital**

Rake Lane, North Shields
Tyne and Wear, NE29 8NH
Phone: 0191 259 6660
Fax: 0191 293 2745

Trust: Northumbria Healthcare
  NHS Trust

The maternity service at North Tyneside delivers around 2000 babies each year. Like other hospitals in Newcastle, the rate of instrumental deliveries is surprisingly high and in particular, forceps are used much more often than in other hospitals. In contrast, very few people have epidurals for pain relief in labour although there is a 24-hour epidural service.

Water births can be supervised if you have one at home. Domino deliveries are offered and home births are also an option although they are relatively infrequent here. Support is provided for women who miscarry and for pregnancies with fetal abnormalities.

Consultant and Midwife Unit

Number of beds	52
Births per midwife	22
Births per bed	0.77
Home births	1%
Amenity Rooms, Price	£23

Obstetrician 24 hours	Yes
Paediatrician 24 hours	Yes
Full Water Birth Service	No

Tests

Routine Triple Testing	Yes
Nuchal Fold Scan	Yes
Fetal Assessment Unit	Yes

Pain Relief

24 hour epidural	Yes
Mobile epidural	No
Pethidine injections	Yes
Water (eg bath)	Yes

Intervention Rates	%	regional average %	national average %
Epidural	19	33	33
Elective Caesarean	7	8	8
Emergency Caesarean	13	12	12
Induction	20	20	20
Forceps	11	4	4
Ventouse	12	6	7
Episiotomy	16	13	14

Northallerton · **Friarage Hospital**

Northallerton
North Yorkshire, DL6 1JG
Phone: 01609 779911
Fax: 01609 777144

Trust: Northallerton Health Services
NHS Trust

Most care at this unit is delivered by midwives, both in the community and in the hospital, except for high-risk women who are cared for by obstetricians. The unit takes a more non-interventionist approach than many other hospitals. The caesarean rate is low and in particular, the rate of elective caesareans is among the lowest in the country.

Epidurals are also used relatively infrequently althoughthe induction rate is above average. Antenatal screening services are more limited than at many hospitals. There is a consultant who specializes in this area, and women are rarely referred elsewhere for this sort of care. Home births are offered but the home birth rate is well below the national average.

Consultant and Midwife Unit

Number of beds	31
Births per midwife	29
Births per bed	0.68
Home births	1%
Amenity Rooms, Price	£30
Obstetrician 24 hours	Yes
Paediatrician 24 hours	No
Full Water Birth Service	Yes

Tests

Routine Triple Testing	No
Nuchal Fold Scan	Yes
Fetal Assessment Unit	No

Pain Relief

24 hour epidural	Yes
Mobile epidural	No
Pethidine injections	Yes
Water (eg bath)	Yes

Intervention Rates	%	regional average %	national average %
Epidural	19	33	33
Elective Caesarean	5	8	8
Emergency Caesarean	11	12	12
Induction	23	20	20
Forceps	4	4	4
Ventouse	7	6	7
Episiotomy	22	13	14

Penrith · **Penrith Hospital**

Bridge Lane, Penrith
Cumbria, CA11 8HY
Phone: 01768 245300
Fax: 01768 245302

Trust: North Cumbria Acute hospitals
NHS Trust

The Penrith Hospital maternity service is a good choice if you are considering home birth, as this option is actively promoted providing you are at low-risk of complications during labour. Women giving birth at the unit are admitted to a two-bedded labour ward, but single rooms are available for hire. Over half of women using the service are cared for in labour by a midwife they know. Water birth is available if you supply your own pool. However, the unit is planning to have its own pool in the near future. Consistent with its low-tech approach, antenatal testing for women is limited. Neither early pregnancy nor anomaly ultrasound scans are routinely carried out. Double testing is offered rather than triple testing.

Midwife Unit

Number of beds	9
Midwives	35
Births	0.26
Home births	-
Amenity Rooms, Price	£35

Obstetrician 24 hours	No
Paediatrician 24 hours	No
Full Water Birth Service	No

Tests

Routine Triple Testing	No
Nuchal Fold Scan	Yes
Fetal Assessment Unit	No

Pain Relief

24 Hour epidural	No
Mobile epidural	No
Pethidine injections	Yes
Water (eg Bath)	Yes

Midwife-led units are adequately equipped to care for women whose pregnancy is progressing normally without complications. As a result, intervention tends to be low in these units. Basic pain relief will be offered, but any woman requesting an epidural during the delivery will need to be transferred to the nearest consultant-led unit. A woman will also be transferred to the obstetric unit if any complications develop during the delivery.

Pontefract · **Pontefract General Infirmary**

Friarwood Lane, Pontefract
West Yorkshire, WF8 1PL
Phone: 01977 600 600
Fax: 01977 606 852

Trust: Pinderfields & Pontefract
 Hospitals NHS Trust

Pontefract General Infirmary will incorporate the services of Pinderfields' maternity unit in February 2002. Pontefract is a good place to have your baby if you want familiar faces around you throughout your hospital stay. Unusually for a large, shared midwife and consultant unit, a partner or friend would typically be allowed to stay with you if you were beginning labour on the antenatal ward overnight. The unit operates team midwifery, in which you are allocated a group of 6-8 midwives. Your team provides you with all care throughout your pregnancy, from booking right through to delivery. The vast majority of women giving birth at the unit are cared for by a midwife they know. Intervention rates in the unit are slightly lower than average although inductions are more frequent.

Consultant and Midwife Unit

Number of beds	37
Births per midwife	28
Births per bed	0.44
Home births	2%
Amenity Rooms, Price	£39

Obstetrician 24 hours	No
Paediatrician 24 hours	Yes
Full Water Birth Service	No

Tests

Routine Triple Testing	No
Nuchal Fold Scan	No
Fetal Assessment Unit	Yes

Pain Relief

24 hour epidural	Yes
Mobile epidural	No
Pethidine injections	Yes
Water (eg bath)	Yes

Intervention Rates	%	regional average %	national average %
Epidural	28	33	33
Elective Caesarean	8	8	8
Emergency Caesarean	11	12	12
Induction	24	20	20
Forceps	3	4	4
Ventouse	5	6	7
Episiotomy	15	13	14

Scarborough · **Scarborough General Hospital**

Woodlands Drive, Scarborough
North Yorkshire, YO12 6QL
Phone: 01723 368 111
Fax: 01723 377 223

Trust: Scarborough & North East
Yorkshire Healthcare NHS Trust

Women are given a named midwife upon booking, who provides the majority of their care. Home births and domino deliveries are also options. Intervention rates are relatively high with an above average elective caesarean rate and one in four women being induced. Antenatal testing services are more restricted. Triple testing is not routinely offered and nuchal fold scans are not available. Facilities for water births are provided, though midwives trained in water births are not always available. There is a Special Care Baby Unit, which has facilities for 10 babies.

An active breastfeeding support group seeks to address the low rates of breastfeeding locally.

Consultant and Midwife Unit

Number of beds	26
Births per midwife	29
Births per bed	0.73
Home births	1%
Amenity Rooms, Price	-
Obstetrician 24 hours	No
Paediatrician 24 hours	No
Full Water Birth Service	No

Tests

Routine Triple Testing	No
Nuchal Fold Scan	No
Fetal Assessment Unit	No

Pain Relief

24 hour epidural	Yes
Mobile epidural	No
Pethidine injections	Yes
Water (eg bath)	Yes

Intervention Rates	%	regional average %	national average %
Epidural	-	33	33
Elective Caesarean	10	8	8
Emergency Caesarean	13	12	12
Induction	25	20	20
Forceps	3	4	4
Ventouse	5	6	7
Episiotomy	12	13	14

South Sheilds · **South Tyneside District Hospital**

Harton Lane, South Shields
Tyne & Wear, NE34 0PL
Phone: 0191 454 8888
Fax: 0191 202 4180

Trust: South Tyneside Health Care
NHS Trust

Although the overall epidural rate is inline with other similar hospital, the availability of epidurals for pain relief in labour is relatively limited with only about one in ten women using this form of pain management. The unit warns that epidurals cannot be guaranteed because anaesthetists are sometimes required for emergencies. The caesarean rate is above average with more frequent use of elective caesareans. Antenatal classes are held in the evenings and at weekends as well as during the week, and groups are organised for ethnic minorities, teenage mothers, and those expecting twins. Midwives also liaise with local schools providing input into sex education programmes.

Consultant and Midwife Unit

Number of beds	35
Births per midwife	26
Births per bed	0.40
Home births	1%
Amenity Rooms, Price	£21

Obstetrician 24 hours	Yes
Paediatrician 24 hours	Yes
Full Water Birth Service	No

Tests

Routine Triple Testing	No
Nuchal Fold Scan	Yes
Fetal Assessment Unit	Yes

Pain Relief

24 hour epidural	Yes
Mobile epidural	No
Pethidine injections	Yes
Water (eg bath)	Yes

Intervention Rates	%	regional average %	national average %
Epidural	34	33	33
Elective Caesarean	10	8	8
Emergency Caesarean	14	12	12
Induction	19	20	20
Forceps	5	4	4
Ventouse	6	6	7
Episiotomy	14	13	14

Hardwick, Stockton-on-Tees
Cleveland, TS19 8PE
Phone: 01642 617617
Fax: 01642 624089

Trust: North Tees and Hartlepool
NHS Trust

The unit offers both midwife-led care for low-risk pregnancies, and shared consultant care for those with high-risk pregnancies. Home births and water births are available for women who are not considered to be at risk of complications during labour.

Intervention rates are average and epidurals are easily available, with a higher than average take-up. A fetal day assessment unit has recently been opened where women with complicated pregnancies can be admitted for the day and undergo investigations and surveillance of their pregnancy.

The unit's team of midwives work in the hospital and in the community and are available to offer support and advice 24hrs a day. This service extends to the postnatal period and is available up until the baby is 28 days old.

Consultant and Midwife Unit

Number of beds	40
Births per midwife	26
Births per bed	0.51
Home births	1%
Amenity Rooms, Price	£17

Obstetrician 24 hours	Yes
Paediatrician 24 hours	Yes
Full Water Birth Service	Yes

Tests

Routine Triple Testing	No
Nuchal Fold Scan	Yes
Fetal Assessment Unit	Yes

Pain Relief

24 hour epidural	Yes
Mobile epidural	No
Pethidine injections	Yes
Water (eg bath)	Yes

Intervention Rates	%	regional average %	national average %
Epidural	37	33	33
Elective Caesarean	6	8	8
Emergency Caesarean	10	12	12
Induction	18	20	20
Forceps	4	4	4
Ventouse	7	6	7
Episiotomy	-	13	14

Kayll Road, Sunderland
Tyne & Wear, SR4 7TP
Phone: 0191 565 6256
Fax: 0191 514 0220

Trust: City Hospitals Sunderland
    NHS Trust

Sunderland Royal Hospital's maternity unit is not based around a traditional labour ward. Instead, at the onset of labour, you would be admitted to one of twenty two dedicated Labour Delivery Recovery Postnatal (LDRP) rooms, where you would stay until transferred home, usually within 24 hours. This avoids the need to transfer you to a postnatal ward after delivery. Mobile epidurals and patient controlled epidurals are available, allowing more control over the level of pain relief. The antenatal screening service is less comprehensive. Alpha feto protein testing, the triple test and nuchal fold scanning are not routinely offered to all women. Intervention rates are below average with relatively few elective caesareans and infrequent use of induction.

Consultant and Midwife Unit

Number of beds	41
Births per midwife	27.6
Births per bed	0.37
Home births	1%
Amenity Rooms, Price	-

Obstetrician 24 hours	Yes
Paediatrician 24 hours	Yes
Full Water Birth Service	No

Tests

Routine Triple Testing	No
Nuchal Fold Scan	No
Fetal Assessment Unit	Yes

Pain Relief

24 hour epidural	Yes
Mobile epidural	Yes
Pethidine injections	Yes
Water (eg bath)	Yes

Intervention Rates	%	regional average %	national average %
Epidural	35	33	33
Elective Caesarean	6	8	8
Emergency Caesarean	12	12	12
Induction	11	20	20
Forceps	5	4	4
Ventouse	6	6	7
Episiotomy	13	13	14

Wakefield · **Pinderfields General Hospital**

Aberford Road, Wakefield
Yorkshire, WF1 4DG
Phone: 01924 201 688
Fax: 01924 814 864

Trust: Pinderfields & Pontefract
   Hospitals NHS Trust

The services at Pinderfields will be moving to Pontefract in February 2002. Inpatient services and hospital deliveries at Pinderfields are carried out by hospital-based midwives. Community-based midwives provide antenatal and postnatal care in GP practices, health centres and in women's homes. Continuity of care is in a little better than most large hospitals, with about one third of women having their baby delivered by a midwife they know. There is a birthing pool at this unit, although there may not always be a midwife trained in water birth deliveries available to supervise.

Triple-testing is only offered to women over 30 or those with a previous history of problems, although it is available on request.

Consultant and Midwife Unit

Number of beds	42
Births per midwife	28
Births per bed	0.70
Home births	1%
Amenity Rooms, Price	£39

Obstetrician 24 hours	No
Paediatrician 24 hours	Yes
Full Water Birth Service	No

Tests

Routine Triple Testing	No
Nuchal Fold Scan	No
Fetal Assessment Unit	Yes

Pain Relief

24 hour epidural	Yes
Mobile epidural	No
Pethidine injections	Yes
Water (eg bath)	Yes

Intervention Rates	%	regional average %	national average %
Epidural	25	33	33
Elective Caesarean	7	8	8
Emergency Caesarean	11	12	12
Induction	24	20	20
Forceps	5	4	4
Ventouse	7	6	7
Episiotomy	18	13	14

Whitby · **Whitby Hospital**

North Yorkshire
YO21 1EE
Phone: 01947 604 851
Fax: 01947 820 568

Trust: Scarborough & North East
Yorkshire Healthcare NHS Trust

This maternity facility is relatively small, with 6 beds and can deliver you either in the unit or in your home. The unit does not offer epidurals, but women can use water, gas and air, opiate injections and TENS machines to aid with pain relief. A water birth facility is being installed, and will be available soon.

Triple testing is only routinely offered to women over 35. Nuchal fold scans are only carried out if medically necessary, although they are available privately.

Support services include antenatal and postnatal helplines, along with a breastfeeding helpline and counsellors. Facilities for partners to stay are available.

Midwife Unit

Number of beds	6
Births per midwife	7
Births per bed	0.10
Home births	8%
Amenity Rooms, Price	-

Obstetrician 24 hours	No
Paediatrician 24 hours	No
Full Water Birth Service	No

Tests	
Routine Triple Testing	No
Nuchal Fold Scan	Yes
Fetal Assessment Unit	No

Pain Relief	
24 hour epidural	No
Mobile epidural	No
Pethidine injections	Yes
Water (eg bath)	Yes

Midwife-led units are adequately equipped to care for women whose pregnancy is progressing normally without complications. As a result, intervention tends to be low in these units. Basic pain relief will be offered, but any woman requesting an epidural during the delivery will need to be transferred to the nearest consultant-led unit. A woman will also be transferred to the obstetric unit if any complications develop during the delivery.

Whitehaven · **West Cumberland Hospital**

Hensingham, Whitehaven
Cumbria, CA28 8JG
Phone: 01946 693181
Fax: 01946 523513

Trust: West Cumbria Healthcare
NHS Trust

The majority of women are put under the care of a particular midwife. they can choose to give birth at home, at hospital or in water. Domino deliveries are also an option.

Wome with more complicated pregnancies are referred to a consultant obstetrician. Consultant clinics are provided in the towns of Millorn, Workington, Maryport and Cockermouth.

Induction rates here are very high with close to one in three women being induced – nearly twice the rate in the nearby Cumberland Infirmary. Rates for caesarean and instrumental delivery are average.

Parent education classes include aquanatal sessions, postnatal groups and special classes for teenagers.

Consultant and Midwife Unit

Number of beds	25
Births per midwife	22.53
Births per bed	0.57
Home births	2%
Amenity Rooms, Price	£25

Obstetrician 24 hours	Yes
Paediatrician 24 hours	Yes
Full Water Birth Service	Yes

Tests

Routine Triple Testing	No
Nuchal Fold Scan	Yes
Fetal Assessment Unit	Yes

Pain Relief

24 hour epidural	Yes
Mobile epidural	No
Pethidine injections	Yes
Water (eg bath)	Yes

Intervention Rates

	%	regional average %	national average %
Epidural	-	33	33
Elective Caesarean	9	8	8
Emergency Caesarean	11	12	12
Induction	31	20	20
Forceps	2	4	4
Ventouse	7	6	7
Episiotomy	6	13	14

York · **York District Hospital**

Wigginton Road, York
Yorkshire, YO31 8HE
Phone: 01904 631 313
Fax: 01904 453 468

Trust: York Health Services
    NHS Trust

York is staffed by five consultant obstetricians, a head of midwifery, two clinical midwifery managers and a team of midwives who each manage about 35 births a year. The unit offers midwife-led care for low-risk women throughout your pregnancy and birth. High-risk women will be put under the care of a consultant. Shared care between GPs and consultants is also available. The delivery suite has eleven delivery rooms, including a birthing pool and active birth room, two obstetric theatres and two high dependency rooms. There is a full pain relief service including mobile epidurals which allow greater feeling and movement.

The unit employs two specialist midwives – a breastfeeding advisor and a diabetic specialist midwife.

Consultant and Midwife Unit

Number of beds	58
Births per midwife	35
Births per bed	0.70
Home births	2%
Amenity Rooms, Price	£45

Obstetrician 24 hours	Yes
Paediatrician 24 hours	Yes
Full Water Birth Service	Yes

Tests

Routine Triple Testing	No
Nuchal Fold Scan	Yes
Fetal Assessment Unit	Yes

Pain Relief

24 hour epidural	Yes
Mobile epidural	Yes
Pethidine injections	Yes
Water (eg bath)	Yes

Intervention Rates	%	regional average %	national average %
Epidural	37	33	33
Elective Caesarean	5	8	8
Emergency Caesarean	14	12	12
Induction	20	20	20
Forceps	3	4	4
Ventouse	7	6	7
Episiotomy	15	13	14

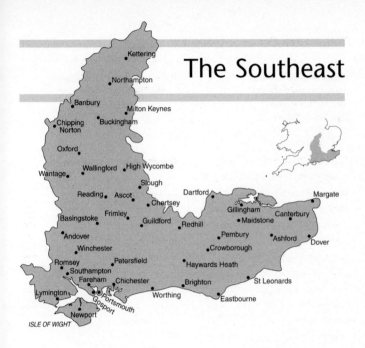

The Southeast

ISLE OF WIGHT

Andover	• Andover War Memorial Community Hospital
Ascot	• Heatherwood Hospital
Ashford	• William Harvey Hospital
Banbury	• Horton Hospital
Basingstoke	• North Hampshire Hospital
Brighton	• Royal Sussex County Hospital
Buckingham	• Stoke Mandeville Hospital
Cantebury	• Kent & Cantebury Hospital
Chertsey	• St Peter's Hospital
Chicester	• St Richard's Hospital
Chipping Norton	• Chipping Norton Community
Crowborough	• Crowborough War Memorial
Dartford	• Darent Valley Hospital
Dover	• Buckland Hospital
Eastbourne	• Eastbourne District General
Fareham	• Blackbrook House Maternity Home
Frimley	• Frimley Park Hospital
Gillingham	• Medway Maritime Hospital
Gosport	• Gosport War Memorial
Guilford	• Royal Surrey County
Haywards Heath	• Princess Royal Hospital
High Wycombe	• Wycombe Hospital
Kettering	• Kettering General Hospital
Lymington	• Lymington Hospital
Maidstone	• Maidstone Hospital
Margate	• Queen Elizabeth the Queen Mother Hospital
Milton Keynes	• Milton Keynes General Hospital
Newport IoW	• St Mary's Hospital
Northampton	• Northampton General Hospital
Oxford	• John Radcliffe Hospital
Pembury	• Pembury Hospital
Petersfield	• Petersfield Hospital
Portsmouth	• St Mary's Hospital
	• St Mary's Hospital (Midwife-led Unit)
Reading	• Royal Berkshire & Battle Hospitals
Redhill	• East Surrey & Crawley Hospitals
Romsey	• Romsey Hospital
St Leonards	• Conquest Hospital
Slough	• Wexham Park Hospital
Southampton	• Hythe Hospital
	• Princess Anne Hospital
	• Wessex Maternity Centre
Wallingford	• Wallingford Community
Wantage	• Wantage Community Hospital
Winchester	• Royal Hampshire County Hospital
Worthing	• Worthing Hospital

Andover · **War Memorial Community Hospital**

Charlton Road, Andover
Hampshire, SP10 3LB
Phone: 01264 358811
Fax: 01264 351424

Trust: Winchester and Eastleigh
Healthcare NHS Trust

Andover Birth Centre is a midwife-led unit with a small team of midwives. About half the women who give birth here are delivered by a midwife they know. This means that you will receive better continuity of care than you would at most large hospitals, although smaller midwife units often manage to ensure that pretty well everybody is looked after in labour by someone they know.

You can also come here for postnatal care after giving birth elsewhere. Alpha-feto protein testing is offered rather than triple testing. If you want a triple test you can have it done privately. Booking scans are not routinely offered.

A water birth pool was recently installed and midwives trained in water birth deliveries are available around the clock.

Midwife Unit

Number of beds	11
Births	144
Midwives	14
Home births	5%
Amenity Rooms, Price	-
Obstetrician 24 hours	No
Paediatrician 24 hours	No
Full Water Birth Service	Yes

Tests

Routine Triple Testing	No
Nuchal Fold Scan	No
Fetal Assessment Unit	No

Pain Relief

24 Hour epidural	No
Mobile epidural	No
Pethidine injections	Yes
Water (eg bath)	Yes

Midwife-led units are adequately equipped to care for women whose pregnancy is progressing normally without complications. As a result, intervention tends to be low in these units. Basic pain relief will be offered, but any woman requesting an epidural during the delivery will need to be transferred to the nearest consultant-led unit. A woman will also be transferred to the obstetric unit if any complications develop during the delivery.

Ascot · Heatherwood Hospital

London Road, Ascot
Berkshire, SL5 8AA
Phone: 01753 633 000
Fax: 01344 874 340

Trust: Heatherwood and Wexham Park
Hospitals NHS Trust

Heatherwood is an unusual maternity unit. It is midwife-led and aims to provide a low-tech home-from-home environment that encourages natural childbirth. However unlike most midwife-led units there is full medical back up with a senior obstetrician and anaesthetist on call 24 hours a day and an obstetrician on site at all times. That means that epidurals are available for pain relief and the unit is capable of dealing with emergency and caesarean deliveries. A large number of planned caesareans are conducted at the hospital and more rarely, emergency caesareans are also performed.

The unit works closely with Wexham Park which deals with more complex pregnancies and has a neonatal intensive care unit on site.

Midwife Unit

Number of beds	16
Births per midwife	32
Births per bed	0.76
Home births	3%
Amenity Rooms, Price	75

Obstetrician 24 hours	Yes
Paediatrician 24 hours	No
Full Water Birth Service	Yes

Tests

Routine Triple Testing	No
Nuchal Fold Scan	Yes
Fetal Assessment Unit	Yes

Pain Relief

24 Hour epidural	Yes
Mobile epidural	Yes
Pethidine injections	Yes
Water (eg bath)	Yes

Intervention Rates	%	regional average	national average
Epidural	35	30	33
Elective Caesarean	13	8	8
Emergency Caesarean	5	13	12
Induction	2	18	20
Forceps	1	4	4
Ventouse	6	7	7
Episiotomy	10	16	14

Ashford · **William Harvey Hospital**

Kennington Road, Willsborough
Ashford
Kent, TN24 0LZ
Phone: 01233 633331
Fax: 01233 616008

Trust: East Kent Hospitals
NHS Trust

The William Harvey Hospital maternity unit offers a shared approach to care, with high-risk women receiving consultant-led care, while midwives work in teams to care for low-risk women. The midwife teams achieve very good continuity of care and three quarters of women are delivered by a midwife they know.

Elective caesareans are performed more often than in most hospitals in contrast with the nearby Kent and Canterbury which has a much lower elective caesarean rate.

Obstetric consultants at the Willliam Harvey are very experienced in delivering breech babies vaginally. Women from the Dover area who give birth here may want to transfer to the Buckland Hospital for postnatal support in a smaller, more homely environment.

Consultant and Midwife Unit

Number of beds	41
Births per midwife	35
Births per bed	0.95
Home births	3%
Amenity Rooms, Price	£25

Obstetrician 24 hours	Yes
Paediatrician 24 hours	Yes
Full Water Birth Service	Yes

Tests

Routine Triple Testing	No
Nuchal Fold Scan	Yes
Fetal Assessment Unit	Yes

Pain Relief

24 hour epidural	Yes
Mobile epidural	No
Pethidine injections	Yes
Water (eg bath)	Yes

Intervention Rates	%	regional average	national average
Epidural	27	30	33
Elective Caesarean	10	8	8
Emergency Caesarean	11	13	12
Induction	19	18	20
Forceps	3	4	4
Ventouse	8	7	7
Episiotomy	15	16	14

Banbury · **The Horton Hospital**

Oxford Road, Banbury
Oxfordshire, OX16 9AL
Phone: 01295 275 500
Fax: 01295 229 055

Trust: Oxford Radcliffe Hospitals
NHS Trust

The unit, much of which as been recently refurbished has six delivery rooms, one with a birthing pool, a bean bag room and an obstetric theatre suite. There are 26 nursing beds, divided into four-bedded wards and single rooms, some with en suite facilities. The special care baby unit has seven cots. There is an antenatal clinic on the ground floor. There is both consultant and midwife-led care with four obstetric consultants in post.

Intervention rates – and in particular the rate of caesarean deliveries – are low for a unit of this type.

The midwives, who provide community cover for the local area, have previously had a heavy workload with over 40 births per midwife per year. However, the unit has since recruited six additional midwives.

Consultant and Midwife Unit

Number of beds	26
Births per midwife	-
Births per bed	0.66
Home births	-
Amenity Rooms, Price	-
Obstetrician 24 hours	Yes
Paediatrician 24 hours	Yes
Full Water Birth Service	Yes

Tests

Routine Triple Testing	No
Nuchal Fold Scan	Yes
Fetal Assessment Unit	No

Pain Relief

24 hour epidural	Yes
Mobile epidural	Yes
Pethidine injections	Yes
Water (eg bath)	Yes

Intervention Rates	%	regional average	national average
Epidural	30	30	33
Elective Caesarean	7	8	8
Emergency Caesarean	11	13	12
Induction	19	18	20
Forceps	5	4	4
Ventouse	7	7	7
Episiotomy	5	16	14

Basingstoke · **North Hampshire Hospital**

Aldermaston Road, Basingstoke
Hampshire, RG24 9NA
Phone: 01256 473202
Fax: 01256 313 164

Trust: North Hampshire Hospitals
    NHS Trust

Care at this maternity unit is shared between midwives and consultants. As with many hospitals in the home counties, midwife staffing levels are stretched with 43 births per year for every midwife.

The caesarean rate is slightly above the national average but the forceps rate is significantly lower than average.

Antenatal classes include weekend groups run especially for fathers, plus groups for mothers who are expecting twins.

Antenatal scanning, including booking ultrasound scans, are not routinely offered to everyone. Triple testing is available but for a charge of £19.

Women with complications in pregnancy can be referred to the fetal assessment unit in Southampton.

Consultant and Midwife Unit

Number of beds	42
ratio of midwives to births	43
Births per bed	0.86
Home births	2%
Amenity Rooms, Price	£31

Obstetrician 24 hours	Yes
Paediatrician 24 hours	Yes
Full Water Birth Service	Yes

Tests

Routine Triple Testing	No
Nuchal Fold Scan	No
Fetal Assessment Unit	No

Pain Relief

24 Hour epidural	Yes
Mobile epidural	No
Pethidine injections	Yes
Water (eg bath)	Yes

Intervention Rates	%	regional average	national average
Epidural	28	30	33
Elective Caesarean	9	8	8
Emergency Caesarean	14	13	12
Induction	17	18	20
Forceps	2	4	4
Ventouse	9	7	7
Episiotomy	15	16	14

Brighton · **Royal Sussex County Hospital**

Eastern Rd, Brighton
East Sussex, BN2 5BE
Phone: 01273 696955
Fax: 01273 664795

Trust: Brighton Health Care
NHS Trust

The maternity unit at the Royal Sussex County Hospital offers team midwifery, which helps to provide better continuity of care. The choices available for care and birth are discussed at the booking, and staff aim to be responsive to each woman's needs. A sign of this is the home birth rate which is much higher than most hospitals of this size.

The unit is extremely busy with over one delivery per labour bed per day.

The pattern of caesarean deliveries suggests women here at least try to give birth naturally. As a result, the elective caesarean rate is well below average. However, so many women end up having emergency caesareans that the overall rate is slightly higher than the national average.

Consultant and Midwife Unit

Number of beds	52
Births per midwife	37
Births per bed	1.22
Home births	8%
Amenity Rooms, Price	£50

Obstetrician 24 hours	Yes
Paediatrician 24 hours	Yes
Full Water Birth Service	Yes

Tests

Routine Triple Testing	Yes
Nuchal Fold Scan	Yes
Fetal Assessment Unit	Yes

Pain Relief

24 hour epidural	Yes
Mobile epidural	No
Pethidine injections	Yes
Water (eg bath)	Yes

Intervention Rates

	%	regional average	national average
Epidural	16	30	33
Elective Caesarean	6	8	8
Emergency Caesarean	17	13	12
Induction	18	18	20
Forceps	7	4	4
Ventouse	8	7	7
Episiotomy	12	16	14

Buckingham · **Stoke Mandeville Hospital**

Mandeville Road, Aylesbury
Buckinghamshire, HP21 8AL
Phone: 01296 315 000
Fax: 01296 316 604

Trust: Stoke Mandeville Hospital
NHS Trust

The unit is adopting team midwifery, and creating five community based teams to facilitate integration between community services and the hospital. Domino care is available on request.

The unit provides a pool, TENS machines and aromatherapy for pain relief. Antenatal classes on offer include evening groups plus dedicated sessions for teenagers and ethnic minorities. Elective caesareans are done less frequently here than in other hospitals and the overall caesarean rate is below average.

Double testing is offered rather than triple testing or nuchal fold scans. There is a fetal assessment unit in the hospital and a 12-cot special care baby unit. There is also a link with the hospital's Spinal Injuries Centre for mothers with spinal injuries.

Consultant and Midwife Unit

Number of beds	40
Births per midwife	38
Births per bed	0.88
Home births	1%
Amenity Rooms, Price	£55

Obstetrician 24 hours	Yes
Paediatrician 24 hours	Yes
Full Water Birth Service	No

Tests

Routine Triple Testing	No
Nuchal Fold Scan	No
Fetal Assessment Unit	Yes

Pain Relief

24 hour epidural	Yes
Mobile epidural	No
Pethidine injections	Yes
Water (eg bath)	Yes

Intervention Rates

	%	regional average	national average
Epidural	32	30	33
Elective Caesarean	6	8	8
Emergency Caesarean	12	13	12
Induction	21	18	20
Forceps	4	4	4
Ventouse	8	7	7
Episiotomy	19	16	14

Canterbury · **Kent & Canterbury Hospital**

Ethelbert Road, Canterbury
Kent, CT1 3NG
Phone: 01227 766 877
Fax: 01227 864 115

Trust: East Kent Hospitals
NHS Trust

The maternity unit operates a team midwifery approach. The teams are kept busy with 39 births per midwife per year. The unit includes a high-risk neonatal referral unit for premature deliveries of over 22 weeks. It also runs early pregnancy and fetal medicine assessment units. The epidural rate is relatively high as is the induction rate. But the overall caesarean rate is significantly below average principally because elective caesareans are done here less often than at other units such as the nearby William Harvey Hospital in Ashford.

The unit caters to partners who want to stay with their spouses before labour, and you can hire an amenity room cheaply at £25 a day. The unit supports acupuncture for pain relief but you will need to arrange the acupunturist yourself.

Consultant and Midwife Unit

Number of beds	36
Births per midwife	39
Births per bed	0.77
Home births	2%
Amenity Rooms, Price	£25

Obstetrician 24 hours	Yes
Paediatrician 24 hours	Yes
Full Water Birth Service	Yes

Tests

Routine Triple Testing	No
Nuchal Fold Scan	Yes
Fetal Assessment Unit	Yes

Pain Relief

24 hour epidural	Yes
Mobile epidural	Yes
Pethidine injections	Yes
Water (eg bath)	Yes

Intervention Rates	%	regional average	national average
Epidural	41	30	33
Elective Caesarean	6	8	8
Emergency Caesarean	12	13	12
Induction	22	18	20
Forceps	4	4	4
Ventouse	10	7	7
Episiotomy	16	16	14

Chertsey · **St Peter's Hospital**

Guildford Road, Chertsey
Surrey, KT16 0PZ
Phone: 01932 872 000
Fax: 01932 874 757

Trust: Ashford and St Peter's Hospital
NHS Trust

The maternity unit at St Peter's Hospital, Chertsey, is a shared consultant midwife-led unit. As with many units in the home counties, recruitment difficulties mean that the midwifery staff are often stretched having to cope with 49 births per year – substantially more than recommended levels.

Intervention rates are relatively high with around one in four women having caesareans. Epidural pain relief is widely used. If you are keen on a water birth, the facilities are available, however midwives trained in water deliveries are not always available around the clock. Home births are offered but the home birth rate is about half the national average.

Consultant and Midwife Unit

Number of beds	63
Births per midwife	49
Births per bed	1.1
Home births	1%
Amenity Rooms, Price	£75

Obstetrician 24 hours	Yes
Paediatrician 24 hours	Yes
Full Water Birth Service	No

Tests

Routine Triple Testing	No
Nuchal Fold Scan	Yes
Fetal Assessment Unit	Yes

Pain Relief

24 hour epidural	Yes
Mobile epidural	Yes
Pethidine injections	Yes
Water (eg bath)	Yes

Intervention Rates

	%	regional average	national average
Epidural	41	30	33
Elective Caesarean	8	8	8
Emergency Caesarean	16	13	12
Induction	23	18	20
Forceps	3	4	4
Ventouse	11	7	7
Episiotomy	-	16	14

Chichester · **St Richard's Hospital**

Chichester
West Sussex, PO19 4SE
Phone: 01243 788122
Fax: 01243 531 267

Trust: Royal West Sussex
NHS Trust

St Richard's Hospital maternity unit offers a choice of where you have your baby. As well as traditional labour rooms, other options include a birthing pool, a 'home-from-home' room, and home births. The 'home-from-home' room is available for women who want a natural birth and contains an en suite bathroom, a small kitchen, soft furnishings and lighting as well as a stereo and television.

Midwives work in teams, which has helped achieve good continuity of care, with 50 per cent of women having their baby delivered by someone they know. Inductions are done much less frequently than in other units and epidurals are not widely used as a means of pain relief. The unit operates a drop-in centre to provide extra support for teenage mothers.

Consultant and Midwife Unit

Number of beds	42
Births per midwife	30
Births per bed	0.64
Home births	3%
Amenity Rooms, Price	£51

Obstetrician 24 hours	Yes
Paediatrician 24 hours	Yes
Full Water Birth Service	Yes

Tests

Routine Triple Testing	No
Nuchal Fold Scan	Yes
Fetal Assessment Unit	Yes

Pain Relief

24 hour epidural	Yes
Mobile epidural	No
Pethidine injections	Yes
Water (eg bath)	Yes

Intervention Rates	%	regional average	national average
Epidural	19	30	33
Elective Caesarean	10	8	8
Emergency Caesarean	13	13	12
Induction	15	18	20
Forceps	5	4	4
Ventouse	6	7	7
Episiotomy	9	16	14

Chipping Norton · **Community Hospital**

Chipping Norton
Oxfordshire, OX7 5AJ
Phone: 01608 628000
Fax: 01608 648 459

Trust: Oxford Radcliffe Hospitals NHS
Trust

Healthy women with straightforward pregnancies, including some expecting their first baby, can choose to give birth at the unit or at home. The unit can also provide antenatal care for women who are intending to deliver at the consultant-led unit in Oxford. Antenatal classes, including aquanatal sessions, are available. Midwives will be called in day or night if a woman is in labour.

The unit offers a full water birth service, aromatherapy and a TENS machine for pain-relief. Your partner can stay with you in the hospital even if you are not properly in labour. Mothers who are giving birth in the consultant unit are encouraged to come back for postnatal help with baby care.

Midwife Unit

Number of beds	5
Births	126
Midwives	5
Home births	7%
Amenity Rooms, Price	-

Obstetrician 24 hours	No
Paediatrician 24 hours	No
Full Water Birth Service	Yes

Tests

Routine Triple Testing	Yes
Nuchal Fold Scan	Yes
Fetal Assessment Unit	No

Pain Relief

24 Hour epidural	No
Mobile epidural	No
Pethidine injections	Yes
Water (eg bath)	Yes

Midwifs-led units are adequately equipped to care for women whose pregnancy is progressing normally without complications. As a result, intervention tends to be low in these units. Basic pain relief will be offered, but any woman requesting an epidural during the delivery will need to be transferred to the nearest consultant-led unit. A woman will also be transferred to the obstetric unit if any complications develop during the delivery.

Crowborough · **War Memorial Hospital**

South View Road, Crowborough
East Sussex, TN 6 1HB
Phone: 01892 652284
Fax: 01892 668877

Trust: Eastbourne Hospitals NHS Trust

Crowborough Birthing Centre (CBC), which is in a separate, but attached wing of the War Memorial Hospital, is a midwife-led unit which has a clean, warm and friendly feel. It is furnished in a non-clinical way with soft furnishings, lighting, catering facilities, TV and audio equipment and a large water birth pool, used by nearly half of the women who give birth at CBC. It takes a completely non-interventionist approach towards birth. Continuity of care is good and three out of four women who deliver here are cared for by a midwife they know. Alternative therapies are welcomed by the midwives: the unit provides aromatherapy and acupuncture to help women cope with pain. Fetal assessment is provided by Eastbourne District General Hospital.

Midwife Unit

Number of beds	8
Births	257
Midwives	8
Home births	-
Amenity Rooms, Price	-

Obstetrician 24 hours	No
Paediatrician 24 hours	No
Full Water Birth Service	Yes

Tests

Routine Triple Testing	Yes
Nuchal Fold Scan	Yes
Fetal Assessment Unit	Yes

Pain Relief

24 Hour epidural	No
Mobile epidural	No
Pethidine injections	Yes
Water (eg bath)	Yes

Midwife-led units are adequately equipped to care for women whose pregnancy is progressing normally without complications. As a result, intervention tends to be low in these units. Basic pain relief will be offered, but any woman requesting an epidural during the delivery will need to be transferred to the nearest consultant-led unit. A woman will also be transferred to the obstetric unit if any complications develop during the delivery.

Dartford · **Darent Valley Hospital**

Darenth Wood Road, Dartford
Kent, DA2 8DA
Phone: 01322 428100
Fax: 01322 283496

Trust: Dartford & Gravesham
NHS Trust

Care is shared between midwives and consultants at this unit. The service can arrange for home births and the number of women who give birth successfully at home is higher than the national average. Water births are also offered, although midwives trained in water birth may not be on hand 24 hours a day. Your partner will not be allowed to stay on the ward with you if you are admitted to the hospital before labour has started, however amenity rooms can be hired cheaply for £22.

The unit has a high rate of medical intervention with about a quarter of women having caesareans. Also, about a quarter of deliveries last year were induced.

There is a range of options including mobile epidurals for pain relief during labour.

Consultant and Midwife Unit

Number of beds	41
Births per midwife	34
Births per bed	0.76
Home births	3%
Amenity Rooms, Price	£22

Obstetrician 24 hours	Yes
Paediatrician 24 hours	Yes
Full Water Birth Service	No

Tests

Routine Triple Testing	Yes
Nuchal Fold Scan	No
Fetal Assessment Unit	Yes

Pain Relief

24 hour epidural	Yes
Mobile epidural	Yes
Pethidine injections	Yes
Water (eg bath)	Yes

Intervention Rates	%	regional average	national average
Epidural	31	30	33
Elective Caesarean	9	8	8
Emergency Caesarean	16	13	12
Induction	24	18	20
Forceps	5	4	4
Ventouse	6	7	7
Episiotomy	17	16	14

Dover · **Buckland Hospital**

Coombe Valley Road, Dover
Kent, CT17 0HD
Phone: 01304 201 624
Fax: 01304 203 565

Trust: East Kent Hospitals NHS Trust

The Buckland Hospital midwifery-led unit provides an alternative to the style of care provided in many larger hospitals. Aromatherapy is offered as a form of pain relief and the unit teaches baby massage. This is a group practice unit – where you will be looked after by the same midwife throughout labour and pregnancy with a second providing back up. Midwives from the unit are also happy to arrange a home birth or a water birth. There is a fetal assessment unit and the unit will arrange nuchal fold scans.

It is possible to hire a private room for £25. Antenatal classes are held in the day and evening, but they are not specifically for women only. The unit also runs a breastfeeding support group.

Midwife Unit

Number of beds	13
Births	169
Midwives	5
Home births	22%
Amenity Rooms, Price	£25
Obstetrician 24 hours	No
Paediatrician 24 hours	No
Full Water Birth Service	Yes

Tests

Routine Triple Testing	No
Nuchal Fold Scan	Yes
Fetal Assessment Unit	Yes

Pain Relief

24 Hour epidural	No
Mobile epidural	No
Pethidine injections	Yes
Water (eg bath)	Yes

Midwife-led units are adequately equipped to care for women whose pregnancy is progressing normally without complications. As a result, intervention tends to be low in these units. Basic pain relief will be offered, but any woman requesting an epidural during the delivery will need to be transferred to the nearest consultant-led unit. A woman will also be transferred to the obstetric unit if any complications develop during the delivery.

Eastbourne · **Eastbourne District General Hospital**

Kings Drive, Eastbourne
East Sussex, BN21 2UD
Phone: 01323 417400
Fax: 01323 414986

Trust: Eastbourne Hospitals
NHS Trust

Eastbourne has a large maternity unit staffed with six consultants providing 24hr emergency cover, as well as supporting clinical care. There is also a special baby care unit on the site. The pattern of medical interventions is interesting with an above average rate of elective caesareans and a below average rate of emergency caesareans suggesting a greater willingness to book women in for caesareans rather than risk an emergency procedure.

Antenatal care, including ultrasound scanning is provided at satellite clinics run in Uckfield, Hailsham, Heathfield, Seaford & Crowborough to save women having to travel into the hospital. Home births are also offered and are done twice as often as in most large hospitals. The unit also runs a breastfeeding clinic.

Consultant and Midwife Unit

Number of beds	46
Births per midwife	27
Births per bed	0.57
Home births	4%
Amenity Rooms, Price	£75

Obstetrician 24 hours	Yes
Paediatrician 24 hours	Yes
Full Water Birth Service	Yes

Tests

Routine Triple Testing	Yes
Nuchal Fold Scan	Yes
Fetal Assessment Unit	Yes

Pain Relief

24 hour epidural	Yes
Mobile epidural	Yes
Pethidine injections	Yes
Water (eg bath)	Yes

Intervention Rates

	%	regional average	national average
Epidural	31	30	33
Elective Caesarean	10	8	8
Emergency Caesarean	11	13	12
Induction	22	18	20
Forceps	2	4	4
Ventouse	5	7	7
Episiotomy	23	16	14

Fareham · **Blackbrook House Maternity Home**

Blackbrook Drive, Fareham
Hampshire, PO14 1PA
Phone: 01329 232 275
Fax: 01329 281887

Trust: Portsmouth Hospitals NHS Trust

Blackbrook House Maternity Home is a ten-bed unit, with just one delivery room. Home births are also offered and account for about one in five births at the unit. As a midwife-led unit, there are no epidurals available, but gas and air, baths and a TENS machine are all offered. You can also be given opiate injections to control pain.

The unit offers evening antenatal classes and women-only classes. If you need to go into hospital before your labour starts your partner will be allowed to stay on the unit.

Booking scans are done 16 weeks rather than 12 and later ultrasound scans are available on request. More complex pregnancies are transferred to nearby Portsmouth Hospital. Support services include counselling. The unit also has links with the National Childbirth Trust.

Midwife Unit

Number of beds	10
Births	116
Midwives	12
Home births	17%
Amenity Rooms, Price	-

Obstetrician 24 hours	No
Paediatrician 24 hours	No
Full Water Birth Service	-

Tests

Routine Triple Testing	Yes
Nuchal Fold Scan	Yes
Fetal Assessment Unit	No

Pain Relief

24 Hour epidural	No
Mobile epidural	No
Pethidine injections	Yes
Water (eg bath)	Yes

Midwife-led units are adequately equipped to care for women whose pregnancy is progressing normally without complications. As a result, intervention tends to be low in these units. Basic pain relief will be offered, but any woman requesting an epidural during the delivery will need to be transferred to the nearest consultant-led unit. A woman will also be transferred to the obstetric unit if any complications develop during the delivery.

Frimley · **Frimley Park Hospital**

Portsmouth Road, Frimley
Surrey, GU16 7UJ
Phone: 01276 604 604
Fax: 01276 604 274

Trust: Frimley Park Hospital
NHS Trust

Women with uncomplicated pregnancies are overseen throughout their labour, pregnancy and postnatal period by one of ten teams of midwives. Domino deliveries are also offered. A separate team of midwives work with women with more complex pregnancies who are under the care of a consultant.

A purpose-built day assessment unit enables day care to be given to women with problem pregnancies without having to admit them to hospital. Nuchal fold scans are offered to all women. Intervention rates are in line with national averages although you are more likely to be induced here than at other units. Your options for pain relief include epidurals and low-dose mobile epidurals which allow greater feeling and movement during labour.

Consultant and Midwife Unit

Number of beds	62
Births per midwife	35
Births per bed	0.70
Home births	2%
Amenity Rooms, Price	£45

Obstetrician 24 hours	Yes
Paediatrician 24 hours	Yes
Full Water Birth Service	Yes

Tests

Routine Triple Testing	No
Nuchal Fold Scan	Yes
Fetal Assessment Unit	Yes

Pain Relief

24 hour epidural	Yes
Mobile epidural	Yes
Pethidine injections	Yes
Water (eg bath)	Yes

Intervention Rates

	%	regional average	national average
Epidural	31	30	33
Elective Caesarean	9	8	8
Emergency Caesarean	12	13	12
Induction	23	18	20
Forceps	4	4	4
Ventouse	4	7	7
Episiotomy	10	16	14

Gillingham · **Medway Maritime Hospital**

Windmill Road, Gillingham
Kent, ME7 5NY
Phone: 01634 830000
Fax: 01634 815811

Trust: The Medway
NHS Trust

This is a new unit, with consultant and midwife care provided by the hospital as well as at home and in local clinics. Home births are offered and the home birth rate is more than double the national average; the unit also provides domino deliveries. You can opt for a water birth but midwives may not always be on hand all day to supervise these.

Intervention rates are above average with a high induction rate. Also, use of epidurals is more widespread than in similar units.

A neonatal/special care baby unit is situated next to the maternity suite.

The unit runs a clinic for women with substance abuse problems as well as a combined diabetic and antenatal clinic.

Consultant and Midwife Unit

Number of beds	60
Births per midwife	33.8
Births per bed	0.87
Home births	5%
Amenity Rooms, Price	£40

Obstetrician 24 hours	Yes
Paediatrician 24 hours	Yes
Full Water Birth Service	No

Tests

Routine Triple Testing	Yes
Nuchal Fold Scan	Yes
Fetal Assessment Unit	Yes

Pain Relief

24 hour epidural	Yes
Mobile epidural	Yes
Pethidine injections	Yes
Water (eg bath)	Yes

Intervention Rates	%	regional average	national average
Epidural	42	30	33
Elective Caesarean	11	8	8
Emergency Caesarean	14	13	12
Induction	24	18	20
Forceps	4	4	4
Ventouse	6	7	7
Episiotomy	17	16	14

Guildford · **Royal Surrey County Hospital**

Egerton Road, Guildford
Surrey, GU2 7XX
Phone: 01483 571 122
Fax: 01483 5645840

Trust: **The Royal Surrey County
Hospital NHS Trust**

If you want an epidural for pain relief you should have no trouble getting one here. This unit has one of the highest epidural rates in the country and has a 24 hour epidural service that does low-dose mobile epidurals.

But the unit also offers alternative forms of pain management including reflexology and aromatherapy which may help you get through labour without anaesthetic drugs.

Intervention rates are broadly in line with national averages although inductions are used more frequently than at other hospitals.

Antenatal care includes a wide range of parentcraft classes such as sessions for grandparents, aquaerobics classes, physical preparation for childbirth and various alternative therapies.

Consultant and Midwife Unit

Number of beds	62
Births per midwife	39
Births per bed	0.86
Home births	3%
Amenity Rooms, Price	£104

Obstetrician 24 hours	Yes
Paediatrician 24 hours	Yes
Full Water Birth Service	Yes

Tests

Routine Triple Testing	No
Nuchal Fold Scan	Yes
Fetal Assessment Unit	Yes

Pain Relief

24 hour epidural	Yes
Mobile epidural	Yes
Pethidine injections	Yes
Water (eg bath)	Yes

Intervention Rates	%	regional average	national average
Epidural	57	30	33
Elective Caesarean	7	8	8
Emergency Caesarean	12	13	12
Induction	23	18	20
Forceps	4	4	4
Ventouse	9	7	7
Episiotomy	13	16	14

Gosport · **War Memorial Hospital**

Bury Road, Gosport
Hampshire, PO12 3PW
Phone: 02392 524 611
Fax: 02392 603201

Trust: Portsmouth Hospitals NHS Trust

The midwives here will deliver your baby in the unit or at your home – about one in ten deliveries is a home birth. If there are any complications in your pregnancy your will probably be referred to Portsmouth.

Pain relief is limited to intramuscular opiate injection, TENS machines and water births.

There are women-only antenatal classes as well as mixed classes. Booking scans are routinely offered at 16 weeks, and later pregnancy scans are given on request.

Support services are provided by counsellors and the National Childbirth Trust.

Midwife Unit

Number of beds	10
Births	204
Midwives	21
Home births	9%
Amenity Rooms, Price	-
Obstetrician 24 hours	No
Paediatrician 24 hours	No
Full Water Birth Service	Yes
Tests	
Routine Triple Testing	Yes
Nuchal Fold Scan	Yes
Fetal Assessment Unit	No
Pain Relief	
24 Hour epidural	No
Mobile epidural	No
Pethidine injections	Yes
Water (eg bath)	Yes

Midwife-led units are adequately equipped to care for women whose pregnancy is progressing normally without complications. As a result, intervention tends to be low in these units. Basic pain relief will be offered, but any woman requesting an epidural during the delivery will need to be transferred to the nearest consultant-led unit. A woman will also be transferred to the obstetric unit if any complications develop during the delivery.

Haywards Heath · **Princess Royal Hospital**

Lewes Road, Haywards Heath
West Sussex, RH16 4EX
Phone: 01444 441 881
Fax: 01444 415 865

Trust: Mid Sussex
NHS Trust

The maternity unit at the Princess Royal Hospital Haywards Heath is a shared midwife and consultant led unit. The unit has a strong midwifery focus. The labour ward is busy with over one birth per delivery bed per day, but there are only rarely problems accommodating women. The maternity unit has six spacious delivery rooms, its own obstetric theatre, a 32 bed antenatal/postnatal ward, a special care baby unit and antenatal clinic and drop in centre.

The caesarean rate is higher than average. Antenatal classes are available in the evening. The unit has a birthing pool and midwives trained in water births are available 24hrs a day. Nuchal fold scans are offered to all women.

Consultant and Midwife Unit

Number of beds	38
Births per midwife	38
Births per bed	1.01
Home births	2%
Amenity Rooms, Price	£43

Obstetrician 24 hours	Yes
Paediatrician 24 hours	Yes
Full Water Birth Service	Yes

Tests

Routine Triple Testing	No
Nuchal Fold Scan	Yes
Fetal Assessment Unit	Yes

Pain Relief

24 hour epidural	Yes
Mobile epidural	No
Pethidine injections	Yes
Water (eg bath)	Yes

Intervention Rates	%	regional average	national average
Epidural	16	30	33
Elective Caesarean	9	8	8
Emergency Caesarean	15	13	12
Induction		18	20
Forceps	4	4	4
Ventouse	5	7	7
Episiotomy	16	16	14

High Wycombe · **Wycombe Hospital**

Queen Alexandra Road, High Wycombe
Buckinghamshire, HP11 2TT
Phone: 01494 526 161
Fax: 01494 425 339

Trust: South Buckinghamshire
NHS Trust

The maternity unit at Wycombe Hospital is a shared midwife and consultant-led unit with a very low caesarean rate – particularly for a hospital in the South East. Both elective and emergency caesarean rates are well below the national average although instrumental deliveries are done just as frequently as elsewhere.

Home births and domino deliveries are offered. Water births are not although you are welcome to bring your own pool to the unit for pain relief.

Antenatal screening is used less than in some other units. Early 12-week ultrasound scans are not routinely offered. Double testing is done rather than triple testing, although nuchal fold scans for Down's syndrome can be arranged for a fee.

Consultant and Midwife Unit

Number of beds	55
Births per midwife	39
Births per bed	0.82
Home births	2%
Amenity Rooms, Price	£42
Obstetrician 24 hours	Yes
Paediatrician 24 hours	Yes
Full Water Birth Service	No

Tests

Routine Triple Testing	No
Nuchal Fold Scan	No
Fetal Assessment Unit	No

Pain Relief

24 hour epidural	Yes
Mobile epidural	No
Pethidine injections	Yes
Water (eg bath)	Yes

Intervention Rates	%	regional average	national average
Epidural	38	30	33
Elective Caesarean	6	8	8
Emergency Caesarean	10	13	12
Induction	22	18	20
Forceps	4	4	4
Ventouse	8	7	7
Episiotomy	20	16	14

Kettering · **Kettering General Hospital**

Rothwell Road, Kettering
Northamptonshire, NN16 8UZ
Phone: 01536 492 000
Fax: 01536 492 295

Trust: Kettering General Hospital
    NHS Trust

This unit aims to maintain a balance between midwife-led care and the involvement of obstetric specialists. Intervention is in line with most large hospitals although inductions are done more often than in most units. Home births are offered but the home birth rate is well below average. In contrast neighbouring Bedford has a much higher rate.

Although the overall epidural rate is in line with the national average this is used mainly for caesareans. Epidurals for pain relief in labour are used for only about one in ten women – much less often than in other hospitals. Mobile epidurals are not available.

Nuchal fold scans are not available but triple testing is offered.

Consultant and Midwife Unit

NNumber of beds	57
Births per midwife	34
Births per bed	0.57
Home births	1%
Amenity Rooms, Price	£30

Obstetrician 24 hours	Yes
Paediatrician 24 hours	Yes
Full Water Birth Service	Yes

Tests

Routine Triple Testing	Yes
Nuchal Fold Scan	No
Fetal Assessment Unit	Yes

Pain Relief

24 hour epidural	Yes
Mobile epidural	No
Pethidine injections	Yes
Water (eg bath)	Yes

Intervention Rates	%	regional average	national average
Epidural	33	30	33
Elective Caesarean	9	8	8
Emergency Caesarean	13	13	12
Induction	25	18	20
Forceps	4	4	4
Ventouse	6	7	7
Episiotomy	24	16	14

Lymington · **Lymington Hospital**

Southampton Road
Lymington, SO41 9ZH
Phone: 01590 677011
Fax: 01590 671787

Trust: Southampton University
Hospitals NHS Trust

The Lymington Hospital maternity service is a good choice if you are anticipating a normal delivery and would like to give birth with a minimum of medical intervention. The unit embarked on caseload midwifery in Autumn 2001, so most women should receive antenatal, intrapartum and postnatal care from their own midwife. Before this, around half of women were cared for in labour by a familiar midwife.

The unit consists of eight single rooms, offering more privacy than a traditional labour ward. Midwives from the unit also attend an above-average number of home births so you should be well supported if you decided to give birth this way. Waterbirth is available 24 hours a day at the unit, and a birthing pool is provided.

Midwife Unit

Number of beds	8
Births	138
Midwives	11
Home births	8%
Amenity Rooms, Price	-

Obstetrician 24 hours	No
Paediatrician 24 hours	No
Full Water Birth Service	Yes

Tests

Routine Triple Testing	No
Nuchal Fold Scan	Yes
Fetal Assessment Unit	No

Pain Relief

24 Hour epidural	No
Mobile epidural	No
Pethidine injections	Yes
Water (eg bath)	Yes

Midwife-led units are adequately equipped to care for women whose pregnancy is progressing normally without complications. As a result, intervention tends to be low in these units. Basic pain relief will be offered, but any woman requesting an epidural during the delivery will need to be transferred to the nearest consultant-led unit. A woman will also be transferred to the obstetric unit if any complications develop during the delivery.

Maidstone · **Maidstone Hospital**

Hermitage Lane, Maidstone
Kent, ME16 9QQ
Phone: 01622 729 000
Fax: 01622 224 114

Trust: Maidstone and Tunbridge Wells
NHS Trust

Continuity of care is reasonably good with about a third of women being looked after in labour by a midwife they know. This is achieved despite relatively stretched staffing levels with 45 births per year for each midwife. Care for straightforward pregnancies is midwife-led and you should not have to see a consultant. The unit is one of the few to have a higher elective caesarean rate then emergency rate. The elective caesarean rate is particularly high.

Both home births and water births are offered. The unit has a particular focus on water births. The home birth rate, however, is below average.

For antenatal scans quadruple testing is offered. You can also get a nuchal fold scan although you will be referred to London for this.

Consultant and Midwife Unit

Number of beds	49
Births per midwife	45
Births per bed	0.96
Home births	1%
Amenity Rooms, Price	£40

Obstetrician 24 hours	Yes
Paediatrician 24 hours	Yes
Full Water Birth Service	Yes

Tests

Routine Triple Testing	Yes
Nuchal Fold Scan	Yes
Fetal Assessment Unit	Yes

Pain Relief

24 hour epidural	Yes
Mobile epidural	Yes
Pethidine injections	Yes
Water (eg bath)	Yes

Intervention Rates	%	regional average	national average
Epidural	18	30	33
Elective Caesarean	13	8	8
Emergency Caesarean	10	13	12
Induction	24	18	20
Forceps	4	4	4
Ventouse	4	7	7
Episiotomy	14	16	14

Margate · **Queen Elizabeth The Queen Mother**

St Peters Road, Margate
Kent, CT9 4AN
Phone: 01843 225544
Fax: 01843 220048

Trust: East Kent Hospitals
NHS Trust

This is a medium sized maternity unit, at which care is shared between midwives and consultants. There is a good midwife to birth ratio and about half the women who give birth here have their baby delivered by a midwife they know. Domino births are available.

The unit includes full water birthing facilities and there are always midwives trained in water births on duty. Intervention rates are low, and although the unit offers a wide range of pain relief, use of epidurals is also relatively low.

Antenatal classes are run both during the day and in the evenings, and women only classes are available. The hospital runs antenatal and postnatal support lines and a breastfeeding help line.

Consultant and Midwife Unit

Number of beds	30
Births per midwife	27
Births per bed	0.59
Home births	1%
Amenity Rooms, Price	-

Obstetrician 24 hours	Yes
Paediatrician 24 hours	Yes
Full Water Birth Service	Yes

Tests

Routine Triple Testing	No
Nuchal Fold Scan	Yes
Fetal Assessment Unit	Yes

Pain Relief

24 hour epidural	Yes
Mobile epidural	No
Pethidine injections	Yes
Water (eg bath)	Yes

Intervention Rates	%	regional average	national average
Epidural	25	30	33
Elective Caesarean	9	8	8
Emergency Caesarean	10	13	12
Induction	14	18	20
Forceps	1	4	4
Ventouse	7	7	7
Episiotomy	17	16	14

Milton Keynes · **General Hospital**

**Standing Way, Eaglestone,
Buckinghamshire, MK6 5LD
Phone: 01908 660 033
Fax: 01908 243 614**

Trust: Milton Keynes General NHS Trust

This hospital has a shared midwife and consultant-led maternity unit, with midwife groups linked to GP practices. The unit's intervention rates fall in line with most of the larger hospitals but use of epidurals is much lower than in other hospitals. This is a busy unit with more than one birth per delivery bed per day. However, more single rooms on the labour ward are planned. Water births are only available for women who choose a home birth and you would need to be responsible for hiring your own pool. Home births are catered for although the home birth rate is below average. Amenity rooms can be hired but cannot be guaranteed as they may be required for other patients. Antenatal screening is more limited than at some hospitals. Nuchal fold scans are not available and triple testing is not routinely offered.

Consultant and Midwife Unit

Number of beds	45
ratio of midwives to births	35
Births per bed	1.24
Home births	1%
Amenity Rooms, Price	£25

Obstetrician 24 hours	Yes
Paediatrician 24 hours	Yes
Full Water Birth Service	Yes

Tests

Routine Triple Testing	No
Nuchal Fold Scan	No
Fetal Assessment Unit	Yes

Pain Relief

24 Hour epidural	Yes
Mobile epidural	Yes
Pethidine injections	Yes
Water (eg bath)	Yes

Intervention Rates	%	regional average	national average
Epidural	15	30	33
Elective Caesarean	9	8	8
Emergency Caesarean	11	13	12
Induction	20	18	20
Forceps	3	4	4
Ventouse	5	7	7
Episiotomy	13	16	14

Newport, IoW · **St Mary's Hospital**

Newport
Isle of Wight, PO30 5TG
Phone: 01983 524 081
Fax: 01983 534 196

Trust: Isle of Wight Healthcare NHS Trust

St Mary's has a high home birth rate and encourages women to take an active role in decision making. The unit operates an integrated midwifery service with midwives working both in the community and at the small informal maternity unit. Staffing levels are higher than most hospitals in the South East and continuity of care is reasonably good with over a third of women being looked after in labour by a midwife they know. The recently upgraded unit has single rooms and small wards. Partners may stay overnight if you have to go into hospital before labour starts. You can attempt a water birth if you bring your own pool. Evening antenatal classes, separate classes for young mothers, and a breastfeeding clinic are available.

Consultant and Midwife Unit

Number of beds	22
Births per midwife	25
Births per bed	0.77
Home births	4%
Amenity Rooms, Price	£48

Obstetrician 24 hours	Yes
Paediatrician 24 hours	Yes
Full Water Birth Service	No

Tests

Routine Triple Testing	No
Nuchal Fold Scan	Yes
Fetal Assessment Unit	Yes

Pain Relief

24 hour epidural	Yes
Mobile epidural	Yes
Pethidine injections	Yes
Water (eg bath)	Yes

Intervention Rates	%	regional average	national average
Epidural	30	30	33
Elective Caesarean	9	8	8
Emergency Caesarean	11	13	12
Induction	19	18	20
Forceps	4	4	4
Ventouse	6	7	7
Episiotomy	12	16	14

Northampton · **Northampton General Hospital**

Cliftonville, Northampton
Northamptonshire, NN1 5BD
Phone: 01604 545 860

Trust: Northamptonshire General
Hospital NHS Trust

This large maternity unit offers a fully integrated service. Domino deliveries are offered so that the midwife who looks after you through your pregnancy can also oversee the delivery of your baby. There are midwives trained in various complementary therapies, including baby massage.

Intervention rates are relatively high and in particular the emergency caesarean rate is much higher than the national average. In contrast elective caesareans are done less frequently than in other units. So women here try to give birth naturally even if many of them end up having caesareans. Support services cater for teenage mothers and women from ethnic minorities.

Consultant and Midwife Unit

Number of beds	52
ratio of midwives to births	35
Births per bed	0.78
Home births	2%
Amenity Rooms, Price	£37

Obstetrician 24 hours	Yes
Paediatrician 24 hours	Yes
Full Water Birth Service	Yes

Tests

Routine Triple Testing	Yes
Nuchal Fold Scan	No
Fetal Assessment Unit	Yes

Pain Relief

24 Hour epidural	Yes
Mobile epidural	No
Pethidine injections	Yes
Water (eg bath)	Yes

Intervention Rates

	%	regional average	national average
Epidural	40	30	33
Elective Caesarean	7	8	8
Emergency Caesarean	17	13	12
Induction	19	18	20
Forceps	3	4	4
Ventouse	6	7	7
Episiotomy	17	16	14

Oxford · **John Radcliffe Hospital**

Headley Way, Headington
Oxfordshire, OX3 9DU
Phone: 01865 741 166
Fax: 01865 741 408

Trust: Oxford Radcliffe Hospitals
NHS Trust

The John Radcliffe says it aims to give women all the facts about childbirth and then support them in their decisions. In practice, this translates into an unusual pattern of care. Overall the caesarean rate is low. But elective caesareans happen more often than would be expected. In contrast the emergency caesarean rate is well below average. This suggests that the unit is good at supporting women trying to give birth naturally. Epidurals are more widely used than at most hospitals and so are inductions. Continuity is good for a large hospital with 50 per cent of women cared for in labour by a midwife they know. Tests for Down's syndrome such as triple testing are not routinely available but can be privately arranged for a fee.

Consultant and Midwife Unit

Number of beds	102
Births per midwife	40
Births per bed	1.10
Home births	3%
Amenity Rooms, Price	£55

Obstetrician 24 hours	Yes
Paediatrician 24 hours	Yes
Full Water Birth Service	Yes

Tests

Routine Triple Testing	No
Nuchal Fold Scan	No
Fetal Assessment Unit	Yes

Pain Relief

24 hour epidural	Yes
Mobile epidural	Yes
Pethidine injections	Yes
Water (eg bath)	Yes

Intervention Rates	%	regional average	national average
Epidural	37	30	33
Elective Caesarean	9	8	8
Emergency Caesarean	9	13	12
Induction	23	18	20
Forceps	6	4	4
Ventouse	7	7	7
Episiotomy	19	16	14

Pembury · **Pembury Hospital**

Tonbridge Road, Pembury
Kent, TN2 4QJ
Phone: 01892 823 535
Fax: 01892 824 267

Trust: Maidstone and Tunbridge Wells
NHS Trust

This unit offers caseload midwifery, in which a patient receives all her care from one named midwife with a named colleague providing backup. The aim is to improve continuity of care and about a third of women here are cared for in labour by a midwife they know. Home births are relatively frequent and water births are offered. Quadruple testing is offered for Down's syndrome but not nuchal fold scans. Overall the caesarean rate is average but unusually, two thirds of caesareans are elective suggesting the unit is relatively happy to plan caesarean deliveries. There are evening antenatal classes, a breastfeeding clinic, and NCT breastfeeding counsellors available on the ward.

Consultant and Midwife Unit

Number of beds	45
Births per midwife	35
Births per bed	0.63
Home births	4%
Amenity Rooms, Price	£66

Obstetrician 24 hours	Yes
Paediatrician 24 hours	Yes
Full Water Birth Service	Yes

Tests

Routine Triple Testing	Yes
Nuchal Fold Scan	No
Fetal Assessment Unit	Yes

Pain Relief

24 hour epidural	Yes
Mobile epidural	No
Pethidine injections	Yes
Water (eg bath)	Yes

Intervention Rates	%	regional average	national average
Epidural	39	30	33
Elective Caesarean	12	8	8
Emergency Caesarean	8	13	12
Induction	18	18	20
Forceps	1	4	4
Ventouse	4	7	7
Episiotomy	17	16	14

Petersfield · **Petersfield Hospital**

Swan Street
Petersfield, GU32 3LB
Phone: 01730 263221
Fax: 02392 866 413

Trust: Portsmouth Hospitals NHS Trust

The maternity unit at Petersfield Hospital is a small midwife-led service. Care can be shared with your GP and about one in three deliveries handled by the unit are home births. The unit only caters for spontaneous vaginal delivery. More complex cases such as breech presentations are referred to the main unit at St Mary's Hospital in Portsmouth.

Your booking scan will be routinely offered at 16 weeks rather than 12, but a later anomaly scan can be done on request. Parent education sessions and antenatal classes are available during the daytime, in the evenings and over the weekends. The unit also runs separate classes for women-only groups.

Midwife Unit

Number of beds	8
Births	94
Midwives	10
Home births	29%
Amenity Rooms, Price	-

Obstetrician 24 hours	No
Paediatrician 24 hours	No
Full Water Birth Service	

Tests

Routine Triple Testing	Yes
Nuchal Fold Scan	Yes
Fetal Assessment Unit	Yes

Pain Relief

24 Hour epidural	No
Mobile epidural	No
Pethidine injections	Yes
Water (eg bath)	Yes

Midwife-led units are adequately equipped to care for women whose pregnancy is progressing normally without complications. As a result, intervention tends to be low in these units. Basic pain relief will be offered, but any woman requesting an epidural during the delivery will need to be transferred to the nearest consultant-led unit. A woman will also be transferred to the obstetric unit if any complications develop during the delivery.

Portsmouth · St Mary's Hospital

Milton Road, Portsmouth
Hampshire, PO3 6AD
Phone: 02392 286 000
Fax: 01705 866 413

Trust: Portsmouth Hospitals
NHS Trust

St Mary's Hospital, Portsmouth, is a shared midwife and consultant led unit. The unit serves a wide and densely populated area along with a number of smaller midwife-led units. These handle uncomplicated deliveries alongside the consultant unit. Intervention rates – in particular the emergency caesarean rate – are relatively high, even after taking into account the fact that many low-risk women go to nearby midwife-led units.

Ultrasound scans are not routinely offered at the time of booking, which is usually around 12 weeks, but they are offered at 16 weeks. The triple test is routinely offered and nuchal fold and anomaly ultrasound scans are available on request.

Consultant and Midwife Unit

Number of beds	68
Births per midwife	26
Births per bed	0.77
Home births	5%
Amenity Rooms, Price	£36

Obstetrician 24 hours	Yes
Paediatrician 24 hours	Yes
Full Water Birth Service	No

Tests	
Routine Triple Testing	Yes
Nuchal Fold Scan	Yes
Fetal Assessment Unit	Yes

Pain Relief	
24 hour epidural	Yes
Mobile epidural	No
Pethidine injections	Yes
Water (eg bath)	Yes

Intervention Rates

	%	regional average	national average
Epidural	24	30	33
Elective Caesarean	8	8	8
Emergency Caesarean	16	13	12
Induction	22	18	20
Forceps	3	4	4
Ventouse	7	7	7
Episiotomy	11	16	14

Portsmouth · **St Mary's Hospital (Midwife Unit)**

Mary Rose Maternity Centre, Milton Road,
Portsmouth, Hampshire, PO3 6AD
Phone: 023 9228 6000
Fax: 023 9286 6413

Trust: The Royal Wolverhampton
Hospitals NHS Trust

The midwife-led unit at St Mary's hospital, Portsmouth, provides low-tech care for women with low-risk pregnancies.

The unit has a high rate of home births and is a good choice if you wish to have your baby at home. Should you choose to have your baby in the unit however, there are single rooms available.

There are water birth facilities and midwives trained in water deliveries are available around the clock. Anomaly ultrasound scans are only available if a consultant thinks it is necessary and you will have to pay for a nuchal fold scan.

If there are unforeseen complications during your delivery you will be transferred to the consultant led unit on the same site.

Midwife Unit

Number of beds	12
Births	670
Midwives	70
Home births	-
Amenity Rooms, Price	-
Obstetrician 24 hours	Yes
Paediatrician 24 hours	Yes
Full Water Birth Service	Yes

Tests

Routine Triple Testing	Yes
Nuchal Fold Scan	No
Fetal Assessment Unit	Yes

Pain Relief

24 Hour epidural	No
Mobile epidural	No
Pethidine injections	Yes
Water (eg bath)	Yes

Midwife-led units are adequately equipped to care for women whose pregnancy is progressing normally without complications. As a result, intervention tends to be low in these units. Basic pain relief will be offered, but any woman requesting an epidural during the delivery will need to be transferred to the nearest consultant-led unit. A woman will also be transferred to the obstetric unit if any complications develop during the delivery.

Reading · **Royal Berkshire & Battle Hospitals**

London Road, Reading
Berkshire, RG1 5AN
Phone: 0118 987 5111
Fax: 0118 987 8883

Trust: Royal Berkshire & Battle
Hospitals NHS Trust

Maternity services at this hospital site deliver approximately 5000 women a year, with a choice of home birth, water birth, specialist obstetrics and midwifery care. There is a well-established community service offering options such as drop-in antenatal and postnatal clinics, parent education and extended postnatal support. Antenatal classes run throughout the week, in the evenings and weekends, and special classes are held for teenage mothers, multiple pregnancies and women preparing for a caesarean. Scans such as nuchal fold are given to women who are considered to need it, not on demand. Pain relief options include mobile epidurals. Availability of epidurals is good. They are used more often than in other hopsitals.

Consultant and Midwife Unit

Number of beds	77
Births per midwife	42
Births per bed	0.70
Home births	2%
Amenity Rooms, Price	£60

Obstetrician 24 hours	Yes
Paediatrician 24 hours	Yes
Full Water Birth Service	Yes

Tests

Routine Triple Testing	No
Nuchal Fold Scan	Yes
Fetal Assessment Unit	No

Pain Relief

24 hour epidural	Yes
Mobile epidural	Yes
Pethidine injections	Yes
Water (eg bath)	Yes

Intervention Rates

	%	regional average	national average
Epidural	45	30	33
Elective Caesarean	8	8	8
Emergency Caesarean	13	13	12
Induction	-	18	20
Forceps	5	4	4
Ventouse	6	7	7
Episiotomy	25	16	14

Redhill · **East Surrey and Crawley Hospitals**

Canada Avenue, Redhill
West Sussex, RH1 5RH
Phone: 01737 768511
Fax: 01737 231 727

Trust: Surrey and Sussex Healthcare
NHS Trust

Continuity of care is good with over one in three women looked after in labour by a midwife they know. Intervention rates are high overall – in particular caesarean deliveries – but forceps are rarely used. Antenatal clinics and classes are available in a variety of community locations, but all hospital births take place at East Surrey Hospital in Redhill.

Most of the delivery rooms in the hospital have bathrooms en suite, and there are five beds for women in early labour. Two wards are available, one for antenatal and postnatal women, and the other for newly delivered mothers. A special care baby unit, equipped with intensive care cots, is close to the delivery suite. If you want a water birth you will have to bring the pool.

Consultant and Midwife Unit

Number of beds	64
Births per midwife	35
Births per bed	0.68
Home births	2%
Amenity Rooms, Price	£80

Obstetrician 24 hours	Yes
Paediatrician 24 hours	Yes
Full Water Birth Service	No

Tests

Routine Triple Testing	Yes
Nuchal Fold Scan	Yes
Fetal Assessment Unit	Yes

Pain Relief

24 hour epidural	Yes
Mobile epidural	No
Pethidine injections	Yes
Water (eg bath)	Yes

Intervention Rates	%	regional average	national average
Epidural	24	30	33
Elective Caesarean	10	8	8
Emergency Caesarean	15	13	12
Induction	18	18	20
Forceps	2	4	4
Ventouse	10	7	7
Episiotomy	20	16	14

Romsey · **Romsey Hospital**

Winchester Hill, Winchester Road
Romsey, SO51 8ZA
Phone: 01794 512343
Fax: 01794 524465

Trust: Southampton University
Hospitals NHS Trust

The Romsey Hospital maternity service is a small home-from-home unit based around a single delivery bed and would be a good choice if you want a natural birth with the minimum of medical intervention during your stay in hospital. The unit's midwives also attend an above average number of home births. The service is not equipped to manage the care of higher risk women. Antenatal screening services are relatively limited and it may also be necessary for some patients to go to the Princess Anne Hospital or the Royal Hampshire County Hospital for some appointments, tests and scans.

Midwife Unit

Number of beds	4
Births	48
Midwives	8
Home births	11%
Amenity Rooms, Price	-

Obstetrician 24 hours	No
Paediatrician 24 hours	No
Full Water Birth Service	No

Tests

Routine Triple Testing	No
Nuchal Fold Scan	No
Fetal Assessment Unit	No

Pain Relief

24 Hour epidural	No
Mobile epidural	No
Pethidine injections	Yes
Water (eg bath)	Yes

Midwife-led units are adequately equipped to care for women whose pregnancy is progressing normally without complications. As a result, intervention tends to be low in these units. Basic pain relief will be offered, but any woman requesting an epidural during the delivery will need to be transferred to the nearest consultant-led unit. A woman will also be transferred to the obstetric unit if any complications develop during the delivery.

St Leonards · **Conquest Hospital**

The Ridge, St Leonard on Sea
East Sussex, TN37 7RD
Phone: 01424 755255
Fax: 01424 758128

Trust: Hastings and Rother
   NHS Trust

The maternity unit at Conquest Hospital opened in 1997. Facilities include a birthing pool and a ROMA birthing wheel. This is an innovatively designed chair, capable of moving in several different directions and providing different postures to help support women women during labour and at birth. Midwives trained in water birth are usually available but this is not guaranteed at all times. If you want an epidural you should get one as epidurals are used very widely at this unit. However home births are done relatively rarely (in contrast to the services offered by the Royal Sussex County Hospital and Eastbourne District General nearby).

Evening antenatal classes are due to begin in the near future, and the unit already runs women-only classes and sessions for teenagers.

Consultant and Materntiy Unit

Number of beds	26
Births per midwife	27
Births per bed	0.51
Home births	1%
Amenity Rooms, Price	£48

Obstetrician 24 hours	Yes
Paediatrician 24 hours	Yes
Full Water Birth Service	No

Tests

Routine Triple Testing	Yes
Nuchal Fold Scan	Yes
Fetal Assessment Unit	Yes

Pain Relief

24 hour epidural	Yes
Mobile epidural	No
Pethidine injections	Yes
Water (eg bath)	Yes

Intervention Rates	%	regional average	national average
Epidural	43	30	33
Elective Caesarean	8	8	8
Emergency Caesarean	15	13	12
Induction	23	18	20
Forceps	4	4	4
Ventouse	7	7	7
Episiotomy	14	16	14

Slough · **Wexham Park Hospital**

Wexham Street, Slough
Berkshire, SL2 4HL
Phone: 01753 633 000
Fax: 01753 634 848

Trust: Heatherwood and Wexham Park
   Hospitals NHS Trust

The maternity unit at Wexham Park works with the unit at Heatherwood – with Wexham park having a particular emphasis on higher risk pregnancies. The unit offers women a choice in the type of care they receive between full consultant care to GP/midwife shared care, low-risk midwifery care to domino as well as home delivery. However, with 51 births per year for every midwife – far more than most hospitals – the staff have a heavy workload to cope with, a problem exacerbated by the difficulties of recruiting midwives in the home counties. Facilities include a special quiet room which has been made available for mothers to breastfeed in privacy if they so wish. The unit has five amenity rooms, available on a fee paying basis, for postnatal recovery.

Consultant and Midwife Unit

Number of beds	59
Births per midwife	51
Births per bed	1.06
Home births	1%
Amenity Rooms, Price	£165

Obstetrician 24 hours	Yes
Paediatrician 24 hours	Yes
Full Water Birth Service	Yes

Tests

Routine Triple Testing	Yes
Nuchal Fold Scan	Yes
Fetal Assessment Unit	Yes

Pain Relief

24 hour epidural	Yes
Mobile epidural	Yes
Pethidine injections	Yes
Water (eg bath)	Yes

Intervention Rates

	%	regional average	national average
Epidural	49	30	33
Elective Caesarean	7	8	8
Emergency Caesarean	17	13	12
Induction	25	18	20
Forceps	6	4	4
Ventouse	8	7	7
Episiotomy	17	16	14

Southampton · **Hythe Hospital**

Beaulieu Road, Hythe
Southampton, SO45 5ZB
Phone: 023 8084 6046
Fax: 023 8042 3245

Trust: Southampton University
Hospitals NHS Trust

This is a small midwife-led unit for low-risk deliveries situated 11 miles from the consultant unit in Southampton. All midwives work in and out of the unit and caseload midwifery, where midwives work in small teams, is now being introduced. This should ensure good continuity of care in a unit that already manages to ensure that two-thirds of women know the midwife who looks after them in labour. Home births are catered for here, and there is a birthing pool on site.

Many diagnostic tests for abnormalities during pregnancy cannot be given here, although the unit will advise you on where you can access this service elsewhere. Antenatal classes include evening sessions and women-only groups.

Midwife Unit

Number of beds	8
Births	115
Midwives	8
Home births	3%
Amenity Rooms, Price	-

Obstetrician 24 hours	No
Paediatrician 24 hours	No
Full Water Birth Service	Yes

Tests

Routine Triple Testing	No
Nuchal Fold Scan	No
Fetal Assessment Unit	Yes

Pain Relief

24 Hour epidural	No
Mobile epidural	No
Pethidine injections	Yes
Water (eg bath)	Yes

Midwife-led units are adequately equipped to care for women whose pregnancy is progressing normally without complications. As a result, intervention tends to be low in these units. Basic pain relief will be offered, but any woman requesting an epidural during the delivery will need to be transferred to the nearest consultant-led unit. A woman will also be transferred to the obstetric unit if any complications develop during the delivery.

Southampton · **Princess Anne Hospital**

Coxford Road, Shirley, Southampton
Hampshire, SO16 6YA
Phone: 023 8077 7222
Fax: 023 8079 4143

Trust: Southampton University
   Hospitals NHS Trust

The Princess Anne Hospital Maternity Unit is part of a large teaching hospital which offers both midwife-led care and an obstetric service. Midwives are organised into teams which look after women throughout their pregancy labour and postnatal period. The unit has four home-from-home style birth rooms; partners are allowed to stay and amenity rooms are available. The caesarean rate is above average but inductions are done relatively infrequently. There are full water birth facilities. Antenatal classes cater to multiple pregnancy and teenagers, although women-only classes are still under consideration. If you want a diagnostic test such as the triple test, you will be referred to other hospitals.

Consultant and Midwife Unit

Number of beds	58
Births per midwife	32.6
Births per bed	0.93
Home births	2%
Amenity Rooms, Price	40

Obstetrician 24 hours	Yes
Paediatrician 24 hours	Yes
Full Water Birth Service	Yes

Tests

Triple Testing	Yes
Nuchal Fold Scan	Yes
Fetal Assessment Unit	Yes

Pain Relief

24 Hour epidural	Yes
Mobile epidural	No
Pethidine injections	Yes
Water (eg bath)	Yes

Intervention Rates

	%	regional average	national average
Epidural	39	30	33
Elective Caesarean	9	8	8
Emergency Caesarean	16	13	12
Induction	13	18	20
Forceps	4	4	4
Ventouse	9	7	7
Episiotomy	-	16	14

Southampton · **Wessex Maternity Centre**

Mansbridge Road, West End,
Southampton, SO18 3HW
Tel: 02380 464721
Fax: 02380 470735

Private Hospital

At the Wessex, every mother is guaranteed two known midwives throughout her pregnancy. One of these will be there through labour and birth. The unit's midwives work together with your GP to deliver care.

The unit consists of two delivery rooms and six postnatal rooms complete with ensuite bathrooms, double beds and televisions. These rooms offer a high level of comfort with midwifery staff on hand to offer support in the early postnatal period, and some women transfer to them after giving birth at home or at a nearby consultant unit such as the Princess Anne Hospital. Because all of the unit's accommodation is single rooms, partners are allowed to stay.

Antenatal tests such as the triple test and nuchal fold scans are not offered through this service, but may be available as part of your NHS care.

Midwife Unit

Number of beds	8
Births	86
Midwives	5
Home births	8%
Amenity Rooms, Price	-

Obstetrician 24 hours	No
Paediatrician 24 hours	No
Full Water Birth Service	Yes

Tests

Routine Triple Testing	No
Nuchal Fold Scan	No
Fetal Assessment Unit	Yes

Pain Relief

24 hour epidural	No
Mobile epidural	No
Pethidine injections	Yes
Water (eg bath)	Yes

Midwife-led units are adequately equipped to care for women whose pregnancy is progressing normally without complications. As a result, intervention tends to be low in these units. Basic pain relief will be offered, but any woman requesting an epidural during the delivery will need to be transferred to the nearest consultant-led unit. A woman will also be transferred to the obstetric unit if any complications develop during the delivery.

Wallingford · **Wallingford Community Hospital**

Reading Road, Wallingford
Oxfordshire, OX10 9DU
Phone: 01491 698500
Fax: 01491 826602

Trust: Oxford Radcliffe Hospitals
NHS Trust

This maternity unit has a relaxed atmosphere and a non-interventionist approach to childbirth. Active birth is promoted and upright, alternative positions encouraged, as well as using the pool, rocking chair, beanbag or mattresses. Soft lighting and music also enhance the environment. Pain relief is available in the form of aromatherapy, TENS, gas and air and pethidine. There is no epidural service. Almost one in five women who are attached to this unit choose to give birth at home. There is also a full water birth service.

Not all pregnancy tests are available at Wallingford; for triple testing or nuchal fold scans, you will need to get the tests done privately at the John Radcliffe Hospital.

Midwife Unit

Number of beds	4
Births	212
Midwives	6
Home births	16%
Amenity Rooms, Price	-

Obstetrician 24 hours	No
Paediatrician 24 hours	No
Full Water Birth Service	Yes

Tests

Routine Triple Testing	No
Nuchal Fold Scan	No
Fetal Assessment Unit	No

Pain Relief

24 Hour epidural	No
Mobile epidural	No
Pethidine injections	Yes
Water (eg bath)	Yes

Midwife-led units are adequately equipped to care for women whose pregnancy is progressing normally without complications. As a result, intervention tends to be low in these units. Basic pain relief will be offered, but any woman requesting an epidural during the delivery will need to be transferred to the nearest consultant-led unit. A woman will also be transferred to the obstetric unit if any complications develop during the delivery.

Wantage · **Wantage Community Hospital**

Garston Lane, Wantage
Oxfordshire, OX12 7AS
Phone: 01235 403801
Fax: 01235 205 822

Trust: Oxford Radcliffe Hospitals
   NHS Trust

This maternity unit is run by a small team of midwives offering family-centred, one-to-one care within a friendly and safe environment. If a baby needs assistance at birth, the midwives are trained to use the resuscitation equipment in the unit. Any women with complications will be transferred to the John Radcliffe Maternity Unit.

Antenatal classes include aquanatal and women-only sessions. Antental scans are not always routinely offered; for example, nuchal fold scans are not available, and triple testing is only available privately.

Although there is no epidural service a variety of pain relief can be given including aromatherapy and Meptid - a painkiller which does not affect a baby's breathing in the way pethidine might.

Midwife Unit

Number of beds	3
Births	73
Midwives	4
Home births	14%
Amenity Rooms, Price	-
Obstetrician 24 hours	No
Paediatrician 24 hours	No
Full Water Birth Service	

Tests

Routine Triple Testing	No
Nuchal Fold Scan	No
Fetal Assessment Unit	No

Pain Relief

24 Hour epidural	No
Mobile epidural	No
Pethidine injections	No
Water (eg bath)	Yes

Midwife-led units are adequately equipped to care for women whose pregnancy is progressing normally without complications. As a result, intervention tends to be low in these units. Basic pain relief will be offered, but any woman requesting an epidural during the delivery will need to be transferred to the nearest consultant-led unit. A woman will also be transferred to the obstetric unit if any complications develop during the delivery.

Winchester · **Royal Hampshire County Hospital**

Romsey Rd, Winchester
Hampshire, SO22 5DG
Phone: 01962 863535
Fax: 01962 824 228

Trust: Winchester and Eastleigh
Healthcare NHS Trust

Care in this unit is shared between obstetric and midwifery services. It seems to favour a less interventionist approach with a relativley low caesarean and induction rate. Home births are offered and the home birth rate is better than at most large hospitals. Domino deliveries are also offered. However as with many units in the South East midwife staffing levels are stretched with 40 births per year for every midwife.

Antenatal classes include aquanatal for women only, and active birth classes are held in the evenings. There are full water birth facilities. Nuchal scans are not offered here, and triple testing is only available privately for a fee. However amniocentesis can be arranged at 14 weeks.

Consultant and Midwife Unit

Number of beds	45
Births per midwife	40
Births per bed	0.85
Home births	3%
Amenity Rooms, Price	£42

Obstetrician 24 hours	Yes
Paediatrician 24 hours	Yes
Full Water Birth Service	Yes

Tests

Routine Triple Testing	No
Nuchal Fold Scan	No
Fetal Assessment Unit	Yes

Pain Relief

24 hour epidural	Yes
Mobile epidural	No
Pethidine injections	Yes
Water (eg bath)	Yes

Intervention Rates	%	regional average	national average
Epidural	-	30	33
Elective Caesarean	8	8	8
Emergency Caesarean	10	13	12
Induction	17	18	20
Forceps	6	4	4
Ventouse	6	7	7
Episiotomy	15	16	14

Worthing · **Worthing Hospital**

Lyndhurst Road, Worthing
West Sussex, BN43 6TQ
Phone: 01903 205111
Fax: 01273 463 690

Trust: Worthing and Southlands
Hospitals NHS Trust

The unit can offer both midwife-led care for low-risk pregnancies, and shared consultant care for those with high-risk pregnancies. The unit offers home births, and water birth facilities have recently been refurbished. Amenity rooms are sometimes available.

Intervention rates are broadly average. A fetal day assessment unit has recently been established where women with complicated pregnancies can be admitted for the day and undergo investigations and surveillance of their pregnancy. A full range of antenatal tests are available, including nuchal fold scans which are used to screen for Down's. The unit's team of midwives work in the hospital and outside, in local clinics and your home. They are available to offer support and advice 24hrs a day.

Consultant and Midwife Unit

Number of beds	41
Births per midwife	35
Births per bed	0.69
Home births	2%
Amenity Rooms, Price	-

Obstetrician 24 hours	Yes
Paediatrician 24 hours	Yes
Full Water Birth Service	Yes

Tests

Routine Triple Testing	Yes
Nuchal Fold Scan	Yes
Fetal Assessment Unit	Yes

Pain Relief

24 hour epidural	Yes
Mobile epidural	No
Pethidine injections	Yes
Water (eg bath)	Yes

Intervention Rates

	%	regional average	national average
Epidural	34	30	33
Elective Caesarean	8	8	8
Emergency Caesarean	12	13	12
Induction	21	18	20
Forceps	3	4	4
Ventouse	7	7	7
Episiotomy	-	16	14

The Southwest

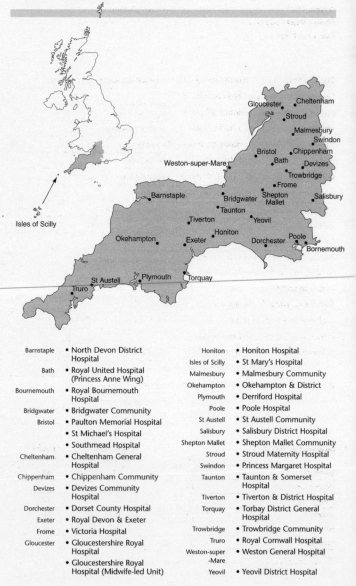

Barnstaple	• North Devon District Hospital	Honiton	• Honiton Hospital
Bath	• Royal United Hospital (Princess Anne Wing)	Isles of Scilly	• St Mary's Hospital
		Malmesbury	• Malmesbury Community
Bournemouth	• Royal Bournemouth Hospital	Okehampton	• Okehampton & District
		Plymouth	• Derriford Hospital
Bridgwater	• Bridgwater Community	Poole	• Poole Hospital
Bristol	• Paulton Memorial Hospital	St Austell	• St Austell Community
	• St Michael's Hospital	Salisbury	• Salisbury District Hospital
	• Southmead Hospital	Shepton Mallet	• Shepton Mallet Community
Cheltenham	• Cheltenham General Hospital	Stroud	• Stroud Maternity Hospital
		Swindon	• Princess Margaret Hospital
Chippenham	• Chippenham Community	Taunton	• Taunton & Somerset Hospital
Devizes	• Devizes Community Hospital		
		Tiverton	• Tiverton & District Hospital
Dorchester	• Dorset County Hospital	Torquay	• Torbay District General Hospital
Exeter	• Royal Devon & Exeter		
Frome	• Victoria Hospital	Trowbridge	• Trowbridge Community
Gloucester	• Gloucestershire Royal Hospital	Truro	• Royal Cornwall Hospital
		Weston-super-Mare	• Weston General Hospital
	• Gloucestershire Royal Hospital (Midwife-led Unit)	Yeovil	• Yeovil District Hospital

Barnstaple · **North Devon District Hospital**

Raleigh Park, Barnstaple
Devon, EX31 4JB
Phone: 01271 322 577
Fax: 01271 311 541

Trust: Northern Devon Healthcare
NHS Trust

The maternity unit at North Devon District Hospital is a shared consultant midwife led unit, with almost 90 per cent of women having a midwife as their lead professional. However, more than half of the births at the unit occur with intervention. The unit has a day assessment unit, which reduces inpatient delays for tests and scans. Ultrasound scanning and screening tests such as triple tests are routinely offered to women. You can be referred for a nuchal fold scans if you need one. The unit's home birth rate is high and rising. Water births are also available and midwives are increasingly able to offer domino deliveries to women who request it. Intervention rates are broadly average althought you are less likely to be induced here than elsewhere.

Consultant and Midwife Unit

Number of beds	30
Births per midwife	30
Births per bed	0.46
Home births	4%
Amenity Rooms, Price	£35

Obstetrician 24 hours	No
Paediatrician 24 hours	No
Water Birth Offered	Yes

Tests

Routine Triple Testing	Yes
Nuchal Fold Scan	Yes
Fetal Assessment Unit	Yes

Pain Relief

24 hour epidural	Yes
Mobile epidural	No
Pethidine injections	Yes
Water (eg bath)	Yes

Intervention Rates	%	regional average %	national average %
Epidural	33	34	33
Elective Caesarean	10	7	8
Emergency Caesarean	13	10	12
Induction	13	19	20
Forceps	3	3	4
Ventouse	7	7	7
Episiotomy	15	12	14

Bath · **Royal United Hospital**

Combe Park, Bath
Somerset, BA1 3NG
Phone: 01225 428 331
Fax: 01225 824 395

Trust: Royal United Hospital Bath
 NHS Trust

The maternity unit at the Royal United Hospital is one of the largest in the country and one of the most unusual. It works jointly with local midwife led units around Bath to offer women a real choice. Consultant-led care at the main hospital is available for women who want epidurals or who have more complex pregnancies. Midwife teams also work from GP surgeries around Bath to give a midwife-led service to women who would prefer this. These teams are also very experienced in home births and domino births. Water births can be done, but you will need to bring your own pool. Intervention rates are low. Antenatal classes are arranged for evenings and weekends and there are strong postnatal support services to help with issues such as breastfeeding or post-natal depression.

Consultant and Midwife Unit

Number of beds	44
Births per midwife	33
Births per bed	1.06
Home births	3%
Amenity Rooms, Price	-

Obstetrician 24 hours	Yes
Paediatrician 24 hours	Yes
Water Birth Offered	Yes

Tests

Routine Triple Testing	No
Nuchal Fold Scan	No
Fetal Assessment Unit	No

Pain Relief

24 hour epidural	Yes
Mobile epidural	Yes
Pethidine injections	Yes
Water (eg bath)	Yes

Intervention Rates

	%	regional average %	national average %
Epidural	17	34	33
Elective Caesarean	-	7	8
Emergency Caesarean	-	10	12
Induction	16	19	20
Forceps	3	3	4
Ventouse	8	7	7
Episiotomy	-	12	14

Bournemouth · **Royal Bournemouth Hospital**

Castle Lane East, Bournemouth
Dorset, BH7 7DW
Phone: 01202 303 626
Fax: 01202 704 077

Trust: Royal Bournemouth and
Christchurch Hospitals NHS Trust

This is a midwife led unit that is geared up only for natural deliveries. There are obstetricians working in the hospital and occassionally ceaseareans are performed in an emergency. But in general, you would be transferred to Poole if you required a caesarean delivery or other medical interventions. Domino system deliveries are offered and most women get looked after in labour by a midwife they know. Water births are also done. The low-tech nature of the unit means that water, intramuscular opiate injection (pethadine), TENS machines and entonox (gas & air) are the only methods of pain relief available during labour. There is no epidural service.

If you want a home birth, the unit is well-experienced in providing this service.

Midwife Unit

Number of beds	20
Births per midwife	18
Births per bed	0.57
Home births	9%
Amenity Rooms, Price	30

Obstetrician 24 hours	Yes
Paediatrician 24 hours	No
Water Birth Offered	Yes

Tests

Routine Triple Testing	No
Nuchal Fold Scan	Yes
Fetal Assessment Unit	Yes

Pain Relief

24 Hour epidural	No
Mobile epidural	No
Pethidine injections	Yes
Water (eg bath)	Yes

Intervention Rates	%	regional average %	national average %
Epidural	0	34	33
Elective Caesarean	0	7	8
Emergency Caesarean	1	10	12
Induction	4	19	20
Forceps	2	3	4
Ventouse	1	7	7
Episiotomy	6	12	14

Bridgwater · **Bridgwater Community Hospital**

Salmon Parade, Bridgwater
Somerset, TA6 5AH
Phone: 01278 451 501
Fax: 01278 444 896

Trust: Taunton and Somerset
NHS Trust

The maternity service at Bridgwater Community Hospital is based around a single delivery bed on the Mary Stanley Wing. The service is midwife-led and around one fifth of the midwives' workload is made up of home births so you they should be well set up to support you if you want a home birth. Waterbirths are not offered at the unit, but if you want to have a water birth at home, a midwife trained in this would be available.

Routine triple testing for Down's syndrome is not offered, but double testing is available. Those requiring nuchal fold scans will need to be referred to Bristol. Because numbers using the service are small, antenatal care is personalised and flexible. Antenatal classes are held in the evenings and on weekdays and can be arranged at weekends for defined groups.

Midwife Unit	
Number of beds	8
Births	98
Midwives	5
Home births	18
Amenity Rooms, Price	–
Obstetrician 24 hours	No
Paediatrician 24 hours	No
Water Birth Offered	No

Tests	
Routine Triple Testing	No
Nuchal Fold Scan	Yes
Fetal Assessment Unit	Yes

Pain Relief	
24 Hour epidural	No
Mobile epidural	No
Pethidine injections	Yes
Water (eg bath)	Yes

Midwife-led units are adequately equipped to care for women whose pregnancy is progressing normally without complications. As a result, intervention tends to be low in these units. Basic pain relief will be offered, but any woman requesting an epidural during the delivery will need to be transferred to the nearest consultant-led unit. A woman will also be transferred to the obstetric unit if any complications develop during the delivery.

Bristol · **Paulton Memorial Hospital**

Salisbury Road, Paulton
Bristol, BS39 7SB
Phone: 01761 412315
Fax: 01761 408117

Trust: Wiltshire and Swindon
Healthcare NHS Trust

The maternity unit at Paulton Memorial Hospital is a small midwife-led unit, catering for women with uncomplicated pregnancies.

Women can choose to deliver in the hospital or at home, and the service carries out a higher than usual proportion of home births. Evening antenatal classes are available and weekend classes are planned for the near future. A full water birth service is also offered, as is a range of pain management options, including a TENS machine.

Triple testing is not routinely offered. The unit does not offer epidurals. Those requiring them, or women with more complex pregnancies, are referred to Bath or Bristol.

Midwife Unit

Number of beds	9
Births	151
Midwives	5
Home births	5%
Amenity Rooms, Price	-
Obstetrician 24 hours	No
Paediatrician 24 hours	No
Water Birth Offered	Yes

Tests

Routine Triple Testing	No
Nuchal Fold Scan	No
Fetal Assessment Unit	No

Pain Relief

24 Hour epidural	No
Mobile epidural	No
Pethidine injections	Yes
Water (eg bath)	Yes

Midwife-led units are adequately equipped to care for women whose pregnancy is progressing normally without complications. As a result, intervention tends to be low in these units. Basic pain relief will be offered, but any woman requesting an epidural during the delivery will need to be transferred to the nearest consultant-led unit. A woman will also be transferred to the obstetric unit if any complications develop during the delivery.

Bristol · **St Michael's Hospital**

Southwell St
Bristol, BS2 8EG
Phone: 0117 921 5411

Trust: United Bristol Healthcare
NHS Trust

St Michael's provides a regional referral centre to deal with higher risk pregnancies, but for the local population there is also a midwife-led service that manages to achieve a better than average home birth rate. You may be offered midwifery care under the domino system here, and midwives can help you to have a water birth at home, although you will need to organise your own pool.

The unit runs classes throughout the week, and includes a twins and multiple births session.

Testing is fairly comprehensive, although you will not necessarily be offered a booking scan, so ask if you would like one. Intervention rates are average, but inductions are noticeably more frequent here than at other units. Epidurals, in contrast, are less common.

Consultant and Midwife Unit

Number of beds	71
Births per midwife	34
Births per bed	1.00
Home births	3%
Amenity Rooms, Price	£50

Obstetrician 24 hours	Yes
Paediatrician 24 hours	Yes
Water Birth Offered	Yes

Tests

Routine Triple Testing	Yes
Nuchal Fold Scan	Yes
Fetal Assessment Unit	Yes

Pain Relief

24 hour epidural	Yes
Mobile epidural	Yes
Pethidine injections	Yes
Water (eg bath)	Yes

Intervention Rates	%	regional average %	national average %
Epidural	24	34	33
Elective Caesarean	9	7	8
Emergency Caesarean	11	10	12
Induction	26	19	20
Forceps	3	3	4
Ventouse	10	7	7
Episiotomy	13	12	14

Bristol · **Southmead Hospital**

Westbury on Trym
Bristol, BS10 5NB
Phone: 0117 950 5050
Fax: 0117 959 0902

Trust: North Bristol
NHS Trust

Women without complications in pregnancy are offered shared care with the midwife and GP. For women experiencing complications in pregnancy, or those who have had previous medical or obstetric problems, care is shared with a consultant obstetrician, midwife, and GPs. There is a team of hospital based midwives to support these women.

Most women are cared for by a team of 6-7 midwives who provide care throughout pregnancy and labour. A group practice midwifery scheme is currently being piloted which offers women the same midwife throughout pregnancy and birth. There are midwives trained in water births, but this service is only available if you bring your own pool. Epidurals are offered for pain relief and are used more often here than in most units.

Consultant and Midwife Unit

Number of beds	70
Births per midwife	32
Births per bed	0.93
Home births	4%
Amenity Rooms, Price	£55

Obstetrician 24 hours	Yes
Paediatrician 24 hours	Yes
Full Water Birth Service	No

Tests

Routine Triple Testing	Yes
Nuchal Fold Scan	Yes
Fetal Assessment Unit	Yes

Pain Relief

24 hour epidural	Yes
Mobile epidural	No
Pethidine injections	Yes
Water (eg bath)	Yes

Intervention Rates	%	regional average %	national average %
Epidural	45	34	33
Elective Caesarean	8	7	8
Emergency Caesarean	11	10	12
Induction	21	19	20
Forceps	4	3	4
Ventouse	8	7	7
Episiotomy	14	12	14

Cheltenham · **Cheltenham General Hospital**

Sandford Road, Cheltenham
Gloucestershire, GL53 7AN
Phone: 01242 222 222
Fax: 01242 273 516

Trust: East Gloucestershire
NHS Trust

The St Paul's wing at Cheltenham General Hospital has a Maternity Assessment Centre, a facility that enables women with more complex needs in pregnancy to be monitored more closely without being admitted to the hospital. There are two wards for ante- and post-natal care made up of four-bedded bays with their own toilet and bath/shower. Adjacent to the delivery unit is the Special Care Baby Unit. Staff in the maternity unit includes five consultant obstetricians, anaesthetists, paediatricians and specially trained physiotherapists. Booking scans are done at 15 weeks rather than 12 and women are not routinely offered the triple test to screen for Down's syndrome. Nuchal fold scans are not available unless you are willing to pay to have it done privately.

Consultant and Midwife Unit

Number of beds	42
Births per midwife	36
Births per bed	0.88
Home births	2%
Amenity Rooms, Price	-
Obstetrician 24 hours	Yes
Paediatrician 24 hours	Yes
Full Water Birth Service	No

Tests

Routine Triple Testing	No
Nuchal Fold Scan	No
Fetal Assessment Unit	Yes

Pain Relief

24 hour epidural	Yes
Mobile epidural	No
Pethidine injections	Yes
Water (eg bath)	Yes

Intervention Rates

	%	regional average %	national average %
Epidural	32	34	33
Elective Caesarean	7	7	8
Emergency Caesarean	14	10	12
Induction	24	19	20
Forceps	4	3	4
Ventouse	11	7	7
Episiotomy	15	12	14

Chippenham · **Chippenham Community Hospital**

Rawden Hill, Chippenham
Wiltshire, SN15 2AJ
Phone: 01249 447100
Fax: 01249 444511

Trust: Wiltshire and Swindon
  Healthcare NHS Trust

Chippenham Hospital has a small, midwife led facility, dealing with about 300 births a year. The unit is low-tech, with virtually all births being spontaneous vaginal deliveries. Epidurals cannot be performed, but water, gas & air and opiate injection are all available as pain relief.

Water birth is offered at the unit, with pools provided and specially trained midwives available 24 hours a day. Home births can also be arranged by the midwives here. Antenatal, postnatal, parent education and breast feeding groups are all available. Weekend sessions are planned in the near future.

Triple testing is not routinely offered, but nuchal fold scans can be arranged.

Midwife Unit

Number of beds	12
Births	282
Midwives	14
Home births	4%
Amenity Rooms, Price	-

Obstetrician 24 hours	No
Paediatrician 24 hours	No
Full Water Birth Service	Yes

Tests

Routine Triple Testing	No
Nuchal Fold Scan	Yes
Fetal Assessment Unit	No

Pain Relief

24 Hour epidural	No
Mobile epidural	No
Pethidine injections	Yes
Water (eg bath)	Yes

Midwife-led units are adequately equipped to care for women whose pregnancy is progressing normally without complications. As a result, intervention tends to be low in these units. Basic pain relief will be offered, but any woman requesting an epidural during the delivery will need to be transferred to the nearest consultant-led unit. A woman will also be transferred to the obstetric unit if any complications develop during the delivery.

Devizes · **Devizes Community Hospital**

Commercial Road, Devizes
Wiltshire, SN10 1EF
Phone: 01380 723511
Fax: 01380 728117

Trust: Wiltshire & Swindon Healthcare
NHS Trust

With 149 births last year and just 9 beds, the maternity service at Devizes Community Hospital is one of the smallest in the country. It works closely with the Royal United Hospital in Bath and provides an environment that encourages natural childbirth for women with low-risk pregnancies. Unlike most midwife-led units, instrumental deliveries are occasionally performed with both ventouse and forceps being used in a small percentage of deliveries. If more serious complications arise you would be transferred to Bath. You may also be referred to Bath for antenatal screening. The unit has a pool and offers water births.

Midwife Unit

Number of beds	8
Births	149
Midwives	7
Home births	3%
Amenity Rooms, Price	-
Obstetrician 24 hours	No
Paediatrician 24 hours	No
Full Water Birth Service	Yes

Tests

Routine Triple Testing	No
Nuchal Fold Scan	No
Fetal Assessment Unit	No

Pain Relief

24 Hour epidural	No
Mobile epidural	No
Pethidine injections	Yes
Water (eg bath)	Yes

Midwife-led units are adequately equipped to care for women whose pregnancy is progressing normally without complications. As a result, intervention tends to be low in these units. Basic pain relief will be offered, but any woman requesting an epidural during the delivery will need to be transferred to the nearest consultant-led unit. A woman will also be transferred to the obstetric unit if any complications develop during the delivery.

Dorchester · **Dorset County Hospital**

Williams Avenue, Dorchester
Dorset, DT1 2JY
Phone: 01305 251 150
Fax: 01305 254 155

Trust: West Dorset General Hospitals
NHS Trust

The maternity unit at Dorset County Hospital has comfortable accomodation with single rooms which are used for labour, delivery, recovery and postnatal care. This avoids you having to be moved to the postnatal ward when you are exhausted after giving birth. The unit offers shared consultant and midwife led care, with consultants caring for high-risk women. The unit is in the unusual position of having a waiting list of midwives who are keen to join. In general, intervention rates are higher than average but the caesarean rate is falling. Deliveries with forceps, however, are rare. The epidural rate is high but this is because they are often used for caesareans rather than pain relief in labour. Water birth is available, though women need to bring their own pool.

Consultant and Midwife Unit

Number of beds	36
Births per midwife	33
Births per bed	0.29
Home births	2%
Amenity Rooms, Price	-

Obstetrician 24 hours	Yes
Paediatrician 24 hours	Yes
Full Water Birth Service	Yes

Tests

Routine Triple Testing	No
Nuchal Fold Scan	Yes
Fetal Assessment Unit	No

Pain Relief

24 hour epidural	Yes
Mobile epidural	No
Pethidine injections	Yes
Water (eg bath)	Yes

Intervention Rates	%	regional average %	national average %
Epidural	40	34	33
Elective Caesarean	11	7	8
Emergency Caesarean	14	10	12
Induction	24	19	20
Forceps	1	3	4
Ventouse	8	7	7
Episiotomy	10	12	14

Exeter · **Royal Devon & Exeter Hospital**

Barrack Road, Wonford, Exeter
Devon, EX2 5DW
Phone: 01392 411 611
Fax: 01392 402 067

Trust: Royal Devon & Exeter Healthcare
NHS Trust

The area around Exeter offers women the choice of midwife led units in Tiverton, Okehampton and Honiton as well as the service offered by the Royal Devon and Exeter hospital, which can handle more complex deliveries. Home births are also well catered for. The home birth rate at the RD&E is more than twice the national average, so you are unlikely to encounter resistance if you want this. Alternatively, you can opt for a domino delivery, where the midwife who looks after you antenatally can care for you in labour and deliver you. Intervention rates are very much average for a large hospital.

Epidurals are offered and used more often than average. However, mobile epidurals are not offered. There is also a full antenatal testing service for those who need it.

Consultant and Midwife Unit

Number of beds	63
Births per midwife	37
Births per bed	1.47
Home births	5%
Amenity Rooms, Price	£40

Obstetrician 24 hours	Yes
Paediatrician 24 hours	Yes
Full Water Birth Service	Yes

Tests

Routine Triple Testing	No
Nuchal Fold Scan	Yes
Fetal Assessment Unit	Yes

Pain Relief

24 hour epidural	Yes
Mobile epidural	No
Pethidine injections	Yes
Water (eg bath)	Yes

Intervention Rates

	%	regional average %	national average %
Epidural	39	34	33
Elective Caesarean	9	7	8
Emergency Caesarean	11	10	12
Induction	19	19	20
Forceps	3	3	4
Ventouse	9	7	7
Episiotomy	4	12	14

Frome · **Victoria Hospital**

Park Road, Frome
Somerset, BA11 1EY
Phone: 01373 463591
Fax: 01373 462345

Trust: Wiltshire and Swindon
Healthcare NHS Trust

The Victoria Hospital in Frome is a small, midwife-led unit but does have full water birth facilities. It is one of a number of midwife led units around Bath that offer women with low-risk pregnancies a choice of home birth with local midwives in attendance or natural delivery in a local unit rather than the more usual option of giving birth in the Princess Anne Wing of the Royal United Hosital. Antenatal education sessions are currently offered during the daytime and in the evenings, and the unit plans to introduce weekend sessions in the near future. The triple test is not offered to all women, but nuchal fold scans are available to those considered at risk. Unusually for a midwife-led service, staff here are trained to conduct ventouse deliveries and a small number of babies are delivered in this way.

Midwife Unit

Number of beds	10
Births	283
Midwives	12
Home births	8%
Amenity Rooms, Price	-

Obstetrician 24 hours	No
Paediatrician 24 hours	No
Full Water Birth Service	Yes

Tests

Routine Triple Testing	No
Nuchal Fold Scan	Yes
Fetal Assessment Unit	No

Pain Relief

24 Hour epidural	No
Mobile epidural	No
Pethidine injections	Yes
Water (eg bath)	Yes

Midwife-led units are adequately equipped to care for women whose pregnancy is progressing normally without complications. As a result, intervention tends to be low in these units. Basic pain relief will be offered, but any woman requesting an epidural during the delivery will need to be transferred to the nearest consultant-led unit. A woman will also be transferred to the obstetric unit if any complications develop during the delivery.

Gloucester · **Royal Hospital**

Great Western Road, Gloucester
Gloucestershire, GL1 3NN
Phone: 01452 528 555
Fax: 01452 394 737

Trust: Gloucestershire Royal
   NHS Trust

The maternity unit at Gloucestershire Royal Hospital is a shared consultant and midwife led unit. There is also a separate midwife led unit within the hospital which is described separately. Low risk women receive the majority of their care at home or in local clinics under the supervision of a midwife and will only be referred to a consultant if complications arise. The unit aims to avoid unnecessary testing and monitoring or restrictions on your freedom of movement during labour. There is a full epidural service, including mobile epidurals that allow greater sensation and movement during labour. Continuity of care is a priority although most women do not end up with a midwife they know looking after them through their labour and delivery. TENS is also offered as a form of pain relief.

Consultant and Midwife Unit

Number of beds	37
Births per midwife	33
Births per bed	0.80
Home births	1%
Amenity Rooms, Price	£45

Obstetrician 24 hours	Yes
Paediatrician 24 hours	Yes
Full Water Birth Service	Yes

Tests

Routine Triple Testing	No
Nuchal Fold Scan	No
Fetal Assessment Unit	Yes

Pain Relief

24 hour epidural	Yes
Mobile epidural	Yes
Pethidine injections	Yes
Water (eg bath)	Yes

Intervention Rates

	%	regional average %	national average %
Epidural	40	34	33
Elective Caesarean	7	7	8
Emergency Caesarean	11	10	12
Induction	19	19	20
Forceps	4	3	4
Ventouse	11	7	7
Episiotomy	18	12	14

Gloucester · **Royal Hospital (Midwife Unit)**

Great Western Road, Gloucester
Goucestershire, GL1 3NN
Phone: 01452 528555
Fax: 01452 394737

Trust: Gloucestershire Royal NHS Trust

The midwifery led service at Gloucestershire Royal Hospital was set up last year to provide care with minimal intervention for low-risk women. The small unit, based in the hospital alongside the larger consultant led unit, is focussed on promoting normal, natural birth and all babies born at the unit are delivered without interventions. The unit actively promotes natural forms of pain relief, but you can also use entonox (gas & air) and pethidine if you wish. Midwives at the unit support home birth and a significant proportion of their work load is home births. If you choose to have your baby at the unit and then run into complications, you can be easily transferred to the nearby consultant-led unit.

Midwife Unit

Number of beds	17
Births	241
Midwives	7
Home births	-
Amenity Rooms, Price	£45

Obstetrician 24 hours	Yes
Paediatrician 24 hours	Yes
Full Water Birth Service	Yes

Tests

Routine Triple Testing	No
Nuchal Fold Scan	No
Fetal Assessment Unit	No

Pain Relief

24 Hour epidural	No
Mobile epidural	No
Pethidine injections	Yes
Water (eg bath)	Yes

Midwife-led units are adequately equipped to care for women whose pregnancy is progressing normally without complications. As a result, intervention tends to be low in these units. Basic pain relief will be offered, but any woman requesting an epidural during the delivery will need to be transferred to the nearest consultant-led unit. A woman will also be transferred to the obstetric unit if any complications develop during the delivery.

Honiton · **Honiton Hospital**

Marlpits Road, Honiton
Devon, EX14 2DE
Phone: 01404 540540
Fax: 01404 540550

Trust: East Devon PCT

The midwifery unit at Honiton Hospital provides care to women with low-risk pregnancies who have no history of obstetric or relevant medical problems. The small midwifery team provides also domino and home births.

All the usual pain relief required for normal labours can be provided, such as water, TENS, entonox and injections of pethidine if needed. Epidurals are not provided but transfer to the Royal Devon & Exeter Heavitree site can easily be arranged for these.

All routine scans are offered at the Axminster Community Hospital or the Heavitree site at Royal Devon & Exeter. Double testing and other routine blood tests are all offered.

The unit also provides a 24hr telephone advice line for all women with worries or problems.

Midwife Unit

Number of beds	9
Births	141
Midwives	8
Home births	5%
Amenity Rooms, Price	32

Obstetrician 24 hours	No
Paediatrician 24 hours	No
Full Water Birth Service	Yes

Tests

Routine Triple Testing	No
Nuchal Fold Scan	Yes
Fetal Assessment Unit	No

Pain Relief

24 Hour epidural	No
Mobile epidural	No
Pethidine injections	Yes
Water (eg bath)	Yes

Midwife-led units are adequately equipped to care for women whose pregnancy is progressing normally without complications. As a result, intervention tends to be low in these units. Basic pain relief will be offered, but any woman requesting an epidural during the delivery will need to be transferred to the nearest consultant-led unit. A woman will also be transferred to the obstetric unit if any complications develop during the delivery.

Isles of Scilly · **St Mary's Hospital**

Hospital Lane, Isles of Scilly
Cornwall, TR21 0LE
Phone: 01720 422 392
Fax: 01720 422 3134

Trust: West of Cornwall PCT

This is a 14-bed cottage hospital with only two designated maternity beds and one delivery suite. Maternity services are shared by midwives and GPs, and the unit only accepts women for delivery with uncomplicated obstetric histories and pregnancy. For complicated pregnancies or epidurals, they are booked or transferred to the mainland to the Royal Cornwall Hospital in Truro.

Antenatal classes are available on a one-to-one basis, and scans are only available at Royal Cornwall or West Cornwall hospitals. Triple testing and nuchal fold scans are available, but there is a charge for these.

As the unit deals with very small numbers, the women receive individualised postnatal care for up to 28 days.

Midwife Unit

Number of beds	2
Births	11
Midwives	3
Home births	0%
Amenity Rooms, Price	-

Obstetrician 24 hours	No
Paediatrician 24 hours	No
Full Water Birth Service	

Tests

Routine Triple Testing	No
Nuchal Fold Scan	No
Fetal Assessment Unit	Yes

Pain Relief

24 Hour epidural	No
Mobile epidural	No
Pethidine injections	Yes
Water (eg bath)	Yes

Midwife-led units are adequately equipped to care for women whose pregnancy is progressing normally without complications. As a result, intervention tends to be low in these units. Basic pain relief will be offered, but any woman requesting an epidural during the delivery will need to be transferred to the nearest consultant-led unit. A woman will also be transferred to the obstetric unit if any complications develop during the delivery.

Malmesbury · **Malmesbury Community Hospital**

Burton Hill, Malmesbury
Wiltshire, SN16 0EQ
Phone: 01666 823358
Fax: 01666 825026

Trust: Wiltshire & Swindon Healthcare
NHS Trust

Malmesbury Community Hospital has a small maternity unit with six beds. It delivered 132 babies last year in the hospital. This is a low-tech unit not designed to deal with complex births and as a result interventions do not in general happen although forceps and ventouse are each used in less than 1 per cent of deliveries. The nature of the unit also means it does not offer epidurals. However, other pain relief methods such as gas & air are available for use in labour. The small team of midwives should be able to ensure good continuity of care. You will usually be transferred to Bath if complications arise during your pregnancy or labour.

Midwife Unit

Number of beds	5
Births	132
Midwives	8
Home births	1%
Amenity Rooms, Price	-
Obstetrician 24 hours	No
Paediatrician 24 hours	No
Full Water Birth Service	Yes

Tests

Routine Triple Testing	No
Nuchal Fold Scan	No
Fetal Assessment Unit	No

Pain Relief

24 Hour epidural	No
Mobile epidural	No
Pethidine injections	Yes
Water (eg bath)	Yes

Midwife-led units are adequately equipped to care for women whose pregnancy is progressing normally without complications. As a result, intervention tends to be low in these units. Basic pain relief will be offered, but any woman requesting an epidural during the delivery will need to be transferred to the nearest consultant-led unit. A woman will also be transferred to the obstetric unit if any complications develop during the delivery.

Okehampton · **Okehampton & District Hospital**

East Street, Okehampton
Devon, EX20 1AX
Phone: 01837 52188
Fax: 01837 55507

Trust: Mid Devon PCT

This small maternity unit shares antenatal care with GPs, although it is mostly run by midwives who work in teams. You will be looked after by a team of midwives who you should get to know through your pregnancy, one of whom ideally will deliver your baby. If you want a home birth, Okehampton has midwives who have experience of supervising these. You can have a water birth if you want one – there are midwives trained in water births on hand 24 hours a day. However there is not pool at the unit, so you will have to bring your own. Classes are held in the evenings, but no longer during the daytime due to lack of interest. Midwives give support and advice in the early antenatal period (up to 12 weeks) and refer women when necessary to the early pregnancy assessment service.

Midwife Unit

Number of beds	4
Births	61
Midwives	5
Home births	5%
Amenity Rooms, Price	-
Obstetrician 24 hours	No
Paediatrician 24 hours	No
Full Water Birth Service	No

Tests

Routine Triple Testing	No
Nuchal Fold Scan	Yes
Fetal Assessment Unit	Yes

Pain Relief

24 Hour epidural	No
Mobile epidural	No
Pethidine injections	Yes
Water (eg bath)	Yes

Midwife-led units are adequately equipped to care for women whose pregnancy is progressing normally without complications. As a result, intervention tends to be low in these units. Basic pain relief will be offered, but any woman requesting an epidural during the delivery will need to be transferred to the nearest consultant-led unit. A woman will also be transferred to the obstetric unit if any complications develop during the delivery.

Plymouth · **Derriford Hospital**

Derriford Road, Plymouth
Devon, PL6 8DH
Phone: 01752 777 111
Fax: 01752 768 976

Trust: Plymouth Hospitals
NHS Trust

The unit situated in a modern, purpose built block at Derriford Hospital. Staffing levels are good. The pattern of interventions is unusual. Caesarean rates are low – in particular the emergency caesarean rate. You are more likely to be delivered by ventouse than have an emergency caesarean. There is the full range of medical services and epidurals for pain relief are more common than in most hospitals.

Acupuncture is offered by three qualified acupuncture midwives for antenatal and postnatal problems although availability may be limited. There is a neonatal intensive care unit and a transitional care ward where babies that need medical supervision can remain with their mothers.

Consultant and Midwife Unit

Number of beds	69
Births per midwife	29
Births per bed	0.93
Home births	3%
Amenity Rooms, Price	£25

Obstetrician 24 hours	Yes
Paediatrician 24 hours	Yes
Full Water Birth Service	Yes

Tests

Routine Triple Testing	No
Nuchal Fold Scan	Yes
Fetal Assessment Unit	Yes

Pain Relief

24 hour epidural	Yes
Mobile epidural	No
Pethidine injections	Yes
Water (eg bath)	Yes

Intervention Rates

	%	regional average %	national average %
Epidural	46	34	33
Elective Caesarean	6	7	8
Emergency Caesarean	7	10	12
Induction		19	20
Forceps	4	3	4
Ventouse	10	7	7
Episiotomy	18	12	14

Poole · **Poole Hospital**

Longfleet Road, Poole
Dorset, BH15 2JB
Phone: 01202 665 511
Fax: 01202 442 562

Trust: Poole Hospitals
NHS Trust

This large maternity unit offers a comprehensive range of services, from low-risk midwife-led care, including home birth, to consultant-led care for higher-risk deliveries. There is a neonatal intensive care unit at the hospital.

The hospital has a policy of letting your partner stay if you have to go into hospital before your labour starts. Antenatal classes are run for women only, and young mothers. Midwives are organised into teams, which means you will be cared for by a group of midwives through your pregnancy, and ideally one of the team will look after you in labour. However in practice you are more likely to be looked after in labour by someone new. The midwives here have a higher than average workload to deal with.

Consultant and Midwife Unit

Number of beds	59
Births per midwife	40
Births per bed	0.73
Home births	2%
Amenity Rooms, Price	£38

Obstetrician 24 hours	Yes
Paediatrician 24 hours	Yes
Full Water Birth Service	Yes

Tests

Routine Triple Testing	No
Nuchal Fold Scan	Yes
Fetal Assessment Unit	Yes

Pain Relief

24 hour epidural	Yes
Mobile epidural	Yes
Pethidine injections	Yes
Water (eg bath)	Yes

Intervention Rates	%	regional average %	national average %
Epidural	38	34	33
Elective Caesarean	10	7	8
Emergency Caesarean	14	10	12
Induction	19	19	20
Forceps	3	3	4
Ventouse	0	7	7
Episiotomy	11	12	14

St Austell · **St Austell Community Hospital**

Porthpean Road
St Austell
Cornwall, PL26 6AA
Phone: 01726 291 100
Fax: 01726 291 140

Trust: Cornwall Healthcare
NHS Trust

This midwife-led unit has two delivery rooms, one with a birthing pool, which has calming lighting and en suite facilities. Twin bedded rooms will be developed in the near future. The pool can be used for pain relief as well as water births. Not all the midwives are experienced in conducting water births at the present time but the unit is working towards this. There is a four-bedded postnatal room for mothers and babies and a day room with a dining area. The unit estimates that about half of women are cared for in labour by a midwife they already know. Partners can stay if you come into the hospital before your labour begins. Parentcraft classes include yoga sessions. You will be referred for any scans and tests you may need to Royal Cornwall Hospital in Truro. The unit is open for tours on any Sunday at 3pm but phone first.

Midwife Unit

Number of beds	4
Births	187
Midwives	18
Home births	7%
Amenity Rooms, Price	-

Obstetrician 24 hours	No
Paediatrician 24 hours	No
Full Water Birth Service	No

Tests

Routine Triple Testing	Yes
Nuchal Fold Scan	Yes
Fetal Assessment Unit	Yes

Pain Relief

24 Hour epidural	No
Mobile epidural	No
Pethidine injections	Yes
Water (eg bath)	Yes

Midwife-led units are adequately equipped to care for women whose pregnancy is progressing normally without complications. As a result, intervention tends to be low in these units. Basic pain relief will be offered, but any woman requesting an epidural during the delivery will need to be transferred to the nearest consultant-led unit. A woman will also be transferred to the obstetric unit if any complications develop during the delivery.

Salisbury · **Salisbury District Hospital**

Salisbury
Wiltshire, SP2 8BJ
Phone: 01722 336 262
Fax: 01722 330 221

Trust: Salisbury District
NHS Trust

This hospital has a shared midwife and consultant-led maternity unit, with midwife groups linked to GP practices. Domino system care is provided, where a midwife will provide your antenatal care at your home or GP surgery and then also look after you in hospital through your labour. You will be offered advice on different antenatal screening tests, however nuchal scans are only available privately for a fee. You receive a home visit from your named midwife at around 34 weeks who will discuss your birth plan and pain management during labour. Midwives at the unit put an emphasis on advising on breast feeding and other aspects of your baby's wellbeing. Support is also organised for women who are at risk of post-natal depresssion.

Consultant and Midwife Unit

Number of beds	29
Births per midwife	30
Births per bed	0.77
Home births	3%
Amenity Rooms, Price	-

Obstetrician 24 hours	Yes
Paediatrician 24 hours	Yes
Full Water Birth Service	Yes

Tests

Routine Triple Testing	Yes
Nuchal Fold Scan	No
Fetal Assessment Unit	No

Pain Relief

24 hour epidural	Yes
Mobile epidural	No
Pethidine injections	Yes
Water (eg bath)	Yes

Intervention Rates	%	regional average %	national average %
Epidural	37	34	33
Elective Caesarean	7	7	8
Emergency Caesarean	12	10	12
Induction	18	19	20
Forceps	5	3	4
Ventouse	7	7	7
Episiotomy	-	12	14

Shepton Mallet · **Shepton Mallet Community Hospital**

Old Wells Road, Shepton Mallet
Somerset, BA4 4PG
Phone: 01749 342931

Trust: Wiltshire and Swindon
Healthcare NHS Trust

The maternity unit is small, delivering 105 births last year and provides a friendlier environment for women with low-risk pregancies wanting to give birth naturally. For pain relief in labour there is water, gas & air, and intramuscular opiate injections.

Parent education sessions and antenatal classes run in the evenings and during the daytime, with weekend classes to start in the near future.

There is an antenatal helpline as well as a postnatal helpline and breastfeeding helpline all able to offer support and advice to mothers. In addition, there is a breastfeeding clinic and access to breastfeeding counsellors.

Midwife Unit

Number of beds	6
Births	105
Midwives	9
Home births	2%
Amenity Rooms, Price	-
Obstetrician 24 hours	No
Paediatrician 24 hours	No
Full Water Birth Service	Yes

Tests

Routine Triple Testing	No
Nuchal Fold Scan	No
Fetal Assessment Unit	No

Pain Relief

24 Hour epidural	No
Mobile epidural	No
Pethidine injections	Yes
Water (eg bath)	Yes

Midwife-led units are adequately equipped to care for women whose pregnancy is progressing normally without complications. As a result, intervention tends to be low in these units. Basic pain relief will be offered, but any woman requesting an epidural during the delivery will need to be transferred to the nearest consultant-led unit. A woman will also be transferred to the obstetric unit if any complications develop during the delivery.

Stroud · **Stroud Maternity Hospital**

Field Road, Stroud
Gloucestershire, GL5 2JB
Phone: 01453 562 140
Fax: 01453 562 141

Trust: Severn NHS Trust

Stroud Maternity Hospital is a small midwife-led unit open to women with uncomplicated pregnancies who are able to have their babies in a low-tech environment. It is a small unit, with only two delivery beds, nine postnatal beds and a birthing pool. It is suitable if you wish to give birth with a minimum amount of intervention.

As with most smaller units, there is better continuity of care, with virtually everyone here being cared for in labour by a midwife they know. There is a drop-in service if you have problems during pregnancy. Home births are offered and form a good proportion of the units work. Postnatal support is also offered including a twins club.

Midwife Unit

Number of beds	9
Births	293
Midwives	18
Home births	7%
Amenity Rooms, Price	-

Obstetrician 24 hours	No
Paediatrician 24 hours	No
Full Water Birth Service	Yes

Tests

Routine Triple Testing	No
Nuchal Fold Scan	No
Fetal Assessment Unit	Yes

Pain Relief

24 Hour epidural	No
Mobile epidural	No
Pethidine injections	Yes
Water (eg bath)	Yes

Midwife-led units are adequately equipped to care for women whose pregnancy is progressing normally without complications. As a result, intervention tends to be low in these units. Basic pain relief will be offered, but any woman requesting an epidural during the delivery will need to be transferred to the nearest consultant-led unit. A woman will also be transferred to the obstetric unit if any complications develop during the delivery.

Swindon · **Princess Margaret Hospital**

Okus Road, Swindon
Wiltshire, SN1 4JU
Phone: 01793 536 231
Fax: 01793 480 817

Trust: Swindon and Marlborough
NHS Trust

This is a large shared midwife and consultant unit, which offers relatively few home births and no water birth facilities at all, although the latter will be introduced next year.

Services such as a fetal assessment unit are arranged through the nearby John Radcliffe Hospital, and so is access to support services such as breast feeding counsellors. Talk to your GP or midwife about antental screening if you want this – neither abnormality scans nor even the booking scan are routinely offered. Caesareans are performed here more often than in other hospitals and the induction rate is also high. Partners may stay with you overnight if you go into hospital before your labour starts – single amenity rooms are available to hire for £85.

Consultant and Midwife Unit

Number of beds	48
Births per midwife	36
Births per bed	-
Home births	1%
Amenity Rooms, Price	£85

Obstetrician 24 hours	Yes
Paediatrician 24 hours	Yes
Full Water Birth Service	No

Tests

Routine Triple Testing	No
Nuchal Fold Scan	Yes
Fetal Assessment Unit	No

Pain Relief

24 hour epidural	Yes
Mobile epidural	Yes
Pethidine injections	Yes
Water (eg bath)	Yes

Intervention Rates	%	regional average %	national average %
Epidural	48	34	33
Elective Caesarean	10	7	8
Emergency Caesarean	16	10	12
Induction	28	19	20
Forceps	2	3	4
Ventouse	7	7	7
Episiotomy	23	12	14

Taunton · **Taunton & Somerset Hospital**

Musgrove Park, Taunton
Somerset, TA1 5DA
Phone: 01823 333 444
Fax: 01823 336 877

Trust: Taunton and Somerset
NHS Trust

The unit is the main provider of midwifery services in west Somerset. Midwives are organised into teams covering different areas, and the domino system is offered. The unit is experienced in delivering home births and water births – the home birth rate is more than double the national average. For more high-risk pregnancies, fetal and maternal medicine clinics are on site. An epidural service is available, but is mainly used for planned caesarean sections rather than for general pain relief. Double testing and ultrasound scans are available, but for more complex tests you will be referred to a unit in Bristol. Elective caesareans are done less often than in most hospitals but the rate of emergency caesareans is above average. Induction levels are also high.

Consultant and Midwife Unit

Number of beds	45
Births per midwife	22
Births per bed	0.79
Home births	5
Amenity Rooms, Price	£25

Obstetrician 24 hours	Yes
Paediatrician 24 hours	Yes
Full Water Birth Service	Yes

Tests

Routine Triple Testing	No
Nuchal Fold Scan	Yes
Fetal Assessment Unit	Yes

Pain Relief

24 hour epidural	Yes
Mobile epidural	No
Pethidine injections	Yes
Water (eg bath)	Yes

Intervention Rates

	%	regional average %	national average %
Epidural	31	34	33
Elective Caesarean	6	7	8
Emergency Caesarean	15	10	12
Induction	24	19	20
Forceps	2	3	4
Ventouse	3	7	7
Episiotomy	10	12	14

Tiverton · **Tiverton & District Hospital**

Bampton Road, Tiverton
Devon, EX16 6AN
Phone: 01884 253251
Fax: 01884 242784

Trust: Mid Devon PCT

This small midwife-led unit services women with low-risk pregnancies. It has an ultrasonographer on staff and can perform some tests for high-risk pregnancies, saving you what might otherwise be a trip into Exeter. The unit works closely with the consultant unit at the Royal Devon and Exeter and if complications arise you would normally be referred there. Intervention is negligible, and there is an emphasis on alternative methods of pain relief. The midwifery team includes several aromatherapists and aquanatal exercise teachers. Most midwives work both in the unit and the community and are involved in the home birth service. You can also book into the Tiverton unit for postnatal care after delivering in the district general hospital's in Exeter and Taunton.

Midwife Unit

Number of beds	9
Births	115
Midwives	9
Home births	29%
Amenity Rooms, Price	£32

Obstetrician 24 hours	No
Paediatrician 24 hours	No
Full Water Birth Service	No

Tests

Routine Triple Testing	No
Nuchal Fold Scan	Yes
Fetal Assessment Unit	Yes

Pain Relief

24 Hour epidural	No
Mobile epidural	No
Pethidine injections	Yes
Water (eg bath)	Yes

Midwife-led units are adequately equipped to care for women whose pregnancy is progressing normally without complications. As a result, intervention tends to be low in these units. Basic pain relief will be offered, but any woman requesting an epidural during the delivery will need to be transferred to the nearest consultant-led unit. A woman will also be transferred to the obstetric unit if any complications develop during the delivery.

Torquay · **Torbay District General Hospital**

Lawes Bridge, Torquay
Devon, TQ2 7AA
Phone: 01803 614 567
Fax: 01803 616 334

Trust: South Devon Healthcare
NHS Trust

The unit will be refurbished in the near future to include facilities for women with disabilities, and facilities for fathers and families. The unit organises midwife care to try to ensure good levels of continuity of care. Staffing levels are good and all women are offered one-to-one care in labour. If you want a home birth you can expect good support. This unit has the highest home birth rate in the UK for a large hospital. Intervention rates are broadly average with a higher than average rate of elective caesareans and inductions. The unit is has been successfully reducing its instrumental intervention rates. Nuchal fold scans and other tests may be done on request or will be offered according to set clinical criteria.

Consultant and Midwife Unit

Number of beds	28
Births per midwife	27
Births per bed	0.68
Home births	10%
Amenity Rooms, Price	£65
Obstetrician 24 hours	Yes
Paediatrician 24 hours	Yes
Full Water Birth Service	Yes

Tests

Routine Triple Testing	No
Nuchal Fold Scan	Yes
Fetal Assessment Unit	Yes

Pain Relief

24 hour epidural	Yes
Mobile epidural	No
Pethidine injections	Yes
Water (eg bath)	Yes

Intervention Rates	%	regional average %	national average %
Epidural	33	34	33
Elective Caesarean	10	7	8
Emergency Caesarean	12	10	12
Induction	24	19	20
Forceps	3	3	4
Ventouse	8	7	7
Episiotomy	11	12	14

Trowbridge · **Trowbridge Community Hospital**

Adcroft Street, Trowbridge
Wiltshire, BA14 8PH
Phone: 01225 752558
Fax: 01225 751627

Trust: Wiltshire & Swindon Healthcare
NHS Trust

The maternity unit at Trowbridge Community Hospital provides a local service for women with low-risk pregnancies wanting to give birth naturally.

Many women booked at the unit choose to give birth at home, and the unit has plenty of experience of handling such births.

The unit offers water birth, with its own pool; midwives trained in this sort of delivery are available 24 hours a day.

As this is a low-tech unit, epidurals are not offered but other pain relief methods, such as gas & air, are available during labour.

Midwife Unit

Number of beds	10
Births	383
Midwives	18
Home births	6%
Price of Amenity Rooms	-
Obstetrician 24 hours	No
Paediatrician 24 hours	No
Full Water Birth Service	Yes

Tests

Routine Triple Testing	No
Nuchal Fold Scan	No
Fetal Assessment Unit	No

Pain Relief

24 Hour epidural	No
Mobile epidural	No
Pethidine injections	Yes
Water (eg bath)	Yes

Midwife-led units are adequately equipped to care for women whose pregnancy is progressing normally without complications. As a result, intervention tends to be low in these units. Basic pain relief will be offered, but any woman requesting an epidural during the delivery will need to be transferred to the nearest consultant-led unit. A woman will also be transferred to the obstetric unit if any complications develop during the delivery.

Truro · **Royal Cornwall Hospital**

Truro
Cornwall, TR1 3LJ
Phone: 01872 250 000
Fax: 01872 252 708

Trust: Royal Cornwall Hospitals
NHS Trust

You will recieve most of your care from midwives unless complications mean that you need to see an obstetrician. Consultants will see women outside the hospital in local clinics as well as in the main hospital. For uncomplex pregnancies, the domino system is offered, where the midwife will provide antenatal care for you at your home in your local GP surgery and will then also oversee your delivery in hospital. Home births are done frequently so this is also an option. The caesarean rate is low, an in particular elective caesareans are done less freqently than in most hospitals. However epidurals are available for pain relief and are used much more often than in most hospitals. If you have a breech baby, consultants have experience in turning the baby.

Consultant and Midwife Unit

Number of beds	57
Births per midwife	37
Births per bed	0.82
Home births	5%
Amenity Rooms, Price	£31

Obstetrician 24 hours	Yes
Paediatrician 24 hours	Yes
Full Water Birth Service	No

Tests

Routine Triple Testing	No
Nuchal Fold Scan	Yes
Fetal Assessment Unit	Yes

Pain Relief

24 hour epidural	Yes
Mobile epidural	No
Pethidine injections	Yes
Water (eg bath)	Yes

ntervention Rates	%	regional average %	national average %
Epidural	53	34	33
Elective Caesarean	6	7	8
Emergency Caesarean	10	10	12
Induction	-	19	20
Forceps	-	3	4
Ventouse	-	7	7
Episiotomy	9	12	14

Weston-super-Mare · **Weston General Hospital**

Grange Road, Uphill, Weston-super-Mare
Somerset, BS23 4TQ
Phone: 01934 647082
Fax: 01934 647220

Trust: Weston Area NHS Trust

The Weston maternity service has been midwife-led for five years and around 400 deliveries are undertaken either in the unit or at home. This activity covers both the hospital and the community. However, the unit is housed in a large district general hospital and can provide consultant obstetric care for antenatal and postnatal women.

The unit has a good rate of home births, and in general it estimates that approximately half of all women in labour are seen by a midwife they know. The staffing levels are high, which helps ensure a good level of personal care. Pain relief includes complementary methods such as aromatherapy, but no epidurals are given.

Midwife Unit

Number of beds	15
Births	369
Midwives	31
Home births	6%
Price of Amenity Rooms	£32

Obstetrician 24 hours	No
Paediatrician 24 hours	No
Full Water Birth Service	No

Tests

Routine Triple Testing	No
Nuchal Fold Scan	Yes
Fetal Assessment Unit	No

Pain Relief

24 Hour epidural	No
Mobile epidural	No
Pethidine injections	Yes
Water (eg bath)	Yes

Midwife-led units are adequately equipped to care for women whose pregnancy is progressing normally without complications. As a result, intervention tends to be low in these units. Basic pain relief will be offered, but any woman requesting an epidural during the delivery will need to be transferred to the nearest consultant-led unit. A woman will also be transferred to the obstetric unit if any complications develop during the delivery.

Yeovil · **Yeovil District Hospital**

Higher Kingston, Yeovil
Somerset, BA21 4AT
Phone: 01935 475122
Fax: 01935 426 850

Trust: East Somerset
  NHS Trust

The unit aims to ensure a high number of 'normal' deliveries and that is reflected in relatively low levels of interventions such as caesarean deliveries or use of forceps. About three quarters of women at the unit have spontaneous vaginal delivery. If you prefer – and if your pregnancy is straightforward – you can opt to have a midwife rather than a doctor as your main carer. 40 per cent of women now book under midwife-led care although many of them are delivered under the supervision of a doctor.

If you want a water birth, the hospital will help you, but you will have to bring your own pool. The unit has full medical facilities including a special care baby unit with eight cots which is able to care for babies that do not require full neonatal intensive care.

Consultant and Midwife Unit

Number of beds	32
Births per midwife	26
Births per bed	0.64
Home births	2%
Amenity Rooms, Price	£37

Obstetrician 24 hours	No
Paediatrician 24 hours	Yes
Full Water Birth Service	Yes

Tests

Routine Triple Testing	Yes
Nuchal Fold Scan	Yes
Fetal Assessment Unit	No

Pain Relief

24 hour epidural	Yes
Mobile epidural	No
Pethidine injections	Yes
Water (eg bath)	Yes

Intervention Rates	%	regional average %	national average %
Epidural	29	34	33
Elective Caesarean	8	7	8
Emergency Caesarean	9	10	12
Induction	21	19	20
Forceps	4	3	4
Ventouse	8	7	7
Episiotomy	15	12	14

Trent

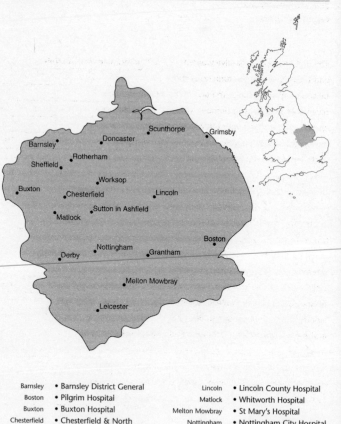

Barnsley	• Barnsley District General	Lincoln	• Lincoln County Hospital
Boston	• Pilgrim Hospital	Matlock	• Whitworth Hospital
Buxton	• Buxton Hospital	Melton Mowbray	• St Mary's Hospital
Chesterfield	• Chesterfield & North Derbyshire Royal Hospital	Nottingham	• Nottingham City Hospital
			• Queen's Medical Center
Derby	• Derby City General Hospital	Rotherham	• Rotherham District General Hospital
Doncaster	• Women's Hospital		
	Doncaster Royal Infirmary	Scunthorpe	• Scunthorpe General Hospital
Grantham	• Grantham & District Hospital	Sheffield	• Royal Hallamshire Hospital (Jessop Wing)
Grimsby	• Grimsby Maternity Hospital		
Leicester	• Leicester General Hospital	Sutton in Ashfield	• King's Mill Hospital
	• Leicester Royal Infirmary	Worksop	• Bassetlaw District General Hospital

Barnsley · **Barnsley District General Hospital**

Gawber Road, Barnsley
South Yorkshire, S75 2EP
Phone: 01226 730000
Fax: 01226 202859

Trust: Barnsley District General
Hospital NHS Trust

The unit attempts to involve women and their families in the running of the unit as much as possible. You are given a 24-hour contact number that allows you to contact your midwife at any time. As far as possible, midwives try to look after women outside the hospital. Higher risk pregnancies are dealt with through daycare clinics which avoid women needing to be admitted to the hospital as an inpatient. Home birth is offered although the number of women delivered at home by this service is still well below the national average. Although a pool is available for use in labour, you will not be able to deliver in the pool. Intervention rates are very much in line with national averages for a large maternity unit although inductions are more common than average.

Consultant and Midwife Unit

Number of beds	39
Births per midwife	25
Births per bed	0.86
Home births	1%
Amenity Rooms, Price	£32

Obstetrician 24 hours	Yes
Paediatrician 24 hours	Yes
Full Water Birth Service	No

Tests

Routine Triple Testing	No
Nuchal Fold Scan	No
Fetal Assessment Unit	Yes

Pain Relief

24 hour epidural	Yes
Mobile epidural	No
Pethidine injections	Yes
Water (eg bath)	Yes

Intervention Rates	%	regional average %	national average %
Epidural	34	31	33
Elective Caesarean	11	9	8
Emergency Caesarean	12	13	12
Induction	23	20	20
Forceps	2	5	4
Ventouse	11	8	7
Episiotomy	-	15	14

Boston · **Pilgrim Hospital**

Sibsey Road, Boston
Lincolnshire, PE21 9QS
Phone: 01205 364801
Fax: 01205 354395

Trust: United Lincolnshire Hospitals
  NHS Trust

Your chances of receiving a high level of personal attention through pregnancy and labour are better at Pilgrim Hospital than at many other units, as midwife staffing levels are significantly above the national average. This can help to reduce stress and increase a woman's ability to manage pain without medical intervention. The epidural rate is marginally below average here. However the emergency caesarean rate is relatively high. Antenatal services include antenatal education sessions held in the evenings and at weekends and women have access to an antenatal support helpline. The triple test is available to all women booked with the service. Women requiring nuchal-fold scans must travel to Queen's Medical Centre in Nottingham.

Consultant and Midwife Unit

Number of beds	40
Births per midwife	21
Births per bed	0.53
Home births	1%
Amenity Rooms, Price	£31

Obstetrician 24 hours	No
Paediatrician 24 hours	Yes
Full Water Birth Service	No

Tests

Routine Triple Testing	Yes
Nuchal Fold Scan	Yes
Fetal Assessment Unit	No

Pain Relief

24 hour epidural	Yes
Mobile epidural	Yes
Pethidine injections	Yes
Water (eg bath)	Yes

Intervention Rates

	%	regional average %	national average %
Epidural	25	31	33
Elective Caesarean	7	9	8
Emergency Caesarean	15	13	12
Induction	14	20	20
Forceps	5	5	4
Ventouse	8	8	7
Episiotomy	4	15	14

Buxton · **Buxton Hospital**

London Road
Buxton, SK17 9NJ
Phone: 01298 22293
Fax: 01298 72653

Trust: Stockport NHS Trust

The Corbar Maternity Unit at Buxton Hospital is a good service to book with if you are considering a homebirth as home births make up a good deal of the unit's workload. The service is midwife-led and has a low-tech approach. For consultant-led care, you should consider the consultant unit at Stepping Hill Hospital.

The unit itself consists of two labour rooms, one of which is fitted with a birthing pool. Water birth is available and done more frequently than in many units. Three-quarters of the women who use the pool for pain relief go on to give birth in the water. A comfortable side room is available where you and your partner can stay in the early stages of labour.

Midwife Unit

Number of beds	8
Births	119
Midwives	14
Home births	14%
Amenity Rooms, Price	-

Obstetrician 24 hours	No
Paediatrician 24 hours	No
Full Water Birth Service	Yes

Tests

Routine Triple Testing	No
Nuchal Fold Scan	No
Fetal Assessment Unit	No

Pain Relief

24 Hour epidural	No
Mobile epidural	No
Pethidine injections	Yes
Water (eg Bath)	Yes

Midwife-led units are adequately equipped to care for women whose pregnancy is progressing normally without complications. As a result, intervention tends to be low in these units. Basic pain relief will be offered, but any woman requesting an epidural during the delivery will need to be transferred to the nearest consultant-led unit. A woman will also be transferred to the obstetric unit if any complications develop during the delivery.

Chesterfield · **Chesterfield & North Derbyshire Royal**

Calow, Chesterfield
Derbyshire, S44 5BL
Phone: 01246 277271
Fax: 01246 276955

Trust: Chesterfield & North Derbyshire
 Royal Hospital NHS

The maternity unit is consultant and midwife-led, and provides a range of alternative services to conventional medical facilities, including aromatherapy, both antenatally and during labour, as well as full water birth facilities. Domino system deliveries are also done. The unit runs active birth classes as well as evening antenatal classes and a debriefing service.

Testing and scanning facilities are fairly comprehensive, although patients requiring CVS are referred to Nottingham. The epidural rate here is significantly above average so you should not have trouble getting an epidural. The caesarean rate is average and forceps are very rarely used.

Consultant and Midwife Unit

Number of beds	47
Births per midwife	31
Births per bed	0.65
Home births	2%
Amenity Rooms, Price	£30
Obstetrician 24 hours	Yes
Paediatrician 24 hours	Yes
Full Water Birth Service	Yes

Tests

Routine Triple Testing	Yes
Nuchal Fold Scan	Yes
Fetal Assessment Unit	Yes

Pain Relief

24 Hour epidural	Yes
Mobile epidural	No
Pethidine injections	Yes
Water (eg Bath)	Yes

Intervention Rates	%	regional average %	national average %
Epidural	47	31	33
Elective Caesarean	7	9	8
Emergency Caesarean	14	13	12
Induction	-	20	20
Forceps	1	5	4
Ventouse	8	8	7
Episiotomy	17	15	14

Derby · **Derby City General Hospital**

Uttoxeter Road, Derby,
Derbyshire DE22 3NE
Phone: 01332 340131
Fax: 01322 290559

Trust: **Southern Derbyshire Acute
Hospitals NHS Trust**

There are plans to build a new unit for Derby, although this won't be confirmed until later this year.

Currently, the unit delivers over 4000 babies a year and also provides antenatal and postnatal services for many women giving birth at other units in the surrounding area.

The unit is a research site linked to the University of Nottingham. If you are concerned about complications arising during your delivery you might feel reassured by booking into a large unit of this type. The unit's obstetricians are experienced in performing external cephalic version and can deliver breech babies. The proportion of breech babies delivered vaginally rather than by caesarean section at the unit is higher than at most units. There is a midwife-led care scheme in development but it is only at the pilot stage.

Consultant and Midwife Unit

Number of beds	62
Births per midwife	30
Births per bed	0.55
Home births	3%
Amenity Rooms, Price	£43
Obstetrician 24 hours	Yes
Paediatrician 24 hours	Yes
Full Water Birth Service	No

Tests

Routine Triple Testing	Yes
Nuchal Fold Scan	No
Fetal Assessment Unit	Yes

Pain Relief

24 hour epidural	Yes
Mobile epidural	No
Pethidine injections	Yes
Water (eg bath)	Yes

Intervention Rates	%	regional average %	national average %
Epidural	31	31	33
Elective Caesarean	8	9	8
Emergency Caesarean	12	13	12
Induction	23	20	20
Forceps	6	5	4
Ventouse	8	8	7
Episiotomy	16	15	14

Doncaster · **Royal Infirmary & Montagu Hospital**

Armthrope Road, Doncaster
South Yorkshire DN2 5LT
Phone: 01302 366 666
Fax: 01302 320 098

Trust: Doncaster Royal & Montagu
Hospital Trust

Continuity of care is better than at many large hospitals but could be improved with about one in five women being delivered by a midwife they know. The unit does, however, offer the domino system, which aims to ensure you know the midwife who looks after you throughout labour and birth. Water birth is offered, and the unit has its own pool with midwives trained in this procedure available around the clock. There are modern purpose built delivery rooms all with en suite facilities and the unit has recently upgraded its assessment and ultrasound departments. The double tests is used rather than the triple test and you would have to look elsewhere if you wanted a nuchal fold translucency scan. Although the episiotomy figure is higher than average, this has since been reduced.

Consultant and Midwife Unit

Number of beds	40
Births per midwife	27
Births per bed	0.99
Home births	1%
Amenity Rooms, Price	£21

Obstetrician 24 hours	Yes
Paediatrician 24 hours	Yes
Full Water Birth Service	Yes

Tests

Routine Triple Testing	No
Nuchal Fold Scan	No
Fetal Assessment Unit	Yes

Pain Relief

24 hour epidural	Yes
Mobile epidural	Yes
Pethidine injections	Yes
Water (eg bath)	Yes

Intervention Rates

	%	regional average %	national average %
Epidural	46	31	33
Elective Caesarean	9	9	8
Emergency Caesarean	12	13	12
Induction	23	20	20
Forceps	3	5	4
Ventouse	10	8	7
Episiotomy	23	15	14

Grantham · **Grantham & District Hospital**

101 Manthorpe Road, Grantham
Lincolnshire, NG31 8DG
Phone: 01476 565232
Fax: 01476 590441

Trust: United Lincolnshire Hospitals
NHS Trust

Grantham & District Hospital's maternity unit is small, with only four delivery beds. Care is midwife-led and as a result the unit is low-tech with minimal levels of intervention.

This means that epidurals are not performed, but water, entonox (gas and air), intramuscular opiate injection (pethadine) and TENS are all available as methods of pain relief. If you are interested in a water birth, trained midwives are available 24hrs a day and there is no need to bring your own pool.

About a third of women cared for by this unit give birth at home. You can access the fetal assessment unit based at the Pilgrim Hospital, Boston.

Midwife Unit

Number of beds	4
Births	98
Midwives	22
Home births	37%
Amenity Rooms, Price	-
Obstetrician 24 hours	No
Paediatrician 24 hours	No
Full Water Birth Service	Yes

Tests

Routine Triple Testing	Yes
Nuchal Fold Scan	No
Fetal Assessment Unit	Yes

Pain Relief

24 Hour epidural	No
Mobile epidural	No
Pethidine injections	Yes
Water (eg Bath)	Yes

Midwife-led units are adequately equipped to care for women whose pregnancy is progressing normally without complications. As a result, intervention tends to be low in these units. Basic pain relief will be offered, but any woman requesting an epidural during the delivery will need to be transferred to the nearest consultant-led unit. A woman will also be transferred to the obstetric unit if any complications develop during the delivery.

Grimsby · **Grimsby Maternity Hospital**

Second Avenue, Nunsthorpe
Grimsby, DN33 1NW
Phone: 01472 874111

Trust: North East Lincolnshire NHS
Trust

Grimsby Maternity Hospital provides shared care between consultants and midwives. If your pregnancy is low-risk, you will be cared for by midwives who are organised into teams that provide your care at the hospital, in local clinics or at home. If you pregnancy is more complex, your care will be managed by consultants in the hospital.

The unit is well staffed and midwives are focused on offering choices in care. A full water birth service is offered with trained midwives available to assist you around the clock.

The caesarean rate is average but almost a quarter of all labours are induced at Grimsby. Ventouse is used far more often than forceps for instrumental deliveries. The hospital is usually able to accommodate single room requests so amenity beds are not necessary.

Consultant and Midwife Unit

Number of beds	40
Births per midwife	26
Births per bed	0.84
Home births	2%
Amenity Rooms, Price	-

Obstetrician 24 hours	Yes
Paediatrician 24 hours	Yes
Full Water Birth Service	Yes

Tests

Routine Triple Testing	No
Nuchal Fold Scan	Yes
Fetal Assessment Unit	Yes

Pain Relief

24 hour epidural	Yes
Mobile epidural	No
Pethidine injections	Yes
Water (eg bath)	Yes

Intervention Rates	%	regional average %	national average %
Epidural	44	31	33
Elective Caesarean	9	9	8
Emergency Caesarean	13	13	12
Induction	23	20	20
Forceps	2	5	4
Ventouse	10	8	7
Episiotomy	18	15	14

Leicester · **Leicester General Hospital**

Gwendolen Road, Leicester
Leicestershire LE5 4PW
Phone: 0116 249 0490
Fax: 0116 258 4666

Trust: University Hospitals of Leicester
 NHS Trust

Leicester General Hospital is a large teaching hospital and care is shared between midwives and consultants. If you have a low-risk pregnancy you will receive all your care from midwives in the community. Domino deliveries are offered as are home births.

A range of daytime antenatal classes are offered, including women-only classes and those for women expecting twins or triplets. Classes also take place in the evenings and weekends. You can also opt for a water birth. The unit has a pool but trained midwives may not always be available. Intervention rates are in line with national averages for this type of unit. The unit practices external cephalic inversion and will sometimes deliver breech babies vaginally.

Consultant and Midwife Unit

Number of beds	65
Births per midwife	33.1
Births per bed	0.84
Home births	-
Amenity Rooms, Price	£41

Obstetrician 24 hours	Yes
Paediatrician 24 hours	No
Full Water Birth Service	No

Tests

Routine Triple Testing	No
Nuchal Fold Scan	No
Fetal Assessment Unit	Yes

Pain Relief

24 hour epidural	Yes
Mobile epidural	Yes
Pethidine injections	Yes
Water (eg bath)	Yes

Intervention Rates	%	regional average %	national average %
Epidural	-	31	33
Elective Caesarean	7	9	8
Emergency Caesarean	12	13	12
Induction	-	20	20
Forceps	5	5	4
Ventouse	6	8	7
Episiotomy	17	15	14

Leicester · **Leicester Royal Infirmary**

Infirmary Square, Leicester
Leicestershire, LE1 5WW
Phone: 0116 254 1414
Fax: 0116 258 5631

Trust: University Hospitals of Leicester
NHS Trust

This large teaching hospital houses a maternity unit providing women with a choice of how they have their baby. The delivery suite has eight delivery rooms for high-risk women, and eight beds for women in early labour or needing close observation. Alternatively there are six midwife-led rooms which are furnished in a more homely style designed to create a relaxed environment for women who want to give birth naturally. Women with uncomplicated pregnancies receive all their care from midwives in the community. More complex cases are overseen by consultants. The unit also has a birthing pool, although trained midwives may not be available. A psychiatric liaison clinic provides support for women with problems such as fear of labour and postnatal depression.

Consultant and Midwife Unit

Number of beds	99
Births per midwife	27.9
Births per bed	0.79
Home births	2%
Amenity Rooms, Price	-

Obstetrician 24 hours	Yes
Paediatrician 24 hours	Yes
Full Water Birth Service	No

Tests

Routine Triple Testing	No
Nuchal Fold Scan	No
Fetal Assessment Unit	Yes

Pain Relief

24 hour epidural	Yes
Mobile epidural	Yes
Pethidine injections	Yes
Water (eg bath)	Yes

Intervention Rates

	%	regional average %	national average %
Epidural	36	31	33
Elective Caesarean	9	9	8
Emergency Caesarean	12	13	12
Induction	18	20	20
Forceps	4	5	4
Ventouse	7	8	7
Episiotomy	14	15	14

Lincoln · **Lincoln County Hospital**

Greetwell Road, Lincoln
Lincolnshire LN2 5QY
Phone: 01522 512512
Fax: 01522 573419

Trust: United Lincolnshire Hospitals
NHS Trust

This is a reasonably large maternity unit sharing care between consultants and midwives. The caesarean delivery rate is above average and the forceps rate is very high. Forceps are used more often than ventouse for instrumental deliveries. However the induction rate is below average.

You may not be offered an ultrasound scan at booking but it may be available if you ask. Nuchal fold scans can also be arranged if requesterd. Anomaly scans at 22-24 weeks are offered to everyone as is triple testing. If you want a water birth, you will need to do it at home and provide your own pool. Trained midwives will supervise.

Consultant and Midwife Unit

Number of beds	60
Births per midwife	31.5
Births per bed	0.76
Home births	1%
Amenity Rooms, Price	£31

Obstetrician 24 hours	Yes
Paediatrician 24 hours	Yes
Full Water Birth Service	No

Tests

Routine Triple Testing	Yes
Nuchal Fold Scan	Yes
Fetal Assessment Unit	Yes

Pain Relief

24 hour epidural	Yes
Mobile epidural	No
Pethidine injections	Yes
Water (eg bath)	Yes

Intervention Rates	%	regional average %	national average %
Epidural	28	31	33
Elective Caesarean	10	9	8
Emergency Caesarean	12	13	12
Induction	18	20	20
Forceps	7	5	4
Ventouse	6	8	7
Episiotomy	16	15	14

Matlock · **Whitworth Hospital**

330 Bakewell Road, Darley Dale
Matlock, DE4 2JD
Phone: 01629 580211
Fax: 01629 583037

Trust: Chesterfield and North
Derbyshire Royal Hospital NHS

The small, midwife-led maternity service at Whitworth hospital is intended to offer home-from-home care in a relaxed environment. This service would be worth considering if you were interested in having a home birth, as midwives from the unit attended an above-average number of these deliveries last year. Like other midwife-led units, Whitworth offers a flexible program of antenatal care. Sessions can be arranged on weekdays, in the evenings and at weekends. You will have to travel for antenatal testing. Ultrasound scanning is done at the Chesterfield and North Derbyshire Royal Hospital.

Midwife Unit

Number of beds	8
Births	84
Midwives	14
Home births	12%
Amenity Rooms, Price	-
Obstetrician 24 hours	No
Paediatrician 24 hours	No
Full Water Birth Service	Yes

Tests

Routine Triple Testing	No
Nuchal Fold Scan	Yes
Fetal Assessment Unit	No

Pain Relief

24 Hour epidural	No
Mobile epidural	No
Pethidine injections	Yes
Water (eg Bath)	Yes

Midwife-led units are adequately equipped to care for women whose pregnancy is progressing normally without complications. As a result, intervention tends to be low in these units. Basic pain relief will be offered, but any woman requesting an epidural during the delivery will need to be transferred to the nearest consultant-led unit. A woman will also be transferred to the obstetric unit if any complications develop during the delivery.

Melton Mowbray · **St Mary's Hospital**

Thorpe Road, Melton Mowbray
Leicestershire, LE13 1SJ
Phone: 01664 854800
Fax: 01664 854888

Trust: University Hospitals of Leicester NHS Trust

The unit is staffed 24hrs a day, seven days a week, so there is always a midwife available to discuss concerns, offer advice and look after labouring women. Other midwives are also available on an on call basis for home births, and the unit is experienced in water births. Staff at the unit are supported by a visiting consultant and local GPs, some of whom are on call should they be required for forceps deliveries. If complications require transfer out of the unit, you can choose any of the local hospitals and a midwife will accompany you.

The unit also supplies antenatal and postnatal care to women who plan to give birth in larger consultant units. Soon after birth, the mother and baby can transfer to St Mary's for postnatal care and support with breastfeeding and parenting skills.

Midwife Unit

Number of beds	10
Births	227
Midwives	15
Home births	20
Amenity Rooms, Price	-

Obstetrician 24 hours	No
Paediatrician 24 hours	No
Full Water Birth Service	Yes

Tests

Routine Triple Testing	No
Nuchal Fold Scan	Yes
Fetal Assessment Unit	No

Pain Relief

24 Hour epidural	No
Mobile epidural	No
Pethidine injections	Yes
Water (eg Bath)	Yes

Midwife-led units are adequately equipped to care for women whose pregnancy is progressing normally without complications. As a result, intervention tends to be low in these units. Basic pain relief will be offered, but any woman requesting an epidural during the delivery will need to be transferred to the nearest consultant-led unit. A woman will also be transferred to the obstetric unit if any complications develop during the delivery.

Nottingham · **Nottingham City Hospital**

Hucknall Road, Nottingham
Nottinghamshire NG5 1PB
Phone: 0115 969 1169
Fax: 0115 962 7788

Trust: Nottingham City Hospital
NHS Trust

Midwife staffing in Nottingham is managed differently to elsewhere in the country. The unit does not manage the community midwifery service, however, sometimes midwives from the community accompany women to the hospital to deliver. Staffing levels are estimated to be about average.

Home births are managed by the community midwifery service which also offers domino deliveries. Intervention rates here are higher than the national average but lower than at the neighbouring Queen's Medical Centre. The unit has hotel facilities with en suite rooms to allow partners to stay. Facilities for women with disabilities include special bathrooms, adjustable couches and cots and electronic beds in the labour suite.

Consultant and Midwife Unit

Number of beds	98
Births per midwife	-
Births per bed	0.88
Home births	-
Amenity Rooms, Price	-

Obstetrician 24 hours	Yes
Paediatrician 24 hours	Yes
Full Water Birth Service	Yes

Tests

Routine Triple Testing	No
Nuchal Fold Scan	Yes
Fetal Assessment Unit	Yes

Pain Relief

24 hour epidural	Yes
Mobile epidural	Yes
Pethidine injections	Yes
Water (eg bath)	Yes

Intervention Rates

	%	regional average %	national average %
Epidural	35	31	33
Elective Caesarean	10	9	8
Emergency Caesarean	13	13	12
Induction	24	20	20
Forceps	6	5	4
Ventouse	8	8	7
Episiotomy	15	15	14

Nottingham · **Queen's Medical Centre**

Clifton Boulevard,
Nottingham, NG7 2UH
Phone: 0115 924 9924
Fax: 0115 849 3331

Trust: Queen's Medical Centre
University Hospital NHS Trust

Maternity services at Queen's Medical Centre are closely linked with the University of Nottingham, and the unit is a centre of teaching and research, taking over the care of women with high-risk pregnancies from around the region. Staffing levels are estimated to be about average.

Intervention rates at Queen's Medical Centre are above average. Around a quarter of women are induced and the same number deliver by caesarean section.

The unit also caters to women with low-risk pregancies who may opt for midwife-led care or shared care, where the community midwife and GP work together. This unit has recently refurbished home-from-home style accommodation designed to create a non-clinical atmosphere for women wanting natural childbirth.

Consultant and Midwife Unit

Number of beds	86
Births per midwife	-
Births per bed	1.06
Home births	-
Amenity Rooms, Price	-

Obstetrician 24 hours	Yes
Paediatrician 24 hours	Yes
Full Water Birth Service	Yes

Tests

Routine Triple Testing	Yes
Nuchal Fold Scan	Yes
Fetal Assessment Unit	Yes

Pain Relief

24 Hour epidural	Yes
Mobile epidural	Yes
Pethidine injections	Yes
Water (eg Bath)	Yes

Intervention Rates	%	regional average %	national average %
Epidural	27	31	33
Elective Caesarean	13	9	8
Emergency Caesarean	14	13	12
Induction	25	20	20
Forceps	6	5	4
Ventouse	9	8	7
Episiotomy	15	15	14

Moorgate Road, Oakwood
Rotherham S60 2UD
Phone: 01709 820000
Fax: 01709 304200

Trust: Rotherham General Hospitals
   NHS Trust

The maternity service at Rotherham District General Hospital offers a full range of care options including shared consultant and midwife care, midwife-led care, and home birth.

Rotherham is a busy unit with more than one delivery per bed each day. However, the unit has recently gained another delivery bed.

Women with uncomplicated pregnancies are encouraged to opt for midwife-led care under a community midwife. Home birth rates are low here but the service is available. Staff at the hospital usually allow your partner to stay with you if you have to go into hospital before your labour has started. Intervention rates are broadly average for a large district general hospital although ventouse deliveries are significanly more common than at other hospitals.

Consultant and Midwife Unit

Number of beds	44
Births per midwife	29.7
Births per bed	1.14
Home births	1%
Amenity Rooms, Price	-

Obstetrician 24 hours	Yes
Paediatrician 24 hours	Yes
Full Water Birth Service	No

Tests

Routine Triple Testing	No
Nuchal Fold Scan	Yes
Fetal Assessment Unit	Yes

Pain Relief

24 hour epidural	Yes
Mobile epidural	No
Pethidine injections	Yes
Water (eg bath)	Yes

Intervention Rates

	%	regional average %	national average %
Epidural	-	31	33
Elective Caesarean	8	9	8
Emergency Caesarean	12	13	12
Induction	21	20	20
Forceps	4	5	4
Ventouse	9	8	7
Episiotomy	-	15	14

Cliff Gardens, Scunthorpe
North Lincolnshire DN15 7BH
Phone: 01724 282282
Fax: 01724 282427

Trust: Scunthorpe and Goole Hospitals
NHS Trust

Scunthorpe General Hospital provides fully integrated team midwifery, with seven teams. Midwives provide most of their services from local centres outside the hospital. While the maternity unit at Scunthorpe General Hospital offers a 24hr epidural service, it is not nearly as widely used as at many hospitals, including near neighbours such as the Castle Hill Hospital, Cottingham and The Maternity Hospital, Hull.

There is also a small midwife-led unit at Goole, 25 miles from Scunthorpe, which works closely with the hospital and caters to women with straighforward pregnancies who can choose to give birth at home or come into the unit. Scunthorpe's high home birth rate reflects partly the number of home births carried out by midwives at Goole. Both units have full water birth facilities.

Consultant and Midwife Unit

Number of beds	35
Births per midwife	40
Births per bed	0.55
Home births	5%
Amenity Rooms, Price	£32

Obstetrician 24 hours	Yes
Paediatrician 24 hours	Yes
Full Water Birth Service	Yes

Tests

Routine Triple Testing	No
Nuchal Fold Scan	Yes
Fetal Assessment Unit	Yes

Pain Relief

24 hour epidural	Yes
Mobile epidural	No
Pethidine injections	Yes
Water (eg bath)	Yes

Intervention Rates	%	regional average %	national average %
Epidural	17	31	33
Elective Caesarean	7	9	8
Emergency Caesarean	14	13	12
Induction	20	20	20
Forceps	4	5	4
Ventouse	5	8	7
Episiotomy	11	15	14

Sheffield · **Royal Hallamshire Hospital**

Tree Root Walk, Sheffield
Yorkshire S10 3SF
Phone: 0114 226 8000
Fax: 0114 270 1403

Trust: Sheffield Teaching Hospital NHS Trust

The Jessop Wing is a new hospital which was formed by the merger of the maternity services at Northern General Hospital and Jessop Hospital for Women. Hospital and community midwife services are integrated and midwife staffing levels are good. The hospital offers one-to-one care during labour which has been shown to improve women's experience of labour and delivery. If appropriate women will be discharged home from the labour ward.

There are two pools available if you wish to use water as a form of pain relief during labour or for water birth. The unit also has a pool available for hire in the community. The unit includes a tertiary neonatal unit, as well as joint clinics for women with diabetes, epilepsy, cardiac, kidney and mental health problems.

Consultant and Midwife Unit

Number of beds	108
Births per midwife	28
Births per bed	0.62
Home births	2%
Amenity Rooms, Price	£29

Obstetrician 24 hours	Yes
Paediatrician 24 hours	Yes
Full Water Birth Service	Yes

Tests

Routine Triple Testing	No
Nuchal Fold Scan	Yes
Fetal Assessment Unit	Yes

Pain Relief

24 hour epidural	Yes
Mobile epidural	Yes
Pethidine injections	Yes
Water (eg bath)	Yes

Intervention Rates

	%	regional average %	national average %
Epidural	49	31	33
Elective Caesarean	9	9	8
Emergency Caesarean	13	13	12
Induction	20	20	20
Forceps	6	5	4
Ventouse	10	8	7
Episiotomy	-	15	14

Sutton in Ashfield · **King's Mill Hospital**

Mansfield Road, Sutton in Ashfield
Nottinghamshire NG17 4JL
Phone: 01623 622515
Fax: 01623 621770

Trust: Sherwood Forest Hospitals
NHS Trust

Maternity services at King's Mill Hospital serve much of the population of mid-Nottinghamshire. The unit is shared midwife and consultant-led, with midwives midwives providing much of the care for low-risk women. Complex cases have 24hr access to an integrated team consisting of midwives, ostetricians and GPs.

Domino deliveries for low-risk women are offered as are homebirths. The unit has a lower than average caesarean rate, particularly for emergency caesareans. The unit does not have water birth facilities. Although the overall epidural rate is above average many of these are used for ceasearean deliveries. Epidurals given in labour for pain relief are used for about one in five labours in line with national averages.

Consultant and Midwife Unit

Number of beds	50
Births per midwife	35
Births per bed	0.46
Home births	1%
Amenity Rooms, Price	-
Obstetrician 24 hours	Yes
Paediatrician 24 hours	Yes
Full Water Birth Service	No

Tests

Routine Triple Testing	No
Nuchal Fold Scan	Yes
Fetal Assessment Unit	Yes

Pain Relief

24 hour epidural	Yes
Mobile epidural	Yes
Pethidine injections	Yes
Water (eg bath)	No

Intervention Rates	%	regional average %	national average %
Epidural	38	31	33
Elective Caesarean	6	9	8
Emergency Caesarean	10	13	12
Induction	17	20	20
Forceps	7	5	4
Ventouse	9	8	7
Episiotomy	13	15	14

Worksop · **Bassetlaw District General Hospital**

Kilton Hill, Worksop
Nottinghamshire S81 0BD
Phone: 01909 500990
Fax: 01909 502246

Trust: Bassetlaw Hospital & Community
Health Services NHS Trust

Bassetlaw is planned to have a structural makeover this year. The unit is relatively small for a district general hospital and has good staffing levels which should help ensure a good level of personal attention.

Intervention rates are higher than at most hospitals with caesarean deliveries and instrumental deliveries being significantly more common than in other hospitals. Epidurals are available for pain relief but used less frequently than in other units.

Full waterbirth facilities are offered by the unit and a dedicated water birth suite has just been built.

Most scans and tests are done on site, but if you require a nuchal fold scan you will be referred to Nottingham or Sheffield.

Consultant and Midwife Unit

Number of beds	30
Births per midwife	28
Births per bed	0.68
Home births	1%
Amenity Rooms, Price	£16

Obstetrician 24 hours	Yes
Paediatrician 24 hours	Yes
Full Water Birth Service	Yes

Tests

Routine Triple Testing	Yes
Nuchal Fold Scan	Yes
Fetal Assessment Unit	No

Pain Relief

24 hour epidural	Yes
Mobile epidural	No
Pethidine injections	Yes
Water (eg bath)	Yes

Intervention Rates

	%	regional average %	national average %
Epidural	25	31	33
Elective Caesarean	9	9	8
Emergency Caesarean	17	13	12
Induction	14	20	20
Forceps	4	5	4
Ventouse	14	8	7
Episiotomy	-	15	14

The West Midlands

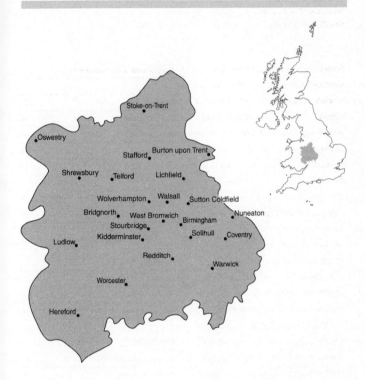

Birmingham	• Birmingham Heartlands		• Royal Shrewsbury Hospital (GP-led Unit)
	• Birmingham Women's Hospital	Solihull	• Solihull Hospital
	• City Hospital	Stafford	• Staffordshire General
Bridgnorth	• Bridgnorth Hospital	Stoke-on-Trent	• North Staffordshire Hospital (Central Delivery Suite)
Burton upon Trent	• Queen's Hospital		• North Staffordshire Hospital (Community Maternity Unit)
Coventry	• Walsgrave Hospital	Stourbridge	• Wordsley Hospital
Hereford	• County Hospital	Sutton Coldfield	• Good Hope District General
Kidderminster	• Kidderminster Hospital	Telford	• Princess Royal Hospital
Lichfield	• Lichfield Victoria Hospital	Walsall	• Manor Hospital
Ludlow	• Ludlow Hospital	Warwick	• Warwick Hospital
Nuneaton	• George Eliot Hospital	West Bromwich	• Sandwell General Hospital
Oswestry	• Robert Jones & Agnes Hunt Orthopaedic & District	Wolverhampton	• New Cross Hospital
Redditch	• Alexandra Hospital	Worcester	• Worcester Royal Infirmary
Shrewsbury	• Royal Shrewsbury Hospital		

Bordesley Green East
Birmingham B9 5SS
Phone: 0121 424 2000
Fax: 0121 424 2336

Trust: Birmingham Heartlands and
Solihull NHS Trust

Birmingham Heartlands Hospital and the Solihull hospital are run as one service, although they have separate entries in this guide. The Solihull site has a low-risk approach while this hospital deals with high-dependency care and has intensive neonatal care on site. As with many inner city maternity units, midwives have a heavy workload. Continuity of care is not as good as in other hospitals. You are unlikely to be delivered by a midwife you know here. Also, home births are very rarely done. Epidural pain management is available but the unit also has more unusual alternatives such as aromatherapy and hypnosis. Triple testing is routinely offered to women over 35 but not to others. Information is available in a range of languages reflecting the local population mix.

Consultant and Midwife Unit

Number of beds	50
Births per midwife	40
Births per bed	-
Home births	0.29%
Amenity Rooms, Price	£50

Obstetrician 24 hours	Yes
Paediatrician 24 hours	Yes
Full Water Birth Service	Yes

Tests

Routine Triple Testing	No
Nuchal Fold Scan	Yes
Fetal Assessment Unit	Yes

Pain Relief

24 hour epidural	Yes
Mobile epidural	Yes
Pethidine injections	Yes
Water (eg bath)	Yes

Intervention Rates

	%	regional average %	national average %
Epidural	36	26	33
Elective Caesarean	9	9	8
Emergency Caesarean	15	13	12
Induction	20	15	20
Forceps	4	3	4
Ventouse	6	6	7
Episiotomy	15	13	14

Edgbaston
Birmingham B15 2TG
Phone: 0121 472 1377
Fax: 0121 627 2602

Trust: Birmingham Women's Health
Care NHS Trust

This is one of a select number of dedicated women's hospitals in the country. It is a regional referral centre providing neonatal intensive care services, a fetal medicine service and a regional genetics service for women who are at risk of carrying genetic diseases. A low tech area is being planned to reduce congestion at the unit. Midwives are organised into teams linked to GPs. Consultants provide 40 hours of cover a week for the department as well as on-call support. The delivery suite has facilities to support all types of delivery, including water birth. Classes include separate sessions for Asian women. The hospital provides specialist antenatal clinics, pre-pregnancy counselling and support for women experiencing bereavement and pregnancy loss.

Consultant and Midwife Unit

Number of beds	98
Births per midwife	33
Births per bed	1.20
Home births	1%
Amenity Rooms, Price	£55

Obstetrician 24 hours	Yes
Paediatrician 24 hours	Yes
Full Water Birth Service	Yes

Tests

Routine Triple Testing	No
Nuchal Fold Scan	No
Fetal Assessment Unit	Yes

Pain Relief

24 hour epidural	Yes
Mobile epidural	No
Pethidine injections	Yes
Water (eg bath)	Yes

Intervention Rates	%	regional average %	national average %
Epidural	26	26	33
Elective Caesarean	11	9	8
Emergency Caesarean	15	13	12
Induction	18	15	20
Forceps	4	3	4
Ventouse	5	6	7
Episiotomy	8	13	14

Birmingham · **City Hospital**

Dudley Road, Winton Green
Birmingham B18 7QH
Phone: 0121 554 3801
Fax: 0121 523 0951

Trust: City Hospital
NHS Trust

City Hospital's busy maternity unit is supported by a sub-regional neonatal unit, allowing extra support for high-risk women. Home birth rates, as in other Birmingham hospitals, are low.

A full range of pain relief services are available, including mobile epidurals. However epidurals are used much less often here than in other hospitals.

If you want a water birth, this will nearly always be available at the time you need it. There is a pool at the unit and, although midwives trained in water birth are not always on site, an on-call system is in operation so midwives trained in water births should be available most of the time.

The hospital runs women-only classes as well as groups for teenagers, Asian mothers and women with multiple pregnancies.

Consultant and Midwife Unit

Number of beds	53
Births per midwife	31
Births per bed	0.62
Home births	0.35%
Amenity Rooms, Price	£70

Obstetrician 24 hours	Yes
Paediatrician 24 hours	Yes
Full Water Birth Service	No

Tests

Routine Triple Testing	No
Nuchal Fold Scan	No
Fetal Assessment Unit	Yes

Pain Relief

24 hour epidural	Yes
Mobile epidural	Yes
Pethidine injections	Yes
Water (eg bath)	Yes

Intervention Rates

	%	regional average %	national average %
Epidural	18	26	33
Elective Caesarean	9	9	8
Emergency Caesarean	12	13	12
Induction	20	15	20
Forceps	3	3	4
Ventouse	5	6	7
Episiotomy	13	13	14

Bridgnorth · **Bridgnorth Hospital**

Northgate, Bridgnorth
Shopshire WV16 4EU
Phone: 01746 762 641
Fax: 01746 766 172

Trust: Royal Shrewsbury Hospital
NHS Trust

This small midwife-led unit has two labour beds and four post-natal beds arranged in two double bedded rooms. Due to its small number of midwives, most patients are familiar with all the staff and vice versa. Midwives qualified to undertake routine scans visit the unit every two weeks. Only low-risk patients are delivered here but if you have your baby in the Royal Shrewsbury Hospital you can come back here for postnatal care. The unit does not take antenatal patients, only women in labour. The unit carries out ultrasound scans at 16 weeks rather than the usual booking scan at 12-14 weeks. The service promotes relaxation techniques as a way of managing pain in addition to more traditional methods. Water births can be done but midwives are not always available to supervise these.

Midwife Unit	
Number of beds	6
Births	85
Midwives	11
Home births	12%
Amenity Rooms, Price	-

Obstetrician 24 hours	No
Paediatrician 24 hours	No
Full Water Birth Service	No

Tests	
Routine Triple Testing	No
Nuchal Fold Scan	Yes
Fetal Assessment Unit	No

Pain Relief	
24 Hour epidural	No
Mobile epidural	No
Pethidine injections	Yes
Water (eg bath)	Yes

Midwife-led units are adequately equipped to care for women whose pregnancy is progressing normally without complications. As a result, intervention tends to be low in these units. Basic pain relief will be offered, but any woman requesting an epidural during the delivery will need to be transferred to the nearest consultant-led unit. A woman will also be transferred to the obstetric unit if any complications develop during the delivery.

Burton upon Trent · **Queen's Hospital**

Belvedere Road, Burton upon Trent
Straffordshire DE13 0RB
Phone: 01283 566 333
Fax: 01283 593006

Trust: Burton Hospitals
NHS Trust

Queen's Hospital has a large, shared midwife and consultant-led maternity unit with an above average proportion of home births. A range of pain-relief methods are available during labour including epidurals. Intervention rates are generally in line with national averages. The episiotomy rate for normal vaginal deliveries is 15.3%.

If you have to be admitted to the hospital before your labour starts, the unit will attempt to accommodate your partner, but this cannot always be guaranteed. Ultrasound scans at 12-14 weeks and 22-24 weeks are offered to all women booked into the unit. Double testing is done, rather than triple testing.

Consultant and Midwife Unit

Number of beds	56
Births per midwife	33
Births per bed	0.94
Home births	3%
Amenity Rooms, Price	£24

Obstetrician 24 hours	Yes
Paediatrician 24 hours	Yes
Full Water Birth Service	No

Tests

Routine Triple Testing	No
Nuchal Fold Scan	No
Fetal Assessment Unit	No

Pain Relief

24 hour epidural	Yes
Mobile epidural	No
Pethidine injections	Yes
Water (eg bath)	Yes

Intervention Rates	%	regional average %	national average %
Epidural	42	26	33
Elective Caesarean	7	9	8
Emergency Caesarean	15	13	12
Induction	21	15	20
Forceps	2	3	4
Ventouse	9	6	7
Episiotomy	-	13	14

Coventry · **Walsgrave Hospital**

Clifford Bridge Road, Walsgrave
Coventry CV2 2DX
Phone: 024 7660 2020
Fax: 024 7662 2197

Trust: The University Hospitals
Coventry and Warwickshire NHS
Trust

Walsgrave is a large and busy maternity unit with shared input from consultants and midwives. The 10-bedded delivery suite is relatively crowded with over one birth per bed per day. However there is a midwife-led unit in the same hospital, which offers an alternative with home-from-home rooms and water birth. Single rooms can be hired in the main unit.

Antenatal classes are available in the evenings and at weekends to fit in with busy lifestyles, and a 'Pals in pregnancy' team operates in the community offering social support to vulnerable pregnant women living in disadvantaged circumstances. Unlike most other services, women booked with Walsgrave are not routinely offered anomaly ultrasound scans.

Consultant and Midwife Unit

Number of beds	84
Births per midwife	30.1
Births per bed	1.14
Home births	2%
Amenity Rooms, Price	£25

Obstetrician 24 hours	Yes
Paediatrician 24 hours	Yes
Full Water Birth Service	No

Tests

Routine Triple Testing	No
Nuchal Fold Scan	No
Fetal Assessment Unit	Yes

Pain Relief

24 hour epidural	Yes
Mobile epidural	No
Pethidine injections	Yes
Water (eg bath)	Yes

Intervention Rates	%	regional average %	national average %
Epidural	23	26	33
Elective Caesarean	10	9	8
Emergency Caesarean	16	13	12
Induction	18	15	20
Forceps	3	3	4
Ventouse	7	6	7
Episiotomy	14	13	14

Hereford · **County Hospital**

Union Walk
Hereford HR1 2ER
Phone: 01432 355 444
Fax: 01432 354 310

Trust: Hereford Hospitals
NHS Trust

Maternity services at County Hospital are shared between consultants and midwives. However, if your pregnancy is low-risk, you will receive most of your antenatal care from midwives. Staffing levels at the unit are good and the home birth rate is above average. If you are unable to attend parent education sessions and antenatal classes during the day, there are evening classes available. These are held in surrounding rural areas as well as in Hereford. Caesareans are performed a great deal less here than in other hospitals – not because there are any fewer elective caesareans – but because of a low emergency caesarean rate. In line with national averages, about one in ten deliveries is instrumental but the ventouse method is much preferred to forceps.

Consultant and Midwife Unit

Number of beds	40
Births per midwife	27.4
Births per bed	0.90
Home births	3%
Amenity Rooms, Price	£32
Obstetrician 24 hours	No
Paediatrician 24 hours	No
Full Water Birth Service	No

Tests

Routine Triple Testing	No
Nuchal Fold Scan	No
Fetal Assessment Unit	No

Pain Relief

24 hour epidural	Yes
Mobile epidural	No
Pethidine injections	Yes
Water (eg bath)	Yes

Intervention Rates	%	regional average %	national average %
Epidural	32	26	33
Elective Caesarean	8	9	8
Emergency Caesarean	10	13	12
Induction	18	15	20
Forceps	2	3	4
Ventouse	9	6	7
Episiotomy	12	13	14

Kidderminster · **Kidderminster Hospital**

Bewdley Road, Kidderminster
Worcestershire DY11 6RJ
Phone: 01562 823 424
Fax: 01562 674 12

Trust: Worcestershire Acute Hospitals
NHS Trust

The Wyre Forest Birth Centre at Kidderminster Hospital caters for women who have a normal pregnancy and for whom a normal birth is anticipated. All midwifes at the facility have undertaken the Advanced Life Support in Obstetrics (ALSO) course, and most have also completed the Advanced Resuscitation of the Newborn (ARNB) course. However in an emergency you could well be transferred elsewhere. Midwife staffing levels are relatively high, and over half of the women delivering at the unit are cared for by a midwife they know. Antenatal classes are held only on weekday evenings, which may not be convenient for all mothers, and some antenatal tests, such as the triple test and nuchal translucency scanning are not routinely available to all women. A TENS machine is available for pain relief.

Midwife Unit

Number of beds	10
Births	175
Midwives	24
Home births	2%
Amenity Rooms, Price	-

Obstetrician 24 hours	No
Paediatrician 24 hours	No
Full Water Birth Service	No

Tests

Routine Triple Testing	No
Nuchal Fold Scan	No
Fetal Assessment Unit	No

Pain Relief

24 Hour epidural	No
Mobile epidural	No
Pethidine injections	Yes
Water (eg bath)	Yes

Midwife-led units are adequately equipped to care for women whose pregnancy is progressing normally without complications. As a result, intervention tends to be low in these units. Basic pain relief will be offered, but any woman requesting an epidural during the delivery will need to be transferred to the nearest consultant-led unit. A woman will also be transferred to the obstetric unit if any complications develop during the delivery.

Lichfield · **Lichfield Victoria Hospital**

Friary Road, Lichfield
Staffordshire WS13 6QN
Phone: 01543 442 000
Fax: 01543 416 729

Trust: South Staffordshire Healthcare
NHS Trust

The Victoria Maternity Unit aims to provide a very different environment from a large hosital. One room has been decorated in a hotel style, another as a fantasy underwater experience while a third – the lavender delivery room – doubles as a complementary therapy room. Delivery rooms have subdued lighting, relaxation music, television, reclining and rocking chairs and ensuite facilities with jacuzzi and aromatherapy diffusers. Partners are welcome and can stay at the unit. About half the women who give birth here are looked after in labour by a midwife they already know. If you want a water birth, staff are available to supervise but you must bring your own pool. Although this is a low-tech unit, gentle induction methods are occasionally used.

Midwife Unit

Number of beds	9
Births	252
Midwives	6
Home births	0%
Amenity Rooms, Price	-

Obstetrician 24 hours	No
Paediatrician 24 hours	No
Full Water Birth Service	No

Tests

Routine Triple Testing	No
Nuchal Fold Scan	No
Fetal Assessment Unit	No

Pain Relief

24 Hour epidural	No
Mobile epidural	No
Pethidine injections	Yes
Water (eg bath)	Yes

Midwife-led units are adequately equipped to care for women whose pregnancy is progressing normally without complications. As a result, intervention tends to be low in these units. Basic pain relief will be offered, but any woman requesting an epidural during the delivery will need to be transferred to the nearest consultant-led unit. A woman will also be transferred to the obstetric unit if any complications develop during the delivery.

Ludlow · **Ludlow Hospital**

Gravel Hill, Ludlow
Shropshire, SY8 1QX
Phone: 01584 872201
Fax: 01584 877908

Trust: Royal Shrewsbury Hospital
   NHS Trust

The Ludlow Hospital maternity service is managed by a combination of GPs and midwives and has just one delivery bed. The service aims to provide relaxed and flexible antenatal and hospital care to women whose pregnancies are low-risk. Antenatal classes are held in the evenings and on weekdays but not at the weekend, and aquanatal groups can be arranged. Antenatal tests are not so readily available if you are booked with the Ludlow Service. The triple test is not routinely offered to all women, though the less reliable alpha feto protein test is available. Similarly, anomaly ultrasound scans are performed, but not early pregnancy scans. For other tests you would be referred to the Royal Shrewsbury Hospital.

GP and Midwife Unit

Number of beds	9
Births	96
Midwives	8
Home births	4%
Amenity Rooms, Price	-

Obstetrician 24 hours	No
Paediatrician 24 hours	No
Full Water Birth Service	No

Tests

Routine Triple Testing	No
Nuchal Fold Scan	Yes
Fetal Assessment Unit	No

Pain Relief

24 Hour epidural	No
Mobile epidural	No
Pethidine injections	Yes
Water (eg bath)	Yes

Midwife-led units are adequately equipped to care for women whose pregnancy is progressing normally without complications. As a result, intervention tends to be low in these units. Basic pain relief will be offered, but any woman requesting an epidural during the delivery will need to be transferred to the nearest consultant-led unit. A woman will also be transferred to the obstetric unit if any complications develop during the delivery.

Nuneaton · **George Eliot Hospital**

College street,
College Hospital, Nuneaton
Warwickshire CV10 7DJ
Phone: 02476 351 351
Fax: 02476 865 175

Trust: George Eliot Hospital
NHS Trust

The maternity unit here has a reputation for friendliness, with a good multi-professional team. The unit does not offer the domino system but community midwives work within GP surgeries and support their own women when in labour. Also, you can be discharged within six hours of giving birth, if you request it and are fit.

Pain management includes TENS machines, aromatherapy and water, as well as more conventional treatments.

Aquanatal and physiotherapy sessions are run alongside usual antenatal classes. There is also a debriefing service where women can review their notes after the birth and understand more clearly the birth of their baby. There is an antenatal assessment unit which you can visit during the day.

Consultant and Midwife Unit

Number of beds	42
Births per midwife	34
Births per bed	0.64
Home births	1%
Amenity Rooms, Price	£31

Obstetrician 24 hours	Yes
Paediatrician 24 hours	Yes
Full Water Birth Service	No

Tests

Routine Triple Testing	No
Nuchal Fold Scan	Yes
Fetal Assessment Unit	Yes

Pain Relief

24 hour epidural	Yes
Mobile epidural	No
Pethidine injections	Yes
Water (eg bath)	Yes

Intervention Rates	%	regional average %	national average %
Epidural	30	26	33
Elective Caesarean	7	9	8
Emergency Caesarean	11	13	12
Induction	19	15	20
Forceps	2	3	4
Ventouse	6	6	7
Episiotomy	17	13	14

Oswestry · **The Robert Jones & Agnes Hunt Hospital**

Oswestry
Shopshire SY10 7AG
Phone: 01691 404 000
Fax: 01691 404 050

Trust: Royal Shrewsbury Hospital
NHS Trust

This is a GP and midwife-led maternity unit, based in the main hospital, dealing with low-risk pregnancies. It is supported by a consultant from the Royal Shrewsbury Hospital. Ultrasonographers visit regularly to perform 16 week scans and the unit has a cardiotocograph to monitor your baby's heart beat, should you become concerned about reduced fetal movement during pregnancy. Triple testing is not routinely offered, but nuchal fold scans are available via the Royal Shrewsbury. The small team of midwives provide a friendly service with three quarters of women being cared for in labour by a midwife they know. Full water birth facilities are available. Midwifes can be contacted 24 hours a day, to offer antenatal and postnatal support.

GP and Midwife Unit

Number of beds	11
Births	92
Midwives	8
Home births	3%
Amenity Rooms, Price	£36

Obstetrician 24 hours	No
Paediatrician 24 hours	No
Full Water Birth Service	Yes

Tests

Routine Triple Testing	No
Nuchal Fold Scan	Yes
Fetal Assessment Unit	Yes

Pain Relief

24 Hour epidural	No
Mobile epidural	No
Pethidine injections	Yes
Water (eg bath)	Yes

Midwife-led units are adequately equipped to care for women whose pregnancy is progressing normally without complications. As a result, intervention tends to be low in these units. Basic pain relief will be offered, but any woman requesting an epidural during the delivery will need to be transferred to the nearest consultant-led unit. A woman will also be transferred to the obstetric unit if any complications develop during the delivery.

Redditch · **Alexandra Hospital**

Woodrow Drive, Redditch
Worcestershire B98 7UB
Phone: 01527 503030
Fax: 01527 517432

Trust: Worcestershire Acute Hospitals
** NHS Trust**

Care here is midwife-led for most low-risk women. High-risk women experience shared care between the midwife, GP and consultant. The unit contains delivery rooms, a birthing-pool room and an antenatal day assessment unit. Most antenatal and postnatal care in the area takes place outside the hospital. Home and domino deliveries are offered, although the home birth rate is below average. A full range of antenatal classes including weekend classes and sessions for teenage mothers, are offered. Intervention rates here are high with a particularly high rate of emergency caesareans and inductions. The forceps rate is also significantly higher than the national average.

Consultant and Midwife Unit

Number of beds	37
Births per midwife	31.33
Births per bed	0.60
Home births	1%
Amenity Rooms, Price	£42

Obstetrician 24 hours	Yes
Paediatrician 24 hours	Yes
Full Water Birth Service	Yes

Tests

Routine Triple Testing	No
Nuchal Fold Scan	No
Fetal Assessment Unit	Yes

Pain Relief

24 hour epidural	Yes
Mobile epidural	Yes
Pethidine injections	Yes
Water (eg bath)	Yes

Intervention Rates	%	regional average %	national average %
Epidural	39	26	33
Elective Caesarean	9	9	8
Emergency Caesarean	16	13	12
Induction	25	15	20
Forceps	7	3	4
Ventouse	5	6	7
Episiotomy	8	13	14

Shrewsbury · **Royal Shrewsbury Hospital**

Mytton Oak Road, Shrewsbury
Shropshire SY3 8XQ
Phone: 01743 261 000
Fax: 01743 261 006

**Trust: Royal Shrewsbury Hospital
NHS Trust**

Royal Shrewsbury Hospital is the only maternity unit in the county that provides consultant-led care. If your pregnancy is low-risk you will be offered a number of other options for your care, to ensure that the majority of women being delivered at the unit are high-risk. For this reason, all home births are dealt with by peripheral maternity units. Consultant clinics are also provided in these units for patients' convenience. The greater use of local midwife-led units in the service reflects perhaps an attitude which is also noticeable in the very low intervention rates here. Taking into account the types of patients looked after here, the unit has the lowest caesarean rate in the country. In particular, elective caesareans are exceptionally infrequent.

Consultant and Midwife Unit

Number of beds	60
Births per midwife	32.5
Births per bed	0.86
Home births	0%
Amenity Rooms, Price	£36

Obstetrician 24 hours	Yes
Paediatrician 24 hours	Yes
Full Water Birth Service	Yes

Tests

Routine Triple Testing	No
Nuchal Fold Scan	Yes
Fetal Assessment Unit	Yes

Pain Relief

24 hour epidural	Yes
Mobile epidural	No
Pethidine injections	Yes
Water (eg bath)	Yes

Intervention Rates

	%	regional average %	national average %
Epidural	21	26	33
Elective Caesarean	3	9	8
Emergency Caesarean	10	13	12
Induction	24	15	20
Forceps	4	3	4
Ventouse	10	6	7
Episiotomy	10	13	14

THE WEST MIDLANDS **407**

Mytton Oak Road, Shrewsbury
Shropshire SY3 8XQ
Phone: 01743 261000
Fax: 01743 261006

Trust: Royal Shrewsbury Hospital
NHS Trust

The Royal Shrewsbury Hospital houses two maternity units, a consultant unit, and a GP-led unit. The GP-led unit provides an environment in which you are encouraged to give birth naturally, but has the assurance that medical assistance is close at hand in the event of complications. This unit also supervises home births and does them frequently. There are two postnatal wards with 12 beds between them, and two single rooms which are available for hire. There are two ensuite delivery rooms and one water birth room. You can ask for a water birth, but the unit does not have midwives trained in water birth available at all times. About one third of women are looked after in labour by a midwife they know. Double testing is used rather than triple testing.

Midwife Unit

Number of beds	16
Births	456
Midwives	14
Home births	6%
Amenity Rooms, Price	£36

Obstetrician 24 hours	Yes
Paediatrician 24 hours	Yes
Full Water Birth Service	No

Tests

Routine Triple Testing	No
Nuchal Fold Scan	Yes
Fetal Assessment Unit	Yes

Pain Relief

24 Hour epidural	No
Mobile epidural	No
Pethidine injections	Yes
Water (eg bath)	Yes

Midwife-led units are adequately equipped to care for women whose pregnancy is progressing normally without complications. As a result, intervention tends to be low in these units. Basic pain relief will be offered, but any woman requesting an epidural during the delivery will need to be transferred to the nearest consultant-led unit. A woman will also be transferred to the obstetric unit if any complications develop during the delivery.

Solihull · **Solihull Hospital**

Lade Lane, Solihull
West Midlands B91 2JL
Phone: 0121 424 2000
Fax: 0121 424 2336

Trust: Birmingham Heartlands and
Solihull NHS Trust

Birmingham Heartlands and Solihull Hospital operates a one-hospital, two-site philosophy. The Solihull site has a low-risk approach, while Birmingham Heartlands takes the higher risk cases. The antenatal care provided by the service is tailored to a local population. Special classes are available for Asian women and teenage mums, and sessions are held in the evenings and at weekends. A full range of antenatal tests is available. Triple tests are only offered routinely to women over 35, whose pregnancies carry a greater risk of chromosome disorders such as Down's Syndrome.

Water birth is offered for deliveries and the unit has its own pool. Midwives are available around the clock to assist you in the pool.

Consultant and Midwife Unit

Number of beds	21
Births per midwife	24
Births per bed	-
Home births	1%
Amenity Rooms, Price	£50

Obstetrician 24 hours	Yes
Paediatrician 24 hours	No
Full Water Birth Service	Yes

Tests

Routine Triple Testing	No
Nuchal Fold Scan	Yes
Fetal Assessment Unit	Yes

Pain Relief

24 hour epidural	Yes
Mobile epidural	Yes
Pethidine injections	Yes
Water (eg bath)	Yes

Intervention Rates	%	regional average %	national average %
Epidural	36	26	33
Elective Caesarean	9	9	8
Emergency Caesarean	15	13	12
Induction	20	15	20
Forceps	4	3	4
Ventouse	6	6	7
Episiotomy	15	13	14

Stafford · **Staffordshire General Hospital**

Weston Road
Stafford ST16 3SA
Phone: 01785 257 731
Fax: 01785 245 211

Trust: Mid Staffordshire General
Hospitals NHS Trust

This unit has made efforts to develop the service with electronically booked admissions – allowing your GP to directly book you an appointment at the hospital – and reducing the length of time women spend in hospital. The midwifery service here is organised in teams – which means you will be looked after through pregnancy and birth by a small group of midwives. Around one in five women delivered here is looked after in labour by a midwife they know from their antental care. Staffing levels are good, with the number of births per midwife well below the average for the region. Intervention rates at this hospital are also low overall with a low rate of elective caesareans.

There is no breastfeeding clinic, but they do provide a breastfeeding liaison midwife.

Consultant and Midwife Unit

Number of beds	27
Births per midwife	23
Births per bed	0.68
Home births	2%
Amenity Rooms, Price	-

Obstetrician 24 hours	Yes
Paediatrician 24 hours	Yes
Full Water Birth Service	No

Tests

Routine Triple Testing	No
Nuchal Fold Scan	Yes
Fetal Assessment Unit	Yes

Pain Relief

24 hour epidural	Yes
Mobile epidural	Yes
Pethidine injections	Yes
Water (eg bath)	Yes

Intervention Rates

	%	regional average %	national average %
Epidural	23	26	33
Elective Caesarean	6	9	8
Emergency Caesarean	11	13	12
Induction	-	15	20
Forceps	2	3	4
Ventouse	8	6	7
Episiotomy	13	13	14

Stoke-on-Trent · **North Staffordshire Hospital**

Royal Infirmary, Princes Road
Stoke-on-Trent ST4 7LN
Phone: 01782 715 444
Fax: 01782 552 001

Trust: North Staffordshire Hospital
NHS Trust

This is the main maternity unit at the North Staffordshire hospital, which also has a separate midwife-led unit. The hospital is a referral centre and takes high-risk cases from a wider area. It has a particularly high caesarean rate – both elective and emergency – however instrumental deliveries are less frequent here than in similar units. Homebirths are offered but not done often. Waterbirths are also an option. A variety of pain management techniques is offered including TENS and epidurals. There are daytime, evening and women only antenatal classes as well as separate classes for partners and husbands. It is not easy for the unit to accommodate your partner if you have to go into hospital before labour starts, but in exceptional circumstances this may be allowed.

Consultant and Midwife Unit

Number of beds	113
Births per midwife	27
Births per bed	0.98
Home births	1%
Amenity Rooms, Price	£26

Obstetrician 24 hours	Yes
Paediatrician 24 hours	Yes
Full Water Birth Service	Yes

Tests

Routine Triple Testing	No
Nuchal Fold Scan	Yes
Fetal Assessment Unit	Yes

Pain Relief

24 hour epidural	Yes
Mobile epidural	No
Pethidine injections	Yes
Water (eg bath)	Yes

Intervention Rates	%	regional average %	national average %
Epidural	31	26	33
Elective Caesarean	11	9	8
Emergency Caesarean	16	13	12
Induction	20	15	20
Forceps	1	3	4
Ventouse	1	6	7
Episiotomy	25	13	14

Stoke-on-Trent · **North Staffordshire Hospital**

Royal Infirmary, Princes Road
Stoke on Trent, ST4 7LN
Phone: 01782 715 444
Fax: 01782 552 001

Trust: North Staffordshire Hospital
NHS Trust

This midwife-led unit offers services for low-risk pregnancies, and aims to provide a 'homely' environment. Two delivery beds are available, sharing an en-suite bathroom and kitchen facilities. Following delivery, women are transferred to the adjoining post-natal ward. Full water birth facilities are on offer, as are a range of supporting services, including genetic counselling and a smoking cessation advisor. Alternative forms of pain management are encouraged including a range of sensory techniques including mats, a pool and coloured lights. However if you decide you need an epidural it may be possible to transfer you to the main unit for this. There are two breastfeeding co-ordinators working at the hospital and a breastfeeding clinic.

Midwife Unit

Number of beds	2
Births	621
Midwives	23
Home births	-
Amenity Rooms, Price	-

Obstetrician 24 hours	Yes
Paediatrician 24 hours	Yes
Full Water Birth Service	Yes

Tests

Routine Triple Testing	No
Nuchal Fold Scan	No
Fetal Assessment Unit	Yes

Pain Relief

24 Hour epidural	No
Mobile epidural	No
Pethidine injections	Yes
Water (eg bath)	Yes

Midwife-led units are adequately equipped to care for women whose pregnancy is progressing normally without complications. As a result, intervention tends to be low in these units. Basic pain relief will be offered, but any woman requesting an epidural during the delivery will need to be transferred to the nearest consultant-led unit. A woman will also be transferred to the obstetric unit if any complications develop during the delivery.

Stourbridge · **Wordsley Hospital**

Stream Road, Wordsley, Stourbridge
West Midlands DY8 5QX
Phone: 01384 456 111
Fax: 01384 244 395

Trust: The Dudley Group of Hospitals
NHS Trust

Wordsley Hospital offers maternity services from a shared midwife and consultant unit. The workload for midwives is relatively high which can sometimes affect the continuity of care your receive. Although the unit does not have a pool, you can have a water birth here if you bring your own pool. The unit is one of the few where elective caesareans are done more often than emergency caesareans. The total number of caesareans is not much higher than at other hospitals but most of them are booked in advance rather than performed as an emergency. Also, epidurals are widely used in the unit as a form of pain relief. Antenatal classes are held over the weekend and in the evenings, as well as during the daytime.

Consultant and Midwife Unit

Number of beds	74
Births per midwife	45.2
Births per bed	0.49
Home births	1%
Amenity Rooms, Price	£33

Obstetrician 24 hours	Yes
Paediatrician 24 hours	Yes
Full Water Birth Service	No

Tests

Routine Triple Testing	No
Nuchal Fold Scan	Yes
Fetal Assessment Unit	Yes

Pain Relief

24 hour epidural	Yes
Mobile epidural	Yes
Pethidine injections	Yes
Water (eg bath)	Yes

Intervention Rates	%	regional average %	national average %
Epidural	41	26	33
Elective Caesarean	12	9	8
Emergency Caesarean	10	13	12
Induction	26	15	20
Forceps	3	3	4
Ventouse	5	6	7
Episiotomy	16	13	14

Sutton Coldfield · **Good Hope District General Hospital**

Rectory Road, Sutton Coldfield
West Midlands B75 7RR
Phone: 0121 378 2211
Fax: 0121 311 1074

Trust: Good Hope Hospital
   NHS Trust

Good Hope District General Hospital aims to offer you choice about how you have your baby. You can opt for midwife-led care, shared care with obstetricians or GPs, a full water birth service, home-from-home birthing rooms, and home birth, though the rate of uptake for this is low. The recently refurbished delivery suite has high dependency facilities and an operating theatre to deal with complicated births. A Parent Education Team offers tours of the unit and guidance about the different choices. Continuity of care seems to be good with 40 per cent of women cared for in labour by a midwife they know from antenatal care – a higher proportion than would be expected at a unit of this size.

Consultant and Midwife Unit

Number of beds	56
Births per midwife	35
Births per bed	0.81
Home births	1%
Amenity Rooms, Price	£60

Obstetrician 24 hours	Yes
Paediatrician 24 hours	Yes
Full Water Birth Service	Yes

Tests

Routine Triple Testing	No
Nuchal Fold Scan	Yes
Fetal Assessment Unit	Yes

Pain Relief

24 hour epidural	Yes
Mobile epidural	Yes
Pethidine injections	Yes
Water (eg bath)	Yes

Intervention Rates

	%	regional average %	national average %
Epidural	23	26	33
Elective Caesarean	8	9	8
Emergency Caesarean	15	13	12
Induction	24	15	20
Forceps	2	3	4
Ventouse	7	6	7
Episiotomy	19	13	14

Telford · **Princess Royal Hospital**

Apley Castle, Telford
Shropshire TF1 6TF
Phone: 01952 641 222
Fax: 01952 243 405

Trust: Princess Royal Hospital
NHS Trust

Women booked into the Wrekin unit at the Princess Royal Hospital are low-risk. Fetal monitoring is available but rarely used, and if problems do occur during labour, women are referred to the consultant-led unit at nearby Royal Shrewsbury Hospital. You can also come to this unit for postnatal care after delivering at the Royal Shrewsbury. The unit estimates that almost a third of patients booked into the unit know the midwife who delivers them. There is a pool here and you can have a water birth, although the unit does not guarantee to have trained midwives on hand. Double testing is offered rather than triple testing for Down's, and for more complex tests and scans you will be referred to the Royal Shrewsbury Hospital.

Midwife Unit

Number of beds	17
Births	413
Midwives	30
Home births	4%
Amenity Rooms, Price	36

Obstetrician 24 hours	No
Paediatrician 24 hours	No
Full Water Birth Service	No

Tests

Routine Triple Testing	No
Nuchal Fold Scan	Yes
Fetal Assessment Unit	Yes

Pain Relief

24 Hour epidural	No
Mobile epidural	No
Pethidine injections	Yes
Water (eg bath)	Yes

Midwife-led units are adequately equipped to care for women whose pregnancy is progressing normally without complications. As a result, intervention tends to be low in these units. Basic pain relief will be offered, but any woman requesting an epidural during the delivery will need to be transferred to the nearest consultant-led unit. A woman will also be transferred to the obstetric unit if any complications develop during the delivery.

Walsall · **Manor Hospital**

Moat Road
Walsall WS2 9PS
Phone: 01922 721172
Fax: 01922 656621

Trust: Walsall Hospitals
  NHS Trust

This purpose built maternity ward has an award-winning security system including guards, video surveillance and electronic tagging for all babies. The wards and delivery suite are designed for maximum comfort and a homely feel – delivery rooms are carpeted and have spa baths for use in labour. The unit does offer epidurals and are used for pain relief in labour as often as in most hospitals. Alternative forms of pain management, such as birthing balls, TENS and reflexology are also on offer. Staffing levels are good but only a very small proportion of women giving birth at the unit are looked after in labour by a midwife they know. Induction is used relatively infrequently here, but the caesarean rate is significantly above the national average.

Consultant, GP and Midwife Unit

Number of beds	46
Births per midwife	30
Births per bed	0.88
Home births	1%
Amenity Rooms, Price	£53

Obstetrician 24 hours	Yes
Paediatrician 24 hours	Yes
Full Water Birth Service	Yes

Tests

Routine Triple Testing	No
Nuchal Fold Scan	Yes
Fetal Assessment Unit	Yes

Pain Relief

24 hour epidural	Yes
Mobile epidural	No
Pethidine injections	Yes
Water (eg bath)	Yes

Intervention Rates	%	regional average %	national average %
Epidural	23	26	33
Elective Caesarean	10	9	8
Emergency Caesarean	14	13	12
Induction	13	15	20
Forceps	3	3	4
Ventouse	6	6	7
Episiotomy	-	13	14

Warwick · **Warwick Hospital**

Lakin Road
Warwick CV34 5BW
Phone: 01926 495 321
Fax: 01926 482 603

Trust: South Warwickshire General Hospitals NHS Trust

The Annie Cay Maternity Unit is a large, purpose-built facility with 'home-from-home' style delivery rooms. Midwives are organised into teams that look after you through pregnancy and labour. However, the workload for midwives is high and the unit estimates that only about one in ten women here get looked after in labour by a midwife they know. There is a popular water birth service and special antenatal classes are organised for this. There are also separate antenatal classes for Asian women. There is a support team for antenatal testing. However triple testing is not routinely offered and if you want a nuchal fold scan or CVS you will have to pay a fee. The service is supported by an 11-cot Special Care Baby Unit that cares for ill or pre-term babies.

Consultant, GP and Midwife Unit

Number of beds	40
Births per midwife	39
Births per bed	0.95
Home births	2%
Amenity Rooms, Price	£27

Obstetrician 24 hours	Yes
Paediatrician 24 hours	Yes
Full Water Birth Service	Yes

Tests

Routine Triple Testing	No
Nuchal Fold Scan	No
Fetal Assessment Unit	Yes

Pain Relief

24 hour epidural	Yes
Mobile epidural	No
Pethidine injections	Yes
Water (eg bath)	Yes

Intervention Rates	%	regional average %	national average %
Epidural	34	26	33
Elective Caesarean	9	9	8
Emergency Caesarean	13	13	12
Induction	18	15	20
Forceps	5	3	4
Ventouse	6	6	7
Episiotomy	19	13	14

West Bromwich · **Sandwell General Hospital**

Lyndon, West Bromwich
West Midlands B71 4HJ
Phone: 0121 553 1831
Fax: 0121 607 3117

Trust: Sandwell Healthcare
NHS Trust

Midwife staffing levels here are good and midwives are organised into teams to try to provide better continuity of care through pregnancy and labour. About one in four women is looked after in labour by a midwife they know. This is in line with most units of this size.

Epidurals are available for pain relief, but they are used less often here than in other hospitals.

The unit gives additional support for women and families with special needs. There is a fetal day assessment unit, which gives women specialised care as an outpatient. A range of services includes a breastfeeding team, multiple birth group, smoking cessation teams and a teenage pregnancy service. Special assistance is offered to women from ethnic minority groups.

Consultant and Midwife Unit

Number of beds	35
Births per midwife	26.6
Births per bed	0.83
Home births	0.2%
Amenity Rooms, Price	£30

Obstetrician 24 hours	Yes
Paediatrician 24 hours	Yes
Full Water Birth Service	No

Tests

Routine Triple Testing	No
Nuchal Fold Scan	Yes
Fetal Assessment Unit	Yes

Pain Relief

24 hour epidural	Yes
Mobile epidural	No
Pethidine injections	Yes
Water (eg bath)	Yes

Intervention Rates

	%	regional average %	national average %
Epidural	16	26	33
Elective Caesarean	11	9	8
Emergency Caesarean	14	13	12
Induction	22	15	20
Forceps	3	3	4
Ventouse	6	6	7
Episiotomy	10	13	14

Wolverhampton · **New Cross Hospital**

Wednesfield Road, Wolverhampton
West Midlands WV10 0QP
Phone: 01902 307 999
Fax: 01902 642 810

Trust: The Royal Wolverhampton
Hospitals Trust

New Cross Hospital is a shared midwife and consultant unit. Some midwives at the unit do work under the domino system, however it is not routinely available for all mothers. Relatively few women are cared for in labour by a midwife they know. Intervention rates at New Cross are average, apart from forceps delivery, which is low. There are no water birth facilities at the hospital. However, midwives trained in water delivery are available 24hrs a day and a water birth is an option if you decide to have your baby at home and hire a pool from the unit. Booking scans and alfa-feto protein testing are offered to all women. The unit runs women only antenatal classes as well as classes for teenagers. Breastfeeding counsellors are available and can provide advice over the phone.

Consultant and Midwife Unit

Number of beds	58
Births per midwife	33
Births per bed	0.98
Home births	1%
Amenity Rooms, Price	£32

Obstetrician 24 hours	Yes
Paediatrician 24 hours	Yes
Full Water Birth Service	No

Tests

Routine Triple Testing	No
Nuchal Fold Scan	Yes
Fetal Assessment Unit	Yes

Pain Relief

24 hour epidural	Yes
Mobile epidural	Yes
Pethidine injections	Yes
Water (eg bath)	Yes

Intervention Rates	%	regional average %	national average %
Epidural	40	26	33
Elective Caesarean	11	9	8
Emergency Caesarean	16	13	12
Induction	-	15	20
Forceps	2	3	4
Ventouse	9	6	7
Episiotomy	13	13	14

Worcester · **Worcester Royal Infirmary**

Ronkswood Branch, Newtown Road
Worcester
Worcestershire WR5 1HN
Phone: 01905 763 333
Fax: 01905 760 787

Trust: Worcestershire Acute Hospitals
NHS Trust

A new hospital is due to open here in March 2002. The unit offers midwife-led care as well as consultant-led care for higher risk women.

The pattern of intervention here is unusual. There is a particularly high caesarean rate – the highest in England – both for elective and emergency caesareans. However other interventions such as induction and instrumental delivery with forceps or ventouse are less frequent than in other large hospitals.

Staffing levels are good and the unit offers the domino system under which the midwife who looks after you through pregnancy oversees your labour. There are women-only antenatal groups. Triple testing is not routinely offered and nuchal scans are not available.

Consultant and GP Care Led Unit

Number of beds	52
Births per midwife	29
Births per bed	0.83
Home births	2%
Amenity Rooms, Price	-

Obstetrician 24 hours	Yes
Paediatrician 24 hours	Yes
Full Water Birth Service	Yes

Tests

Routine Triple Testing	No
Nuchal Fold Scan	No
Fetal Assessment Unit	Yes

Pain Relief

24 hour epidural	Yes
Mobile epidural	Yes
Pethidine injections	Yes
Water (eg bath)	Yes

Intervention Rates

	%	regional average %	national average %
Epidural	37	26	33
Elective Caesarean	13	9	8
Emergency Caesarean	17	13	12
Induction	16	15	20
Forceps	3	3	4
Ventouse	5	6	7
Episiotomy	-	13	14

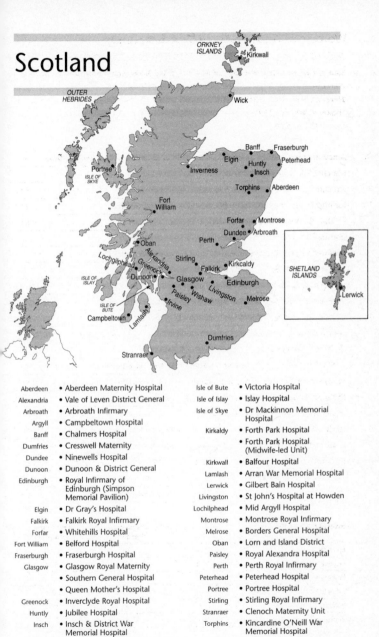

Scotland

Aberdeen	• Aberdeen Maternity Hospital	Isle of Bute	• Victoria Hospital
Alexandria	• Vale of Leven District General	Isle of Islay	• Islay Hospital
Arbroath	• Arbroath Infirmary	Isle of Skye	• Dr Mackinnon Memorial Hospital
Argyll	• Campbeltown Hospital		
Banff	• Chalmers Hospital	Kirkaldy	• Forth Park Hospital
Dumfries	• Cresswell Maternity		• Forth Park Hospital (Midwife-led Unit)
Dundee	• Ninewells Hospital		
Dunoon	• Dunoon & District General	Kirkwall	• Balfour Hospital
Edinburgh	• Royal Infirmary of Edinburgh (Simpson Memorial Pavilion)	Lamlash	• Arran War Memorial Hospital
		Lerwick	• Gilbert Bain Hospital
		Livingston	• St John's Hospital at Howden
Elgin	• Dr Gray's Hospital	Lochilphead	• Mid Argyll Hospital
Falkirk	• Falkirk Royal Infirmary	Montrose	• Montrose Royal Infirmary
Forfar	• Whitehills Hospital	Melrose	• Borders General Hospital
Fort William	• Belford Hospital	Oban	• Lorn and Island District
Fraserburgh	• Fraserburgh Hospital	Paisley	• Royal Alexandra Hospital
Glasgow	• Glasgow Royal Maternity	Perth	• Perth Royal Infirmary
	• Southern General Hospital	Peterhead	• Peterhead Hospital
	• Queen Mother's Hospital	Portree	• Portree Hospital
Greenock	• Inverclyde Royal Hospital	Stirling	• Stirling Royal Infirmary
Huntly	• Jubilee Hospital	Stranraer	• Clenoch Maternity Unit
Insch	• Insch & District War Memorial Hospital	Torphins	• Kincardine O'Neill War Memorial Hospital
Inverness	• Raigmore Hospital	Wick	• Caithness General Hospital
Irvine	• Ayrshire Central Hospital	Wishaw	• Wishaw General Hospital

Aberdeen · **Aberdeen Maternity Hospital**

Cornhill road, Aberdeen
AB25 2ZL
Phone: 01224 840 606

Trust: Grampian University Hospitals
NHS Trust

Aberdeen Maternity Hospital is the regional referral centre for the population of Grampian, Orkney and Shetland as well as the local maternity hospital for women in and around Aberdeen. Women requiring medical attention are flown here in an emergency.

The fact that the unit takes so many high-risk cases from across the north of Scotland is reflected in its relatively high caesarean rate.

The unit offers a choice of pain management options, ranging from epidurals and low-dosage mobile epidurals to a TENS machine.

A full range of antenatal screening tests are offered to all women booked with the service.

Consultant and Midwife Unit

Number of beds	102
Births per midwife	23.8
Births per bed	0.83
Home births	0.4%
Amenity Rooms, Price	£100

Obstetrician 24 hours	Yes
Paediatrician 24 hours	Yes
Full Water Birth Service	Yes

Tests

Routine Triple Testing	Yes
Nuchal Fold Scan	Yes
Fetal Assessment Unit	Yes

Pain Relief

24 hour epidural	Yes
Mobile epidural	Yes
Pethidine injections	Yes
Water (eg bath)	Yes

Intervention Rates

	%	national average %
Epidural	21	29
Elective Caesarean	6	7
Emergency Caesarean	19	13
Induction	21	24
Forceps	5	7
Ventouse	10	6
Episiotomy	12	15

Alexandria · **Vale of Leven District General Hospital**

Main Street, Alexandria
Dunbartonshire G83 0UA
Phone: 01389 754121
Fax: 01389 755948

Trust: Argyll & Clyde Acute Hospitals
 NHS Trust

The type of care you will receive at Vale of Leven District General Hospital depends on whether your pregnancy is judged to be high or low-risk. High-risk bookings are managed by a partnership of three obstetric consultants, GPs and midwives, while low-risk births are typically midwife-led or shared between midwives and GPs. You can choose domino system deliveries or home births as well as hospital delivery. A 19 bedded inpatient wing offers ante/postnatal care. There is also a 6 cot Special Care Baby Unit (SCBU). The proportion of induced births at the unit is significantly above average. The ventouse is used far more often than forceps for instrumental deliveries unlike many other hospitals in Scotland.

Consultant and Midwife Unit

Number of beds	24
Births per midwife	18.4
Births per bed	0.51
Home births	0.1%
Amenity Rooms, Price	-

Obstetrician 24 hours	Yes
Paediatrician 24 hours	Yes
Full Water Birth Service	No

Tests

Routine Triple Testing	No
Nuchal Fold Scan	No
Fetal Assessment Unit	Yes

Pain Relief

24 hour epidural	Yes
Mobile epidural	No
Pethidine injections	Yes
Water (eg bath)	Yes

Intervention Rates	%	national average %
Epidural	37	29
Elective Caesarean	9	7
Emergency Caesarean	13	13
Induction	31	24
Forceps	3	7
Ventouse	10	6
Episiotomy	19	15

Arbroath · **Arbroath Infirmary**

Rosemount Road
Arbroath
DD11 2AD
Phone: 01241 872584

Trust: Tayside University Hospitals NHS Trust

If your pregnancy is straightforward and you are happy to give birth naturally without epidural pain relief, the Arbroath Infirmary provides a good alternative to the main unit in Dundee. Also, local women who plan to deliver in Ninewells Hospital can have their antenatal and postnatal care here. The triple test, early pregnancy ultrasound scans and anomaly ultrasound scans are offered to all women. For some scans and tests you would have to travel to Ninewells Hospital in Dundee, which should provide access to all the services you might need.

In the event of problems developing, such as your labour failing to progress, you would be transferred to Ninewells in Dundee. This happens to about one in five women.

Midwife Unit

Number of beds	6
Births	85
Midwives	10
Home births	0%
Amenity Rooms, Price	-
Obstetrician 24 hours	No
Paediatrician 24 hours	No
Water Birth Offered	No

Tests

Routine Triple Testing	Yes
Nuchal Fold Scan	Yes
Fetal Assessment Unit	No

Pain Relief

24 hour epidural	No
Mobile epidural	No
Pethidine injections	Yes
Water (eg bath)	Yes

Midwife-led units are adequately equipped to care for women whose pregnancy is progressing normally without complications. As a result, intervention tends to be low in these units. Basic pain relief will be offered, but any woman requesting an epidural during the delivery will need to be transferred to the nearest consultant-led unit. A woman will also be transferred to the obstetric unit if any complications develop during the delivery.

Argyll · **Campbeltown Hospital**

Ralston Road
Campbeltown
Argyll
Scotland, PA28 6BP

Trust: Lomond & Argyll Primary Care
NHS Trust

The maternity unit in Campbeltown Hospital is a small modern facility that can offer local women a natural birth experience. Those considered at higher risk would not be suitable for the unit and would probably be advised to book with a consultant and midwife shared facility, such as the Southern General Hospital in Glasgow. If you book with the Campbeltown Service, you will be offered the triple test and an early pregnancy ultrasound scan. Anomaly ultrasound scans, however, are not offered routinely to all women.

More complex procedures, such as nuchal fold scans, amniocentesis and chorionic villus sampling would be available if you needed them, but you would have to travel to the Southern General Hospital.

Midwife Unit

Number of beds	4
Births	6
Midwives	1
Home births	0
Amenity Rooms and Price	-

Obstetrician 24 hours	No
Paediatrician 24 hours	No
Water Birth Offered	No

Tests

Routine Triple Testing	Yes
Nuchal Fold Scan	Yes
Fetal Assessment Unit	No

Pain Relief

24 hour epidural	No
Mobile epidural	No
Pethidine injections	Yes
Water (eg bath)	Yes

Midwife-led units are adequately equipped to care for women whose pregnancy is progressing normally without complications. As a result, intervention tends to be low in these units. Basic pain relief will be offered, but any woman requesting an epidural during the delivery will need to be transferred to the nearest consultant-led unit. A woman will also be transferred to the obstetric unit if any complications develop during the delivery.

Banff · **Chalmers Hospital**

Clunie Street
Banff, AB45 2PS
Phone: 01261 812567
Fax: 01261 818074

Trust: Grampian Primary Care
NHS Trust

This midwife-led unit provides antenatal and postnatal care for women who deliver at the consultant units in Aberdeen and Elgin as well as the women who give birth here. Ultrasound services are available although booking scans are not done as a matter of course for everybody but only if you are unsure of the age of the fetus. A consultant visits monthly to review any problems.

The domino system is available on request but continuity of care through pregnancy and labour is pretty much assured in such a small unit. The unit uses hot packs, a Ten machine, and promotes mobility as a form of pain relief.

Midwife Unit

Number of beds	6
Births	57
Midwives	11
Home births	0%
Amenity Rooms, Price	-
Obstetrician 24 hours	No
Paediatrician 24 hours	No
Full Water Birth Service	No

Tests

Routine Triple Testing	No
Nuchal Fold Scan	Yes
Fetal Assessment Unit	No

Pain Relief

24 Hour epidural	No
Mobile epidural	No
Pethidine injections	Yes
Water (eg bath)	Yes

Midwife-led units are adequately equipped to care for women whose pregnancy is progressing normally without complications. As a result, intervention tends to be low in these units. Basic pain relief will be offered, but any woman requesting an epidural during the delivery will need to be transferred to the nearest consultant-led unit. A woman will also be transferred to the obstetric unit if any complications develop during the delivery.

Dumfries · **Cresswell Maternity Hospital**

Dumfries
DG1 2ES
Phone: 01387 246246

Trust: Dumfries & Galloway Acute &
Maternity Hospitals NHS Trust

Cresswell's maternity unit will soon be moving to a new building on the Dumfries and Galloway Hospital site.

The unit is managed by midwives and consultants, and unusually for a consultant unit, epidurals are not offered for pain relief in labour. However, alternative forms of pain management are offered including water birth, relaxation, aromatherapy and a Ten machine.

Midwives are organised in teams which means you will be looked after by one team throughout your pregnancy and labour. This helps to improve continuity of care – three-quarters of women are cared for in labour by a midwife they know. Domino deliveries are also offered. The unit also organises aquanatal and baby massage classes.

Consultant and Midwife Unit

Number of beds	40
Births per midwife	20
Births per bed	0.68
Home births	1%
Amenity Rooms, Price	-

Obstetrician 24 hours	No
Paediatrician 24 hours	No
Full Water Birth Service	Yes

Tests

Routine Triple Testing	Yes
Nuchal Fold Scan	Yes
Fetal Assessment Unit	Yes

Pain Relief

24 hour epidural	No
Mobile epidural	No
Pethidine injections	Yes
Water (eg bath)	Yes

Intervention Rates	%	national average %
Epidural	0	29
Elective Caesarean	9	7
Emergency Caesarean	14	13
Induction	23	24
Forceps	-	7
Ventouse	-	6
Episiotomy	14	15

Dundee · **Ninewells Hospital**

Dundee
DD4 9NN
Phone: 01382 660111
Fax: 01382 660445

Trust: Tayside University Hospitals
NHS Trust

Ninewells is a regional referral centre for the population of Tayside and northeast Fife, and a number of women transfer from the smaller midwife-led facilities to the main unit if they have more complex pregnancies or if they are keen to have epidural pain relief not always offered in smaller units. The rate of epidural use in this hospital is, perhaps as a result, higher than average. Also, this is one of the rare hospitals that has a significantly higher number of elective caesareans than emergency caesareans.

There are three midwife-led units connected to Ninewells : the Arbroath Infirmay in Arbroath, the Whitehills Hospital in Forfar and the Montrose Royal Infirmary in Montrose. All cater for women wanting natural deliveries without epidural pain relief.

Consultant and Midwife Unit

Number of beds	42
Births per midwife	27
Births per bed	1.1
Home births	0.4%
Amenity Rooms, Price	£30

Obstetrician 24 hours	Yes
Paediatrician 24 hours	Yes
Full Water Birth Service	No

Tests

Routine Triple Testing	Yes
Nuchal Fold Scan	Yes
Fetal Assessment Unit	Yes

Pain Relief

24 hour epidural	Yes
Mobile epidural	No
Pethidine injections	Yes
Water (eg bath)	Yes

Intervention Rates

	%	national average %
Epidural	47	29
Elective Caesarean	13	7
Emergency Caesarean	10	13
Induction	22	24
Forceps	9	7
Ventouse	6	6
Episiotomy	22	15

Dunoon · **Dunoon & District General Hospital**

Sandbank Road, Dunoon
Argyll, PA23 7RL
Phone: 01369 704341
Fax: 01369 702192

Trust: Lomond & Argyll Primary Care NHS Trust

This midwife-led maternity unit at Dunoon and District General Hospital has a small team of midwives who create a user-friendly service. The midwives make great efforts to support home births – which are relatively rare in Scotland. Domino deliveries are also offered.

Water births are possible if you provide your own pool, although there may not always be midwives trained in water birth available at all times. The unit is flexible about postnatal and antenatal visits.

A parent education programme runs over seven weeks, with two classes in the evening. Breastfeeding and reunion groups are also offered.

Midwife Unit

Number of beds	7
Births	28
Midwives	8
Home births	3%
Amenity Rooms, Price	-

Obstetrician 24 hours	No
Paediatrician 24 hours	No
Full Water Birth Service	No

Tests

Routine Triple Testing	Yes
Nuchal Fold Scan	No
Fetal Assessment Unit	No

Pain Relief

24 Hour epidural	No
Mobile epidural	No
Pethidine injections	Yes
Water (eg bath)	Yes

Midwife-led units are adequately equipped to care for women whose pregnancy is progressing normally without complications. As a result, intervention tends to be low in these units. Basic pain relief will be offered, but any woman requesting an epidural during the delivery will need to be transferred to the nearest consultant-led unit. A woman will also be transferred to the obstetric unit if any complications develop during the delivery.

Edinburgh · **Royal Infirmary of Edinburgh**

Lauriston Place, Edinburgh
EH3 9YW
Phone: 0131 5361000
Fax: 0131 5361001

Trust: Lothian University Hospitals
  NHS Trust

The Simpson Memorial Maternity Pavilion at the Royal Infirmary of Edinburgh is the largest maternity unit in Scotland and the only unit in Edinburgh. It is transferring to a new, purpose built hospital in March 2002 and will be the main maternity centre in south-east Scotland.

As a regional referral centre it has a relatively high caesarean rate. These are done much more often as an emergency procedure – usually where a woman has attempted natural delivery but problems have developed – rather than as a planned procedure. Also, forceps are used much more often than in other units. Home births are offered and done more often than by other large Scottish hospitals.

There is a full epidural service including mobile epidurals.

Consultant and Midwife Unit

Number of beds	94
Births per midwife	31
Births per bed	1.17
Home births	0.9%
Amenity Rooms, Price	£83

Obstetrician 24 hours	Yes
Paediatrician 24 hours	Yes
Full Water Birth Service	Yes

Tests

Routine Triple Testing	Yes
Nuchal Fold Scan	No
Fetal Assessment Unit	Yes

Pain Relief

24 hour epidural	Yes
Mobile epidural	Yes
Pethidine injections	Yes
Water (eg bath)	Yes

Intervention Rates

	%	national average %
Epidural	25	29
Elective Caesarean	7	7
Emergency Caesarean	17	13
Induction	20	24
Forceps	10	7
Ventouse	3	6
Episiotomy	10	15

Elgin · **Dr Gray's Hospital**

Elgin, Moray
IV30 1SN
Phone: 01343 543 131

Trust: Grampian University Hospitals
NHS Trust

Three obstetric consultants work at this shared-care unit, one of which is named to each expectant mother. Each consultant will routinely see you two to three times during your pregnancy, including the booking appointment at which a dating scan is offered. There is not 24-hour obstetric cover on the labour ward but consultants are on call and close to the unit. Midwife staffing levels are good and domino deliveries are offered.

Epidurals are not offered for pain relief. To get one you would need to go to either Raigmore, Inverness or Aberdeen maternity unit. The unit runs postnatal support groups for women to share experiences. Breastfeeding counsellors are also available.

Consultant and Midwife Unit

Number of beds	26
Births per midwife	21.6
Births per bed	0.47
Home births	2%
Amenity Rooms, Price	£50

Obstetrician 24 hours	No
Paediatrician 24 hours	No
Full Water Birth Service	

Tests

Routine Triple Testing	No
Nuchal Fold Scan	Yes
Fetal Assessment Unit	Yes

Pain Relief

24 hour epidural	No
Mobile epidural	No
Pethidine injections	Yes
Water (eg bath)	Yes

Intervention Rates

	%	national average %
Epidural	-	29
Elective Caesarean	7	7
Emergency Caesarean	9	13
Induction	28	24
Forceps	5	7
Ventouse	8	6
Episiotomy	-	15

Falkirk · **Falkirk Royal Infirmary**

Major's Loan, Falkirk
FK1 5QE
Phone: 01324 624000
Fax: 01324 616068

Trust: Forth Valley Acute Hospitals
NHS Trust

Care is shared between obstetricians, teams of midwives and GP surgeries. You will be assigned to a team of midwives who will work with your GP to look after you through pregnancy and delivery. Intervention rates are low here. In particular elective caesareans are rare. Epidurals are available for pain relief and even though there is not a 24 hour service many women who give birth here do get epidurals to manage the pain. Home births can be done but are not done often. Water births can be arranged but women need to organize their own pool. Neonatal special care and intensive care provision is available on site with middle grade paediatric staff supporting this facility. Close links exist with neonatal and paediatric units in Glasgow and Edinburgh.

Consultant and Midwife Unit

Number of beds	42
Births per midwife	15
Births per bed	0.51
Home births	0.1%
Amenity Rooms, Price	£45

Obstetrician 24 hours	Yes
Paediatrician 24 hours	Yes
Full Water Birth Service	No

Tests

Routine Triple Testing	No
Nuchal Fold Scan	Yes
Fetal Assessment Unit	Yes

Pain Relief

24 hour epidural	No
Mobile epidural	No
Pethidine injections	Yes
Water (eg bath)	Yes

Intervention Rates

	%	national average %
Epidural	22	29
Elective Caesarean	5	7
Emergency Caesarean	12	13
Induction	20	24
Forceps	4	7
Ventouse	5	6
Episiotomy	14	15

Forfar · **Whitehills Hospital**

Forfar
Angus DD8 3DY
Phone: 01307 464551

Trust: Tayside Univeristy Hospitals NHS Trust

The Whitehills unit has two delivery beds and is staffed by at least one midwife between 8.00am and 5.00pm. Outside these hours, two midwives are available on call. The unit also provides antenatal and postnatal care for women delivered in Dundee. Discharge after birth is usually quick – most go home six hours after the birth. In the event of a complication in your delivery at the Whitehills Hospital maternity unit, midwives are advised by telephone by an obstetric consultant at Ninewells Hospital in Dundee. If necessary, you would be transferred to the consultant unit to complete the birth. There is a maternity day care unit here but for some tests or investigations you might have to travel to Ninewells Hospital.

Midwife Unit

Number of beds	2
Births	51
Midwives	6
Home births	4%
Amenity Rooms, Price	-

Obstetrician 24 hours	No
Paediatrician 24 hours	No
Water Birth Offered	No

Tests

Routine Triple Testing	Yes
Nuchal Fold Scan	Yes
Fetal Assessment Unit	No

Pain Relief

24 hour epidural	No
Mobile epidural	No
Pethidine injections	Yes
Water (eg bath)	Yes

Midwife-led units are adequately equipped to care for women whose pregnancy is progressing normally without complications. As a result, intervention tends to be low in these units. Basic pain relief will be offered, but any woman requesting an epidural during the delivery will need to be transferred to the nearest consultant-led unit. A woman will also be transferred to the obstetric unit if any complications develop during the delivery.

Fort William · **Belford Hospital**

Belford Road
Fort William, PH33 6BS
Phone: 01397 702481
Fax: 01397 792772

Trust: Highland Acute Hospitals
NHS Trust

This midwifery-led unit operates an 'open door' policy, allowing women 24hr access to advice and a friendly ear. This ensures that all women have access to the advice of a midwife regardless of their location. Set up by midwives in 1998, the unit attempts to create a homely atmosphere and be flexible about meeting different women's wishes. The small unit is able to provide good continuity of care – almost every women who gives birth here knows the midwife who delivers her. Domino deliveries are an option as are home births which are done relatively frequently. You may also request a water birth at home. Antenatal class arrangements are flexible and provide one-to-one sessions. Complications are referred to Inverness.

Midwife Unit

Number of beds	6
Births	38
Midwives	8
Home births	5%
Amenity Rooms, Price	-
Obstetrician 24 hours	No
Paediatrician 24 hours	No
Full Water Birth Service	Yes

Tests

Routine Triple Testing	Yes
Nuchal Fold Scan	Yes
Fetal Assessment Unit	Yes

Pain Relief

24 Hour epidural	No
Mobile epidural	No
Pethidine injections	Yes
Water (eg bath)	Yes

Midwife-led units are adequately equipped to care for women whose pregnancy is progressing normally without complications. As a result, intervention tends to be low in these units. Basic pain relief will be offered, but any woman requesting an epidural during the delivery will need to be transferred to the nearest consultant-led unit. A woman will also be transferred to the obstetric unit if any complications develop during the delivery.

Fraserburgh · **Fraserburgh Hospital**

Lochpots Road, Fraserburgh
Aberdeenshire, AB43 9WF
Phone: 01346 513151
Fax: 01346 514548

Trust: Grampian Primary Care
  NHS Trust

Fraserburgh Maternity Unit is staffed by a small team of midwives who provide antenatal care, postnatal care and care through labour and delivery. The unit caters for women with uncomplicated pregnancies who want to give birth naturally. Difficult pregnancies are referred to Aberdeen Maternity Hospital. As with many small units, the level of personal care is better than in larger hospitals – one-to-one care in labour is pretty well guaranteed and almost everyone who gives birth here knows the midwife who delivers them. Domino deliveries are offered. Antenatal classes are provided throughout the week and at weekends, and partners, friends and relatives are welcome to attend. Support services include a breastfeeding clinic.

Midwife Unit

Number of beds	6
Births	78
Midwives	10
Home births	1%
Amenity Rooms, Price	-

Obstetrician 24 hours	No
Paediatrician 24 hours	No
Full Water Birth Service	No

Tests

Routine Triple Testing	Yes
Nuchal Fold Scan	No
Fetal Assessment Unit	Yes

Pain Relief

24 Hour epidural	No
Mobile epidural	No
Pethidine injections	Yes
Water (eg bath)	Yes

Midwife-led units are adequately equipped to care for women whose pregnancy is progressing normally without complications. As a result, intervention tends to be low in these units. Basic pain relief will be offered, but any woman requesting an epidural during the delivery will need to be transferred to the nearest consultant-led unit. A woman will also be transferred to the obstetric unit if any complications develop during the delivery.

Glasgow · **Princess Royal Maternity Hospital**

146-163 Rottenrow,
Glasgow, G4 0NA
Phone: 0141 2115400
Fax: 0141 2115399

Trust: North Glasgow University
**   Hospitals NHS Trust**

Formally known as the Glasgow Royal Maternity hospital, this is a largest of three large maternity units in Glasgow, with 14 delivery beds.

The hospital has the highest induction rate in the UK with 40 per cent of women being induced. In contrast, the Southern General only induces 23 per cent of women.

Staffing levels are good but continuity of care is not yet provided so few women are delivered by a midwife they know.

Home births are performed very rarely. Water birth is offered and a pool has recently been installed at the unit.

A full range of pain relief is offered and occasionally mobile epidurals are also available. Over half of all women delivering vaginally had an epidural.

Consultant and Midwife Unit

Number of beds	85
Births per midwife	21
Births per bed	0.93
Home births	0.3%
Amenity Rooms, Price	-

Obstetrician 24 hours	Yes
Paediatrician 24 hours	Yes
Full Water Birth Service	No

Tests

Routine Triple Testing	No
Nuchal Fold Scan	Yes
Fetal Assessment Unit	Yes

Pain Relief

24 hour epidural	Yes
Mobile epidural	Yes
Pethidine injections	Yes
Water (eg bath)	Yes

Intervention Rates	%	national average %
Epidural	45	29
Elective Caesarean	7	7
Emergency Caesarean	15	13
Induction	40	24
Forceps	9	7
Ventouse	5	6
Episiotomy	9	15

Glasgow · **Southern General Hospital**

1345 Govan Road,
Glasgow, G51 4TF
Phone: 0141 201 1100
Fax: 0141 201 2999

Trust: South Glasgow University Hospitals NHS Trust

Southern General makes an interesting contrast to the Princess Royal Maternity Hospital – intervention rates are much lower with far fewer caesareans and inductions.

A range of different methods of conventional and complementary pain relief are available as well as epidurals which are widely used.

The unit routinely offers triple testing, though women must pay for nuchal scans which are done at The Queen Mother's Hospital.

Parent education sessions, antenatal classes, women only classes, minority language and classes for grandparents are all available. There is a breastfeeding clinic and access to breastfeeding counsellors.

Consultant and Midwife Unit

Number of beds	67
Births per midwife	20
Births per bed	0.78
Home births	0.6%
Amenity Rooms, Price	-

Obstetrician 24 hours	Yes
Paediatrician 24 hours	Yes
Full Water Birth Service	No

Tests

Routine Triple Testing	No
Nuchal Fold Scan	No
Fetal Assessment Unit	Yes

Pain Relief

24 hour epidural	Yes
Mobile epidural	No
Pethidine injections	Yes
Water (eg bath)	Yes

Intervention Rates	%	national average %
Epidural	45	29
Elective Caesarean	7	7
Emergency Caesarean	10	13
Induction	23	24
Forceps	6	7
Ventouse	7	6
Episiotomy	-	15

Glasgow · **The Queen Mother's Hospital**

Yorkhill, Glasgow
G3 8SJ
Phone: 0141 2010550
Fax: 0141 2010836

Trust: Yorkhill NHS Trust

Rates for forceps-assisted deliveries at The Queen Mother's Hospital in Glasgow are among the highest in the country, though this may be influenced by the unit's special interest in the management of high-risk pregnancies. The caesarean rate – and in particular the elective caesarean rate – is also high. There is a neonatal paediatric unit with 10 intensive care cots and 18 special care cots. The proximity of the Royal Hospital for Sick Children provides access to a wide range of highly specialised paediatric services. The fetal medicine and ultrasound departments provide sophisticated investigations including fetal blood sampling.

If your pregnancy is low-risk, care would be managed largely by midwives in a separate four-bed labour suite and medical intervention in the birth would be much less likely.

Consultant and Midwife Unit

Number of beds	84
Births per midwife	19
Births per bed	0.71
Home births	0.4%
Amenity Rooms, Price	-

Obstetrician 24 hours	Yes
Paediatrician 24 hours	Yes
Full Water Birth Service	

Tests

Routine Triple Testing	No
Nuchal Fold Scan	Yes
Fetal Assessment Unit	Yes

Pain Relief

24 hour epidural	Yes
Mobile epidural	Yes
Pethidine injections	Yes
Water (eg bath)	Yes

Intervention Rates

	%	national average %
Epidural	34	29
Elective Caesarean	10	7
Emergency Caesarean	15	13
Induction	-	24
Forceps	13	7
Ventouse	5	6
Episiotomy	-	15

438 GOOD BIRTH GUIDE

Greenock · **Inverclyde Royal Hospital**

Larkfield Road, Greenock
Renfrewshire PA16 0XN
Phone: 01475 633777
Fax: 01475 636753

Trust: Argyll & Clyde Acute Hospitals
  NHS Trust

The facility is a small, compact unit, offering a service which is fully integrated with community provision, and community midwives spend one day a week in the labour ward.

Home births are not undertaken often but you do have the option of domino care. Epidurals are available for pain relief but the service is only 24 hours Monday to Thursday, so it is, perhaps, not suprising that the number of women having epidurals is below average. The caesarean rate is much lower than average – in particular the emergency caesarean rate. Inductions however are widespread with nearly a third of women being induced. Antenatal classes include one-to-one sessions. The unit offers short hospital stays. Double testing for Down's is offered rather than triple testing.

Consultant and Midwife Unit

Number of beds	30
Births per midwife	16.9
Births per bed	0.45
Home births	0.2%
Amenity Rooms, Price	£15

Obstetrician 24 hours	Yes
Paediatrician 24 hours	Yes
Full Water Birth Service	No

Tests

Routine Triple Testing	No
Nuchal Fold Scan	Yes
Fetal Assessment Unit	Yes

Pain Relief

24 hour epidural	No
Mobile epidural	No
Pethidine injections	Yes
Water (eg bath)	Yes

Intervention Rates

	%	national average %
Epidural	26	29
Elective Caesarean	6	7
Emergency Caesarean	7	13
Induction	30	24
Forceps	5	7
Ventouse	7	6
Episiotomy	12	15

Huntly · **Jubilee Hospital**

Bleachfield Street
Huntly, AB54 8EX
Phone: 01466 792116
Fax: 01466 794544

Trust: Grampian Primary Care
NHS Trust

The Huntly maternity unit is a midwife-led service for women with uncomplex pregnancies who want to give birth naturally. However postnatal care, with consultant supervision, is provided for all risk categories, so if you give birth elsewhere you can return here for postnatal care. There is only one delivery bed and only a handful of births take place in the unit each year. Several more births are handled as home births by the unit. Water births can be supervised if you hire your own pool. Both midwife and consultant antenatal clinics and parenting classes take place at the unit. Weekend classes may be arranged. The unit has a comprehensive breastfeeding support service.

Midwife Unit

Number of beds	4
Births	20
Midwives	10
Home births	17%
Amenity Rooms, Price	-

Obstetrician 24 hours	No
Paediatrician 24 hours	No
Full Water Birth Service	No

Tests

Routine Triple Testing	Yes
Nuchal Fold Scan	Yes
Fetal Assessment Unit	No

Pain Relief

24 Hour epidural	No
Mobile epidural	No
Pethidine injections	Yes
Water (eg bath)	Yes

Midwife-led units are adequately equipped to care for women whose pregnancy is progressing normally without complications. As a result, intervention tends to be low in these units. Basic pain relief will be offered, but any woman requesting an epidural during the delivery will need to be transferred to the nearest consultant-led unit. A woman will also be transferred to the obstetric unit if any complications develop during the delivery.

Insch · **Insch & District War Memorial Hospital**

Rannes Street
Insch, AB51 3UL
Phone: 01464 820213
Fax: 01464 820233

Trust: Grampian Primary Care
NHS Trust

This small maternity unit looks after women with low-risk pregnancies who can give birth in the unit or at home without the need for any medical intervention or epidural pain relief. Postnatal care is also provided for local people who give birth elsewhere. Water births can be done but you would be required to hire your own pool. You may also have a domino delivery, with discharge after birth taking place within six hours. Antenatal classes can be arranged at weekends if a woman is over 36 weeks pregnant and has failed to attend any sessions, otherwise classes take place in the evenings. Only health visitor sessions take place during the daytime. The unit's breastfeeding support service includes a twice-monthly breastfeeding support group.

Midwife Unit

Number of beds	3
Births	20
Midwives	10
Home births	13%
Amenity Rooms, Price	-

Obstetrician 24 hours	No
Paediatrician 24 hours	No
Full Water Birth Service	No

Tests

Routine Triple Testing	Yes
Nuchal Fold Scan	Yes
Fetal Assessment Unit	No

Pain Relief

24 Hour epidural	No
Mobile epidural	No
Pethidine injections	Yes
Water (eg bath)	Yes

Midwife-led units are adequately equipped to care for women whose pregnancy is progressing normally without complications. As a result, intervention tends to be low in these units. Basic pain relief will be offered, but any woman requesting an epidural during the delivery will need to be transferred to the nearest consultant-led unit. A woman will also be transferred to the obstetric unit if any complications develop during the delivery.

Inverness · **Raigmore Hospital**

Old Perth Road, Inverness
IV2 3UJ
Phone: 01463 704000
Fax: 01463 711322

Trust: Highland Acute Hospitals
NHS Trust

Raigmore is the main maternity unit for a large area of the highlands. Staffing levels are good, and you can request a domino delivery but home births are very rarely undertaken – not surprising, perhaps, in view of the local geography. Water birth is available with a purpose-built facility at the unit, but only on a limited basis as not all midwives in the unit are trained in water deliveries.

Parent education sessions include special classes for teenagers and for second time mothers. The unit has a breastfeeding support group which offers advice to mothers and there is also access to breastfeeding counsellors. Antenatal testing is limited. Triple testing is not routine and nuchal fold scans are not available.

Consultant and Midwife Unit

Number of beds	60
Births per midwife	29.1
Births per bed	0.63
Home births	0.1%
Amenity Rooms, Price	£20

Obstetrician 24 hours	Yes
Paediatrician 24 hours	Yes
Full Water Birth Service	No

Tests

Routine Triple Testing	No
Nuchal Fold Scan	No
Fetal Assessment Unit	No

Pain Relief

24 hour epidural	Yes
Mobile epidural	No
Pethidine injections	Yes
Water (eg bath)	Yes

Intervention Rates	%	national average %
Epidural	36	29
Elective Caesarean	8	7
Emergency Caesarean	15	13
Induction	17	24
Forceps	6	7
Ventouse	5	6
Episiotomy	19	15

Irvine · **Ayrshire Central Hospital**

Kilwinning Road, Irvine
Ayrshire KA12 8SS
Phone: 01294 274191
Fax: 01294 278680

Trust: Ayrshire and Arran Acute
 Hospitals NHS Trust

Women booked with the Ayrshire Central Hospital maternity service may have their hospital care delivered by a team of midwives and consultants in a traditional setting, or by midwives only in a small four-bedded side unit. The midwife unit is designed to feel homely – steel trolleys and medical equipment are absent. In contrast the consultant unit has full medical facilities including a neonatal unit. In the midwife unit, the emphasis is on allowing women freedom of movement during labour and you will be encouraged to be up and about for as long as possible during labour. It is possible to walk round the grounds, which include a secluded garden. If you decide you need an epidural – or if an emergency arises – you can be transfered to the main consultant unit.

Consultant and Midwife Unit

Number of beds	72
Births per midwife	18.5
Births per bed	0.89
Home births	0.1%
Amenity Rooms, Price	-

Obstetrician 24 hours	Yes
Paediatrician 24 hours	Yes
Full Water Birth Service	Yes

Tests

Routine Triple Testing	Yes
Nuchal Fold Scan	No
Fetal Assessment Unit	Yes

Pain Relief

24 hour epidural	Yes
Mobile epidural	Yes
Pethidine injections	Yes
Water (eg bath)	Yes

Intervention Rates

	%	national average %
Epidural	33	29
Elective Caesarean	8	7
Emergency Caesarean	13	13
Induction	26	24
Forceps	7	7
Ventouse	2	6
Episiotomy	12	15

Isle of Bute · **Victoria Hospital**

High Street, Rothesay
Isle of Bute, PA20 9JJ
Phone: 01700 503938
Fax: 01700 502865

Trust: Lomond and Argyll Primary Care
NHS Trust

This is a small GP maternity unit with one delivery bed. Deliveries are low-risk; high-risk women are booked to deliver in the Rankin Unit at Inverclyde Royal Hospital. Each of the hospital-based midwives has her own caseload of women and works as part of a small team, so all women know the midwife who delivers their baby. Occasionally, high-risk women deliver on the island due to unforeseen circumstances. The unit's guide deems that any woman over 5cm dilated should not be transferred to the mainland. For a number of antenatal screens and tests women are referred to Inverclyde. There is a very flexible antenatal class service, with classes available any time on request. The health visitor provides breastfeeding counselling.

Midwife Unit

Number of beds	3
Births	9
Midwives	5
Home births	0%
Amenity Rooms, Price	-

Obstetrician 24 hours	No
Paediatrician 24 hours	No
Full Water Birth Service	No

Tests

Routine Triple Testing	Yes
Nuchal Fold Scan	Yes
Fetal Assessment Unit	No

Pain Relief

24 Hour epidural	No
Mobile epidural	No
Pethidine injections	Yes
Water (eg bath)	Yes

Midwife-led units are adequately equipped to care for women whose pregnancy is progressing normally without complications. As a result, intervention tends to be low in these units. Basic pain relief will be offered, but any woman requesting an epidural during the delivery will need to be transferred to the nearest consultant-led unit. A woman will also be transferred to the obstetric unit if any complications develop during the delivery.

Isle of Islay · **Islay Hospital**

Gortanvogle Road, Bowmore
Isle of Islay, PA43 7JD
Phone: 01496 810219
Fax: 01496 810754

Trust: Lomond & Argyll Primary Care
    NHS Trust

This maternity unit is one of the smallest in the UK, with just five births taking place there last year. Care is GP-led, and the unit has just one bed. Despite its size, the unit does offer an antenatal testing service that includes triple testing and booking ultrasound scans. Antenatal classes are flexible and include women-only groups.

Midwife Unit

Number of beds	1
Births	5
Midwives	6
Home births	0%
Amenity Rooms, Price	-
Obstetrician 24 hours	No
Paediatrician 24 hours	No
Full Water Birth Service	No

Tests

Routine Triple Testing	Yes
Nuchal Fold Scan	No
Fetal Assessment Unit	No

Pain Relief

24 Hour epidural	No
Mobile epidural	No
Pethidine injections	Yes
Water (eg bath)	No

Midwife-led units are adequately equipped to care for women whose pregnancy is progressing normally without complications. As a result, intervention tends to be low in these units. Basic pain relief will be offered, but any woman requesting an epidural during the delivery will need to be transferred to the nearest consultant-led unit. A woman will also be transferred to the obstetric unit if any complications develop during the delivery.

Isle of Skye · **Dr Mackinnon Memorial Hospital**

Broadford
Isle of Skye, IV49 9AA
Phone: 01471 822137
Fax: 01471 822022

Trust: Highland Primary Care
NHS Trust

Currently care is shared between midwives and GPs here, and a midwife-led service is planned for 2002. This very small unit delivered 6 babies last year, and has only one delivery bed. Continuity of care is inevitably good with such a small unit. Partners are allowed to stay if you need to go in to hospital before labour begins. In the event of complications women can be transferred to Inverness.

Midwife Unit

Number of beds	1
Births	6
Midwives	-
Home births	-
Amenity Rooms, Price	-

Obstetrician 24 hours	No
Paediatrician 24 hours	No
Full Water Birth Service	No

Tests

Routine Triple Testing	No
Nuchal Fold Scan	No
Fetal Assessment Unit	No

Pain Relief

24 hour epidural	No
Mobile epidural	No
Pethidine injections	Yes
Water (eg bath)	Yes

Midwife-led units are adequately equipped to care for women whose pregnancy is progressing normally without complications. As a result, intervention tends to be low in these units. Basic pain relief will be offered, but any woman requesting an epidural during the delivery will need to be transferred to the nearest consultant-led unit. A woman will also be transferred to the obstetric unit if any complications develop during the delivery.

Kircaldy · **Forth Park Hospital**

30 Bennochy Road, Kirkcaldy
Fife KY2 5RA
Phone: 01592 643355
Fax: 01592 642376

Trust: Fife Acute hospitals NHS Trust

Forth Park has both a consultant-led unit for higher risk deliveries and a midwife-led unit (covered separately) for women with uncomplicated pregnancies. Intervention rates for the hospital are in line with averages, although epidurals are used less frequently than in most similar hospitals.

The unit has 11 beds plus a further 5 observation beds. Antenatal classes run during the daytime and in the evenings. There are women only classes as well as special classes for teenagers and women expecting multiple births. There is a full water birth service with a pool.

Consultant and Midwife Unit

Number of beds	16
Births per midwife	17.8
Births per bed	0.92
Home births	1%
Amenity Rooms, Price	£30

Obstetrician 24 hours	Yes
Paediatrician 24 hours	Yes
Full Water Birth Service	Yes

Tests

Routine Triple Testing	No
Nuchal Fold Scan	No
Fetal Assessment Unit	Yes

Pain Relief

24 hour epidural	Yes
Mobile epidural	No
Pethidine injections	Yes
Water (eg bath)	Yes

Intervention Rates

	%	national average %
Epidural	18	29
Elective Caesarean	7	7
Emergency Caesarean	12	13
Induction	23	24
Forceps	7	7
Ventouse	3	6
Episiotomy	16	15

Kirkcaldy · **Forth Park Hospital**

30 Bennochy Road, Kirkcaldy
Fife, KY2 5RA
Phone: 01592 643355
Fax: 01592 642376

Trust: Fife Acute Hospitals
NHS Trust

Forth Park Hospital's midwife-led unit is a separate unit that provides care to low-risk women. There is no medical presence within the unit, which is managed and run by midwives. All the deliveries are spontaneous with no inductions or epidurals. Very few home births are attached to this unit, but the domino system is offered. If any complications arise during labour, you will be transferred to the obstetric unit. Pain relief includes gas and air and the use of a Ten machine. But if you want an epidural you would again have to transfer to the main consultant unit.

Midwife Unit

Number of beds	5
Births	936
Midwives	51
Home births	1%
Amenity Rooms, Price	£30
Obstetrician 24 hours	Yes
Paediatrician 24 hours	Yes
Full Water Birth Service	Yes

Tests

Routine Triple Testing	No
Nuchal Fold Scan	No
Fetal Assessment Unit	Yes

Pain Relief

24 Hour epidural	No
Mobile epidural	No
Pethidine injections	Yes
Water (eg bath)	Yes

Midwife-led units are adequately equipped to care for women whose pregnancy is progressing normally without complications. As a result, intervention tends to be low in these units. Basic pain relief will be offered, but any woman requesting an epidural during the delivery will need to be transferred to the nearest consultant-led unit. A woman will also be transferred to the obstetric unit if any complications develop during the delivery.

Kirkwall · **Balfour Hospital**

New Scapa Road, Kirkwall
Orkney, KW15 1BH
Phone: 01856 885400
Fax: 01856 885413

Healthboard: Orkney Health Board

Based in Orkney, this is one of the very few maternity units that performs caesarean deliveries despite not having obstetric consultants on staff. The unit is small, and care is provided by midwives and GPs. Midwives are committed to supporting women in pregnancy and labour towards an active, natural birth. To help make the mother more comfortable during labour there is a bath, a body/birthing ball, a floor mat and a birthing chair available. Spinals can only be offered for caesarean sections, not for those in labour. For complicated pregnancies you may be referred to the consultant-led units at Aberdeen or Inverness. Postnatal support including breastfeeding advice is available via phone from the unit and community visits can be arranged.

Midwife Unit

Number of beds	8
Births	90
Midwives	8
Home births	3%
Amenity Rooms, Price	-

Obstetrician 24 hours	No
Paediatrician 24 hours	No
Full Water Birth Service	

Tests

Routine Triple Testing	No
Nuchal Fold Scan	Yes
Fetal Assessment Unit	No

Pain Relief

24 Hour epidural	No
Mobile epidural	No
Pethidine injections	Yes
Water (eg bath)	Yes

Intervention Rates	%	national average %
Epidural	21	29
Elective Caesarean	16	7
Emergency Caesarean	6	13
Induction	1	24
Forceps	2	7
Ventouse	1	6
Episiotomy	4	15

Lamlash · **Arran War Memorial Hospital**

Lamlash
Isle of Arran, KA27 8LF
Phone: 01770 600777
Fax: 01770 600445

Trust: Ayrshire & Arran Primary Care
NHS Trust

Arran War Memorial Hospital can only manage low-risk deliveries, as transfers off the island in the event of complications or an emergency can be difficult. A helicopter transfer to a nearby mainland hospital can usually be arranged, but this is dependent on the weather. Because of this, all antenatal women booking with the service are first screened by a visiting obstetric consultant, and those in risk groups leave the island to stay near their hospital of choice at 38 weeks gestation. The unit is very small, with just one delivery bed. A consultant visits the island every six weeks to carry out antenatal ultrasound scans, which are offered to all women. Nuchal fold scans, chorionic villus sampling, and amniocentesis are available by referral to Ayrshire Central Hospital.

Midwife Unit

Number of beds	2
Births	9
Midwives	5
Home births	0%
Amenity Rooms, Price	-

Obstetrician 24 hours	No
Paediatrician 24 hours	No
Full Water Birth Service	No

Tests

Routine Triple Testing	No
Nuchal Fold Scan	Yes
Fetal Assessment Unit	No

Pain Relief

24 Hour epidural	No
Mobile epidural	No
Pethidine injections	Yes
Water (eg bath)	Yes

Midwife-led units are adequately equipped to care for women whose pregnancy is progressing normally without complications. As a result, intervention tends to be low in these units. Basic pain relief will be offered, but any woman requesting an epidural during the delivery will need to be transferred to the nearest consultant-led unit. A woman will also be transferred to the obstetric unit if any complications develop during the delivery.

Lerwick · **Gilbert Bain Hospital**

Lerwick
Shetland, ZE1 0TB
Phone: 01595 743000
Fax: 01595 696608

Healthboard: Shetland Health Board

Like the Balfour Hospital in Orkney, this hospital has no obstetric consultants but will from time to time perform caesareans – although only in emergencies. In general higher risk cases are transferred to Aberdeen and there is an air ambulance service for this. Midwives work an on-call rota for duties including escorting women by air-ambulance to Aberdeen. For straightforward deliveries midwives provide care throughout pregnancy, labour and postnatally, both in hospital and in the community. You can also be delivered at home.

Midwife Unit

Number of beds	9
Births	158
Midwives	8
Home births	6%
Amenity Rooms, Price	-

Obstetrician 24 hours	No
Paediatrician 24 hours	No
Full Water Birth Service	No

Tests

Routine Triple Testing	Yes
Nuchal Fold Scan	Yes
Fetal Assessment Unit	No

Pain Relief

24 Hour epidural	No
Mobile epidural	No
Pethidine injections	Yes
Water (eg bath)	Yes

Intervention Rates	%		national average %
Epidural	6	-	29
Elective Caesarean	0	-	7
Emergency Caesarean	5	-	13
Induction	15	-	24
Forceps	0	-	7
Ventouse	6	-	6
Episiotomy	18	-	15

Livingston · St John's Hospital at Howden

Howden Road West, Livingston
West Lothian EH54 6PP
Phone: 01506 419666
Fax: 01506 416484

Trust: West Lothian Healthcare
NHS Trust

The shared midwife and consultant unit in St John's Hospital at Howden has many characteristics in common with other large Scottish maternity departments. The induction rate is high, with 28 per cent of women induced. Forceps are used far more often than the ventouse suction pump for instrumental deliveries, and home births happen very infrequently.

For pain relief there are some interesting alternatives. For example, hypnotherapy is offered as a way of managing pain. There is a TENS machine. Epidurals are also available and are used fairly widely. Alpha feto protein testing is offered to all but you will not necessarily be offered an ultrasound scan or more complex tests such as triple testing. Nuchal fold scans can be accessed by referral to Edinburgh or Glasgow.

Consultant and Midwife Unit

Number of beds	44
Births per midwife	32.5
Births per bed	0.70
Home births	0.2%
Amenity Rooms, Price	-

Obstetrician 24 hours	Yes
Paediatrician 24 hours	Yes
Full Water Birth Service	Yes

Tests

Routine Triple Testing	No
Nuchal Fold Scan	Yes
Fetal Assessment Unit	Yes

Pain Relief

24 hour epidural	Yes
Mobile epidural	No
Pethidine injections	Yes
Water (eg bath)	Yes

Intervention Rates

	%	national average %
Epidural	32	29
Elective Caesarean	8	7
Emergency Caesarean	13	13
Induction	28	24
Forceps	6	7
Ventouse	2	6
Episiotomy	-	15

Lochilphead · **Mid Argyll Hospital**

Blarbuie Road, Lochgilphead
Argyll, PA31 8JZ
Phone: 01546 602952
Fax: 01546 606500

Trust: Lomond & Argyll Primary Care
NHS Trust

Mid Argyll Hospital is a GP and midwife-led maternity unit with two beds. The unit covers rural Argyll, an area of 400 square miles and provides a service for women with uncomplicated pregnancies who can give birth without medical intervention. Almost a quarter of women have home births.

Many women who receive antenatal care at the unit end up delivering at Vale of Leven Hospital, approximately 80 miles away, where a combined gynaecological and antenatal service is also available.

Mid Argyll provides a local, personalised service and everybody who gives birth here knows the midwives who look after them. Your partner is welcome to stay with you whenever you go into hospital.

Some antenatal tests are carried out at Vale of Leven.

Midwife Unit

Number of beds	3
Births	21
Midwives	4
Home births	19%
Amenity Rooms, Price	-
Obstetrician 24 hours	No
Paediatrician 24 hours	No
Full Water Birth Service	Yes

Tests

Routine Triple Testing	Yes
Nuchal Fold Scan	Yes
Fetal Assessment Unit	Yes

Pain Relief

24 Hour epidural	No
Mobile epidural	No
Pethidine injections	Yes
Water (eg bath)	Yes

Midwife-led units are adequately equipped to care for women whose pregnancy is progressing normally without complications. As a result, intervention tends to be low in these units. Basic pain relief will be offered, but any woman requesting an epidural during the delivery will need to be transferred to the nearest consultant-led unit. A woman will also be transferred to the obstetric unit if any complications develop during the delivery.

Montrose · **Montrose Royal Infirmary**

66 Bridge Street
Montrose
Angus DD10 8AJ

Trust: Tayside University Hospitals NHS Trust

Despite having only two delivery beds, at least one midwife is on duty 24-hours a day at the Montrose Royal Infirmary maternity unit. A second midwife is always available on call, and all women delivering at the unit are attended by two midwives. This means that if problems arise in labour and you have to be transferred to Ninewells Hospital, you will be accompanied by one of your midwives. This happens to about one in ten women. The unit also provides antenatal and postnatal support to women who have their baby at Ninewells. There is a maternity day care service at the unit but for more complex tests or investigations you would be referred to Ninewells.

Midwife Unit

Number of beds	6
Births	85
Midwives	10
Home births	2%
Amenity Rooms, Price	-

Obstetrician 24 hours	No
Paediatrician 24 hours	No
Water Birth Offered	No

Tests

Routine Triple Testing	Yes
Nuchal Fold Scan	Yes
Fetal Assessment Unit	No

Pain Relief

24 hour epidural	No
Mobile epidural	No
Pethidine injections	Yes
Water (eg bath)	Yes

Midwife-led units are adequately equipped to care for women whose pregnancy is progressing normally without complications. As a result, intervention tends to be low in these units. Basic pain relief will be offered, but any woman requesting an epidural during the delivery will need to be transferred to the nearest consultant-led unit. A woman will also be transferred to the obstetric unit if any complications develop during the delivery.

Melrose · **Borders General Hospital**

Melrose
Roxburghshire TD6 9BS
Phone: 01896 826000
Fax: 01896 823476

Trust: Borders General Hospital
NHS Trust

The maternity unit is situated adjacent to the special care baby unit and paediatric ward. This unit is well equipped to deal with the whole spectrum of maternity care. Midwife staffing levels are good and the unit is able to provide one-to-one care in labour. You also get a chance to have a debriefing session with the midwife afterwards.

Intervention rates are much in line with national averages although forceps deliveries and episiotomies are more frequent.

There is a 24-hour epidural service for pain relief in labour although, in practice, epidurals are used far less often here than in other hospitals. There is a pregnancy assessment unit which can investigate and monitor any problems during the pregnancy.

Consultant and Midwife Unit

Number of beds	22
Births per midwife	27
Births per bed	0.55
Home births	0.3%
Amenity Rooms, Price	£33
Obstetrician 24 hours	Yes
Paediatrician 24 hours	Yes
Full Water Birth Service	Yes

Tests

Routine Triple Testing	Yes
Nuchal Fold Scan	No
Fetal Assessment Unit	Yes

Pain Relief

24 hour epidural	Yes
Mobile epidural	No
Pethidine injections	Yes
Water (eg bath)	Yes

Intervention Rates

	%	national average %
Epidural	18	29
Elective Caesarean	6	7
Emergency Caesarean	14	13
Induction	22	24
Forceps	11	7
Ventouse	6	6
Episiotomy	24	15

Oban · **Lorn and Islands District General Hospital**

Glengallon Road, Oban
Argyll, PA34 4HH
Phone: 01631 567500
Fax: 01631 567134

Trust: Argyll & Clyde Acute Hospitals
NHS Trust

Lorn and Islands' midwife-led maternity unit is small, looking after families within a very rural area in excess of 2,000 square miles, including some islands. It provides antenatal and postnatal care to women from the area who deliver elsewhere as well as delivering some of the more straightforward pregnancies in the unit. The unit is 85 miles away from the nearest consultant unit, so deals only with uncomplicated births. A consultant holds a clinic at Lorn and Islands once a week. Any antenatal testing needed is carried out at the womans chosen consultant-led unit. The care which is provided to women in labour is individualised, relaxed, and low-tech.

Midwife Unit

Number of beds	6
Births	49
Midwives	7
Home births	0%
Amenity Rooms, Price	-

Obstetrician 24 hours	No
Paediatrician 24 hours	No
Full Water Birth Service	No

Tests

Routine Triple Testing	Yes
Nuchal Fold Scan	Yes
Fetal Assessment Unit	No

Pain Relief

24 Hour epidural	No
Mobile epidural	No
Pethidine injections	Yes
Water (eg bath)	Yes

Midwife-led units are adequately equipped to care for women whose pregnancy is progressing normally without complications. As a result, intervention tends to be low in these units. Basic pain relief will be offered, but any woman requesting an epidural during the delivery will need to be transferred to the nearest consultant-led unit. A woman will also be transferred to the obstetric unit if any complications develop during the delivery.

Paisley · **Royal Alexandra Hospital**

Corsebar Road, Paisley
Renfrewshire PA2 9PN
Phone: 0141 8879111
Fax: 0141 8876701

Trust: Argyll & Clyde Acute Hospitals
NHS Trust

The unit has a good staffing ratio of 23 births to each midwife which helps allow it to provide one-to-one midwife support in labour – where you have one midwife solely looking after you. This is something many large hospitals cannot manage. Midwives are organised as teams, one of which will aim to provide continuity of care through pregnancy, labour and afterwards. Home births are hardly ever performed.

This hospital has the highest rate of caesarean interventions in Scotland with about 26 per cent of women delivering that way.

Aromatherapy is offered as one alternative to more medical forms of pain relief. Epidurals are also available. The unit has a drug abuse advice service and a special needs midwife.

Consultant and Midwife Unit

Number of beds	40
Births per midwife	23
Births per bed	0.58
Home births	0.03%
Amenity Rooms, Price	-

Obstetrician 24 hours	Yes
Paediatrician 24 hours	Yes
Full Water Birth Service	No

Tests

Routine Triple Testing	Yes
Nuchal Fold Scan	No
Fetal Assessment Unit	Yes

Pain Relief

24 hour epidural	Yes
Mobile epidural	No
Pethidine injections	Yes
Water (eg bath)	Yes

Intervention Rates	%	national average %
Epidural	24	29
Elective Caesarean	-	7
Emergency Caesarean	-	13
Induction	23	24
Forceps	6	7
Ventouse	7	6
Episiotomy	-	15

Taymount Terrace, Perth
PH1 1NX
Phone: 01738 623311
Fax: 01738 473206

Trust: Tayside University Hospitals
    NHS Trust

The future of Perth Maternity Unit, located in Perth Royal Infirmary, is currently under review and options include closing the unit or making it a midwife-led service only. As it stands, the unit undertakes all births except for pre-term birth and where the baby may require intensive care.

Intervention rates are lower than average here – in particular forceps are less often used.

The midwife service is integrated and covers care through pregnancy labour and afterwards.

A full range of antenatal tests and scans are done. For more complex tests you will be referred to Ninewells hospital in Dundee.

The unit runs aquanatal classes and groups for teenagers and multiple births.

Consultant and Midwife Unit

Number of beds	20
Births per midwife	24
Births per bed	0.67
Home births	1%
Amenity Rooms, Price	£30

Obstetrician 24 hours	Yes
Paediatrician 24 hours	Yes
Full Water Birth Service	No

Tests

Routine Triple Testing	Yes
Nuchal Fold Scan	Yes
Fetal Assessment Unit	Yes

Pain Relief

24 hour epidural	Yes
Mobile epidural	No
Pethidine injections	Yes
Water (eg bath)	Yes

Intervention Rates

	%	national average %
Epidural	31	29
Elective Caesarean	7	7
Emergency Caesarean	12	13
Induction	19	24
Forceps	4	7
Ventouse	6	6
Episiotomy	7	15

Peterhead · **Peterhead Hospital**

Links Terrace
Peterhead, AB42 2XB
Phone: 01779 478234
Fax: 01779 478111

Trust: Grampian Primary Care
NHS Trust

This small unit – with just two delivery beds and four postnatal beds – provides midwife-led care for women with uncomplicated natural deliveries.

The midwife who books in a woman will see her for the duration of her pregnancy and postnatal care but will give her a choice of where she would like to give birth. Many choose to have their baby at Peterhead because of the relaxed atmosphere in the unit. Women with specialist needs are advised to be delivered in Aberdeen Maternity Hospital. There is a homely atmosphere in Peterhead and the midwives aim to build good relationships with women during their pregnancies. There are good support services including a miscarriage group, a counselling service, a breastfeeding support group and a drop-in service.

Midwife Unit

Number of beds	6
Births	120
Midwives	7
Home births	0%
Amenity Rooms, Price	-
Obstetrician 24 hours	No
Paediatrician 24 hours	No
Full Water Birth Service	No

Tests

Routine Triple Testing	Yes
Nuchal Fold Scan	Yes
Fetal Assessment Unit	Yes

Pain Relief

24 Hour epidural	No
Mobile epidural	No
Pethidine injections	Yes
Water (eg bath)	Yes

Midwife-led units are adequately equipped to care for women whose pregnancy is progressing normally without complications. As a result, intervention tends to be low in these units. Basic pain relief will be offered, but any woman requesting an epidural during the delivery will need to be transferred to the nearest consultant-led unit. A woman will also be transferred to the obstetric unit if any complications develop during the delivery.

Portree · **Portree Hospital**

Portree
IV51 9BZ
Phone: 01478 613200
Fax: 01478 613526

Trust: Highland Primary Care NHS Trust

Portree hospital is a small, 13-bed Community Hospital with one maternity bed for low-risk births. There are approximately 10 deliveries carried out annually in the unit, usually with the assistance of the GP, as well as a couple of home births. In the event of an emergency, midwives are trained in resuscitation, and both mother and baby can be stabilised during transfer to the nearest consultant obstetric unit in Inverness – 120 miles away – where specialist tests are also carried out. Water births are an option, but midwives are not specifically trained and women must provide their own pool.

Maternity Unit

Number of beds	1
Births	10
Midwives	5
Home births	17%
Amenity Rooms, Price	-

Obstetrician 24 hours	No
Paediatrician 24 hours	No
Full Water Birth Service	

Tests

Routine Triple Testing	Yes
Nuchal Fold Scan	Yes
Fetal Assessment Unit	No

Pain Relief

24 Hour epidural	No
Mobile epidural	No
Pethidine injections	Yes
Water (eg bath)	Yes

Midwife-led units are adequately equipped to care for women whose pregnancy is progressing normally without complications. As a result, intervention tends to be low in these units. Basic pain relief will be offered, but any woman requesting an epidural during the delivery will need to be transferred to the nearest consultant-led unit. A woman will also be transferred to the obstetric unit if any complications develop during the delivery.

Stirling · **Stirling Royal Infirmary**

Livilands
Stirling, FK8 2AU
Phone: 01786 434000
Fax: 01786 450588

Trust: Forth Valley Acute Hospitals NHS Trust

Midwife staffing levels are high in relation to the number of births in the unit and, with midwives largely organised in teams, continuity of care is good. Three quarters of women who give birth here know the midwife who delivers their baby. An individualised care plan for each mother is discussed on a one-to-one basis at an early stage in the pregnancy. Domino deliveries are an option. Epidurals are available for pain relief however there is no dedicated service available 24 hours a day. Despite this, epidurals are quite widely used. Interventions are generally average although inductions are used less frequently than similar units. Water births can be done but you must supply your own birthing pool.

Consultant and Midwife Unit

Number of beds	37
Births per midwife	15
Births per bed	0.62
Home births	0.4%
Amenity Rooms, Price	£45

Obstetrician 24 hours	Yes
Paediatrician 24 hours	Yes
Full Water Birth Service	No

Tests

Routine Triple Testing	No
Nuchal Fold Scan	Yes
Fetal Assessment Unit	Yes

Pain Relief

24 hour epidural	No
Mobile epidural	No
Pethidine injections	Yes
Water (eg bath)	Yes

Intervention Rates

	%	national average %
Epidural	34	29
Elective Caesarean	7	7
Emergency Caesarean	16	13
Induction	14	24
Forceps	5	7
Ventouse	9	6
Episiotomy	23	15

Stranraer · **Clenoch Maternity Unit**

Dalrymple Hospital, Stranraer
Wigtownshire, DG9 7DH
Phone: 01776 702323

Trust: Dumfries & Galloway Acute &
Maternity Hospitals NHS Trust

This is a small midwife-led unit situated west of Dumfries and Galloway. The nearest consultant unit is in Dumfries, 78 miles away.

The unit practices team midwifery – where you are looked after throughout pregnancy, labour and afterwards by a team of midwives.

Many more women are booked into the unit for antenatal care than actually deliver at the unit. Only women who are considered as low-risk will deliver at the unit.

Each month, three consultant clinics and three consultant gynaecology clinics are held at the unit. Local women have 24hr access to the service for support and advice.

Antenatal classes can be arranged with midwives, and include a father's night. The unit plans to install a birthing pool in the near future.

Midwife Unit

Number of beds	8
Births	100
Midwives	10
Home births	1%
Amenity Rooms, Price	-

Obstetrician 24 hours	No
Paediatrician 24 hours	No
Full Water Birth Service	No

Tests

Routine Triple Testing	Yes
Nuchal Fold Scan	No
Fetal Assessment Unit	No

Pain Relief

24 Hour epidural	No
Mobile epidural	No
Pethidine injections	Yes
Water (eg bath)	Yes

Midwife-led units are adequately equipped to care for women whose pregnancy is progressing normally without complications. As a result, intervention tends to be low in these units. Basic pain relief will be offered, but any woman requesting an epidural during the delivery will need to be transferred to the nearest consultant-led unit. A woman will also be transferred to the obstetric unit if any complications develop during the delivery.

Torphins · **Kincardine O'Neill War Memorial Hospital**

Torphins
Aberdeenshire, AB31 4FQ
Phone: 01339 882302
Fax: 01339 882580

Trust: Grampian Primary Care
NHS Trust

This maternity unit is a small, midwife-led service. It strongly adheres to the named midwife concept and, where possible, one or two midwives care for each patient before, during and after birth. Women with uncomplicated pregnancies can be delivered in the unit or at home. For pain management options are limited but there is gas & air, pethidine injections and a Ten machine. There are trained midwives available to supervise water births but you will need to bring your own pool for this.

Midwife Unit

Number of beds	5
Births	40
Midwives	6
Home births	7%
Amenity Rooms, Price	-
Obstetrician 24 hours	No
Paediatrician 24 hours	No
Full Water Birth Service	No

Tests

Routine Triple Testing	Yes
Nuchal Fold Scan	Yes
Fetal Assessment Unit	No

Pain Relief

24 Hour epidural	No
Mobile epidural	No
Pethidine injections	Yes
Water (eg bath)	Yes

Midwife-led units are adequately equipped to care for women whose pregnancy is progressing normally without complications. As a result, intervention tends to be low in these units. Basic pain relief will be offered, but any woman requesting an epidural during the delivery will need to be transferred to the nearest consultant-led unit. A woman will also be transferred to the obstetric unit if any complications develop during the delivery.

Wick · **Caithness General Hospital**

Bankhead Road, Wick
Caithness, KW1 5NS
Phone: 01955 605050
Fax: 01955 604606

Trust: Highland Acute Hospitals
NHS Trust

Caithness General Hospital has a small obstetric maternity unit, which covers a large catchment area in Caithness and north Sunderland. It is located 110 miles away from the nearest tertiary unit with special care baby facilities. Home births here are rare, all women give birth in the unit. There are no water birth facilities either. Antenatal education includes one-to-one sessions and women-only groups. Partners may be accommodated in a single room with patients. Caesareans are performed less frequently here than in larger obstetric hospitals. However forceps are used in more than one in ten births – much more frequently than the ventouse suction pump. Epidurals for pain relief are available but are only rarely used for pain relief in labour, with most being used for caesarean deliveries.

Consultant and Midwife Unit

Number of beds	14
Births per midwife	15
Births per bed	0.33
Home births	0%
Amenity Rooms, Price	-

Obstetrician 24 hours	No
Paediatrician 24 hours	No
Full Water Birth Service	No

Tests

Routine Triple Testing	No
Nuchal Fold Scan	Yes
Fetal Assessment Unit	No

Pain Relief

24 hour epidural	Yes
Mobile epidural	No
Pethidine injections	Yes
Water (eg bath)	Yes

Intervention Rates

	%	national average %
Epidural	23	29
Elective Caesarean	5	7
Emergency Caesarean	10	13
Induction	20	24
Forceps	11	7
Ventouse	4	6
Episiotomy	14	15

Wishaw · **Wishaw General Hospital**

Netherton Street, Wishaw
Lanarkshire, ML2 OEF
Phone: 01698 361100

Trust: Salisbury District
NHS Trust

This unit aims to maintain a balance between midwife-led care and the involvement of obstetric specialists. Midwives provide most of the care for low-risk pregnancies. The unit includes 21 home-from-home style rooms where you can be admitted, deliver your baby and then recover before being discharged home without having to be first transferred to a postnatal ward. There are also seven traditional delivery rooms in the high-risk ward.

Intervention rates in the unit are slightly lower than average and in particular instrumental deliveries happen relatively infrequently. There is a well equipped neonatal unit designed to limit the need for mothers to be transferred elsewhere.

Consultant and Midwife Unit

Number of beds	86
Births per midwife	27.5
Births per bed	-
Home births	0.2%
Amenity Rooms, Price	-
Obstetrician 24 hours	Yes
Paediatrician 24 hours	Yes
Full Water Birth Service	Yes

Tests

Routine Triple Testing	No
Nuchal Fold Scan	No
Fetal Assessment Unit	Yes

Pain Relief

24 hour epidural	Yes
Mobile epidural	No
Pethidine injections	Yes
Water (eg bath)	Yes

Intervention Rates

	%	national average %
Epidural	-	29
Elective Caesarean	8	7
Emergency Caesarean	11	13
Induction	23	24
Forceps	5	7
Ventouse	5	6
Episiotomy	-	15

Wales

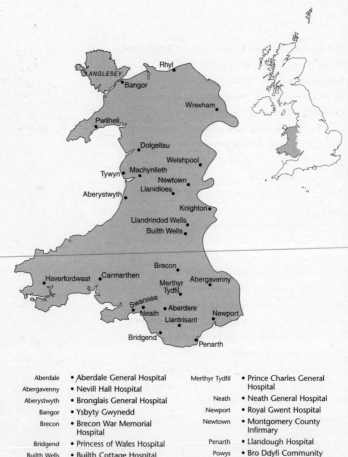

Aberdale	• Aberdale General Hospital	Merthyr Tydfil	• Prince Charles General Hospital
Abergavenny	• Nevill Hall Hospital		
Aberystwyth	• Bronglais General Hospital	Neath	• Neath General Hospital
Bangor	• Ysbyty Gwynedd	Newport	• Royal Gwent Hospital
Brecon	• Brecon War Memorial Hospital	Newtown	• Montgomery County Infirmary
Bridgend	• Princess of Wales Hospital	Penarth	• Llandough Hospital
Builth Wells	• Builth Cottage Hospital	Powys	• Bro Ddyfi Community Hospital
Carmarthen	• West Wales General Hospital		
		Pwllheli	• Bryn Beryl Hospital
Dolgellau	• Dolgellau & Barmouth	Rhyl	• Clan Clwyd District General Hospital
Haverfordwest	• Withybush General Hospital		
Knighton	• Knighton Hospital	Swansea	• Singleton Hospital
Llandrindod Wells	• Llandrindod Wells Hospital	Tywyn	• Tywyn & District War Memorial Hospital
Llanidloes	• Llanidloes War Memorial Hospital		
		Welshpool	• Victoria Memorial Hospital
Llantrisant	• Royal Glamorgan Hospital	Wrexham	• Wrexham Maelor Hospital

Aberdare · **Aberdare General Hospital**

Abernant Road, Aberdare
Mid Glamorgan, CF44 0RF
Phone: 01685 872411
Fax: 01685 882741

Trust: North Glamorgan
NHS Trust

This small unit provides a friendly service run by a small team of midwives. The accomodation consists of five rooms and a family suite. Continuity of care in such a small unit is inevitably good and you will get to know the midwives looking after you. Home birth is also an option. Antenatal classes are run in the evening and cater to women only, couples and teenagers. The unit offers double testing. If you require a nuchal fold scan you will be referred to the maternity unit at Prince Charles General Hospital. You would also go to Prince Charles General if complications arose. There is no epidural service here but the unit provides alternatives in pain management such as a TENS machine and aromatherapy.

Midwife Unit

Number of beds	5
Births	165
Midwives	8
Home births	2%
Amenity Rooms, Price	-
Obstetrician 24 hours	No
Paediatrician 24 hours	No
Full Water Birth Service	No

Tests

Routine Triple Testing	No
Nuchal Fold Scan	Yes
Fetal Assessment Unit	Yes

Pain Relief

24 Hour epidural	No
Mobile epidural	No
Pethidine injections	Yes
Water (eg Bath)	Yes

Midwife-led units are adequately equipped to care for women whose pregnancy is progressing normally without complications. As a result, intervention tends to be low in these units. Basic pain relief will be offered, but any woman requesting an epidural during the delivery will need to be transferred to the nearest consultant-led unit. A woman will also be transferred to the obstetric unit if any complications develop during the delivery.

Abergavenny · **Nevill Hall Hospital**

Brecon Road, Abergavenny
Gwent NP7 7EG
Phone: 01873 732732
Fax: 01873 859168

Trust: Gwent Healthcare NHS Trust

The maternity unit at Nevill Hall Hospital serves an area stretching from the industrial valley of South Wales to the Brecon Beacon National Park and the Wye Valley.

This is a busy unit where occasionally all delivery beds are occupied. If this happens, babies can be delivered in a first stage or admission room. Care is shared between midwives and consultants, however midwives will provide the majority of your care if you have a low-risk pregnancy. It is a small unit, with only four delivery beds. Facilities include a fetal and early pregnancy assessment unit, and aquanatal classes. Domino deliveries are offered – a system which should ensure continuity of care through your pregnancy and labour. Triple tests are not routinely offered and nuchal fold scans are not available.

Consultant and Midwife Unit

Number of beds	31
Births per midwife	23
Births per bed	1.08
Home births	2%
Amenity Rooms, Price	-

Obstetrician 24 hours	Yes
Paediatrician 24 hours	Yes
Full Water Birth Service	No

Tests

Routine Triple Testing	No
Nuchal Fold Scan	No
Fetal Assessment Unit	Yes

Pain Relief

24 hour epidural	Yes
Mobile epidural	No
Pethidine injections	Yes
Water (eg bath)	Yes

Intervention Rates

	%	national average %
Epidural	11	26
Elective Caesarean	11	10
Emergency Caesarean	14	13
Induction	28	21
Forceps	-	2
Ventouse	-	7
Episiotomy	8	10

Aberystwyth · **Bronglais General Hospital**

Ceredigion
Dyfed SY23 1ER
Phone: 01970 623 131
Fax: 01970 635 923

Trust: Ceredigion and Mid Wales
NHS Trust

The maternity unit at Bronglais General Hospital is a small unit, with midwives providing the majority of care for low-risk women. Intervention rates are low compared with the national average. Midwives work under the domino system and provide a home delivery service over a large rural area. The home birth rate is high for this type of unit suggesting good support for this option. All forms of pain management are available including epidurals. You will be offered a range of diagnostic tests and scans, but this will not routinely include an ultrasound scan on booking. However scans can be arranged at 18 weeks if you need one. There is good support if you choose to breast feed. The unit achieves a higher than average breast-feeding rate.

Consultant and Midwife Unit

Number of beds	14
Births per midwife	21
Births per bed	0.33
Home births	4%
Amenity Rooms, Price	£25

Obstetrician 24 hours	Yes
Paediatrician 24 hours	Yes
Full Water Birth Service	No

Tests

Routine Triple Testing	Yes
Nuchal Fold Scan	Yes
Fetal Assessment Unit	No

Pain Relief

24 hour epidural	Yes
Mobile epidural	No
Pethidine injections	Yes
Water (eg bath)	Yes

Intervention Rates

	%	national average %
Epidural	19	26
Elective Caesarean	8	10
Emergency Caesarean	9	13
Induction	15	21
Forceps	2	2
Ventouse	7	7
Episiotomy	14	10

Bangor · Ysbyty Gwynedd

Penrhosgarnedd, Bangor
Gwynedd LL57 2PW
Phone: 01248 384 384
Fax: 01248 370 629

Trust: North West Wales
NHS Trust

The maternity service at Ysbyty Gwynedd cares for women from a large area of North West Wales and it is a referral centre for high risk pregnancies. Induction rates and ventouse rates are higher than average. Domino deliveries are offered which help to ensure that you are looked after by a midwife you know throughout your pregnancy and labour. Water births are not offered, but the unit does have a pool which can be used to help ease pain during labour. Antenatal screening services are limited. The unit does double testing rather than triple testing and early-pregnancy ultrasound scans are not routinely offered. Nuchal fold scans are not available.

The unit does have a water birth pool, but it is used for pain relief in labour rather than for deliveries.

Consultant and Midwife Unit

Number of beds	30
Births per midwife	25.9
Births per bed	0.61
Home births	3%
Amenity Rooms, Price	£33

Obstetrician 24 hours	Yes
Paediatrician 24 hours	Yes
Full Water Birth Service	No

Tests

Routine Triple Testing	No
Nuchal Fold Scan	No
Fetal Assessment Unit	No

Pain Relief

24 hour epidural	Yes
Mobile epidural	No
Pethidine injections	Yes
Water (eg bath)	Yes

Intervention Rates

	%	national average %
Epidural	25	26
Elective Caesarean	8	10
Emergency Caesarean	13	13
Induction	27	21
Forceps	3	2
Ventouse	10	7
Episiotomy	14	10

Brecon · **Brecon War Memorial Hospital**

Cerrigcochion Road, Brecon
Powys, LD3 7NS
Phone: 01874 622 443
Fax: 01874 622 443

Trust: Powys Healthcare
NHS Trust

Brecon War Memorial Hospital is a small midwife-led unit that provides care for low-risk women. Until last year, the unit offered GP-led care and was set up to perform interventions such as ceaserean section deliveries. However it now provides a low-tech environment where intervention is minimal. Epidural pain relief is not offered. Single rooms are available for hire but the unit will let your partner stay with you if you have to go into hospital before going into labour, so long as the other mothers don't object. The unit has above average home birth rates so should be well set-up to support you if you want to have your baby at home. Some of the midwives are trained in water births, but you will have to set up your own pool at home if you want this.

Midwife Unit

Number of beds	6
Births	111
Midwives	7
Home births	5%
Amenity Rooms, Price	-

Obstetrician 24 hours	No
Paediatrician 24 hours	No
Full Water Birth Service	No

Tests

Routine Triple Testing	No
Nuchal Fold Scan	No
Fetal Assessment Unit	No

Pain Relief

24 Hour epidural	No
Mobile epidural	No
Pethidine injections	Yes
Water (eg Bath)	Yes

Midwife-led units are adequately equipped to care for women whose pregnancy is progressing normally without complications. As a result, intervention tends to be low in these units. Basic pain relief will be offered, but any woman requesting an epidural during the delivery will need to be transferred to the nearest consultant-led unit. A woman will also be transferred to the obstetric unit if any complications develop during the delivery.

Bridgend · **Princess of Wales Hospital**

Coitoi Road, Bridgend
Glamorgan CF31 1RQ
Phone: 01656 752 752

Trust: Bro Morgannwg
NHS Trust

There is a very good chance you will get looked after throughout your pregnancy and labour by one midwife who you will get to know well. The midwives here provide a group practice which means midwives are assigned to care for you throughout your pregnancy and labour helping to ensure better continuity of care. Over two thirds of women are looked after in labour by a midwife they know. Also, you should get one-to-one care in labour. For those women who have been assessed as likely to have a complicated pregnancy, obstetric support is available. However, elective caesareans are much less common here than at other units.

Methods of pain relief offered include reflexology. The unit provides aquanatal classes and maternity support groups.

Consultant and Midwife Unit

Number of beds	33
Births per midwife	23.7
Births per bed	0.72
Home births	2%
Amenity Rooms, Price	£24

Obstetrician 24 hours	Yes
Paediatrician 24 hours	Yes
Full Water Birth Service	No

Tests

Routine Triple Testing	Yes
Nuchal Fold Scan	Yes
Fetal Assessment Unit	No

Pain Relief

24 hour epidural	Yes
Mobile epidural	No
Pethidine injections	Yes
Water (eg bath)	Yes

Intervention Rates

	%	national average %
Epidural	31	26
Elective Caesarean	6	10
Emergency Caesarean	14	13
Induction	13	21
Forceps	4	2
Ventouse	4	7
Episiotomy	7	10

Builth Wells · **Builth Cottage Hospital**

Hospital Road, Builth Wells
Powys, LD2 3HE
Phone: 01982 552 221
Fax: 01982 552 398

Trust: Powys Healthcare
NHS Trust

This hospital is a small, intimate maternity unit, with just thirty births in the past year and a small staff, which means you will inevitably get to know the midwives looking after you fairly well. Partners are welcome to stay if you have to go into the hospital early. There are no water birth facilities but if you want to give birth this way, the midwives will support you if you set up a pool in your own home. About one in ten births handled by the unit is a home birth.

Antenatal classes are offered in the evenings rather than the daytime. Most tests are given if you need them although triple testing is not routinely offered. Nuchal fold scans can be arranged but only if you pay for a private service.

Midwife Unit

Number of beds	2
Births	30
Midwives	2
Home births	3%
Amenity Rooms, Price	-

Obstetrician 24 hours	No
Paediatrician 24 hours	No
Full Water Birth Service	No

Tests

Routine Triple Testing	No
Nuchal Fold Scan	No
Fetal Assessment Unit	No

Pain Relief

24 Hour epidural	No
Mobile epidural	No
Pethidine injections	Yes
Water (eg Bath)	Yes

Midwife-led units are adequately equipped to care for women whose pregnancy is progressing normally without complications. As a result, intervention tends to be low in these units. Basic pain relief will be offered, but any woman requesting an epidural during the delivery will need to be transferred to the nearest consultant-led unit. A woman will also be transferred to the obstetric unit if any complications develop during the delivery.

Cardiff · **University Hospital of Wales**

Heath Park, Cardiff
CF14 4XW
Phone: 029 2074 7747
Fax: 029 2074 2968

Trust: Cardiff and Vale
NHS Trust

University Hospital of Wales is a tertiary maternity unit which means that it has the expertise to deal with more complex pregnancies. Services include a fetal medicine unit and specialist care for maternal medical problems. The service also offers low-risk midwife-led care, but despite this only around one half of all births occur without medical intervention. Caesarean section rates, including elective caesareans, are above average, reflecting in part the higher number of more complex pregancies.

Midwife staffing levels are lower than the UK average. This is currently under review, as the service has reported difficulty in providing one-to-one care in labour. The chance of being cared for in labour by a midwife you have met before is lower here than at many smaller units.

Consultant and Midwife Unit

Number of beds	40
Births per midwife	36
Births per bed	0.71
Home births	1%
Amenity Rooms, Price	-

Obstetrician 24 hours	Yes
Paediatrician 24 hours	Yes
Full Water Birth Service	No

Tests

Routine Triple Testing	No
Nuchal Fold Scan	Yes
Fetal Assessment Unit	Yes

Pain Relief

24 hour epidural	Yes
Mobile epidural	No
Pethidine injections	Yes
Water (eg bath)	Yes

Intervention Rates

	%	national average %
Epidural	30	26
Elective Caesarean	11	10
Emergency Caesarean	19	13
Induction	-	21
Forceps	5	2
Ventouse	9	7
Episiotomy	8	10

Carmarthen · **West Wales General Hospital**

Glangwili, Carmarthen
Dyfed SA31 2AF
Phone: 01267 235151
Fax: 01267 237662

Trust: **Carmarthenshire
NHS Trust**

The maternity unit shares care between midwives and consultants and there is a special care baby unit. Accommodation is single rooms and four bedded bays. There are good staffing levels of midwives here.

All mothers have a named midwife as part of a team of four midwives who are responsible for the woman's care including the delivery.

The unit has a high rate of home births despite being relatively large. Intervention rates are broadly average for a unit of this size.

If you would like to have a women-only antenatal class, the hospital will provide this on a one-to-one basis. Check with the unit on which scans will be made available to you; your booking ultrasound will be done at 15 weeks here rather than 12.

Consultant and Midwife Unit

Number of beds	32
Births per midwife	21
Births per bed	0.85
Home births	5%
Amenity Rooms, Price	£26

Obstetrician 24 hours	Yes
Paediatrician 24 hours	Yes
Full Water Birth Service	No

Tests

Routine Triple Testing	No
Nuchal Fold Scan	No
Fetal Assessment Unit	Yes

Pain Relief

24 hour epidural	Yes
Mobile epidural	No
Pethidine injections	Yes
Water (eg bath)	Yes

Intervention Rates	%	national average %
Epidural	37	26
Elective Caesarean	11	10
Emergency Caesarean	14	13
Induction	-	21
Forceps	2	2
Ventouse	5	7
Episiotomy	12	10

Dolgellau · **Dolgellau & Barmouth Hospital**

Dolgellau
Gwynedd, LL40 1NP
Phone: 01341 422479
Fax: 01341 423684

Trust: North West Wales
NHS Trust

The Dolgellau & Barmouth Hospital maternity unit has just one labour bed and is run by a small team of midwives. This allows for a friendly flexible service. Antenatal classes and appointments can be arranged on weekdays, evenings and weekends to suit individual needs. With only 18 births a year, the unit is usually able to provide two midwives to look after you during labour – many large hospitals are unable even to ensure that you have one midwife to yourself during labour. You go to Bangor to have antenatal tests such as alpha-feto protein testing and anomaly ultrasound scans. Other antenatal tests, such as the triple test and nuchal fold translucency scans are not routinely offered. After the birth, you are provided with 24hr access to a named midwife for support.

Midwife Unit

Number of beds	5
Births	18
Midwives	3
Home births	0%
Amenity Rooms, Price	-

Obstetrician 24 hours	No
Paediatrician 24 hours	No
Full Water Birth Service	Yes

Tests

Routine Triple Testing	No
Nuchal Fold Scan	No
Fetal Assessment Unit	No

Pain Relief

24 Hour epidural	No
Mobile epidural	No
Pethidine injections	Yes
Water (eg Bath)	Yes

Midwife-led units are adequately equipped to care for women whose pregnancy is progressing normally without complications. As a result, intervention tends to be low in these units. Basic pain relief will be offered, but any woman requesting an epidural during the delivery will need to be transferred to the nearest consultant-led unit. A woman will also be transferred to the obstetric unit if any complications develop during the delivery.

Haverfordwest · **Withybush General Hospital**

Fishguard Road, Haverfordwest
Pembrokeshire SA61 2PZ
Phone: 01437 764 545
Fax: 01437 773 353

Trust: Pembrokeshire and Derwen NHS Trust

In this relatively large unit, staffing levels are good and a third of women in labour will be cared for by a midwife they already know. You also have a choice of a domino delivery but the service is limited. Antenatal classes are offered at all times including weekends, as are women only and aquanatal classes. The unit does not do routine triple testing but you are offered the double test and can have a nuchal fold scan. Elective caesarean rates are high and forceps rates very low. Homebirths are done regularly and full waterbirth facilities are offered. The unit has experience in delivering breech babies vaginally, but normally advises women that a caesarean would be a safer option. Your partner should be able to stay with you if you need to go into hospital before labour has started.

Consultant and Midwife Unit

Number of beds	26
Births per midwife	22.8
Births per bed	0.78
Home births	4%
Amenity Rooms, Price	-

Obstetrician 24 hours	No
Paediatrician 24 hours	Yes
Full Water Birth Service	Yes

Tests

Routine Triple Testing	No
Nuchal Fold Scan	Yes
Fetal Assessment Unit	Yes

Pain Relief

24 hour epidural	Yes
Mobile epidural	No
Pethidine injections	Yes
Water (eg bath)	Yes

Intervention Rates

	%	national average %
Epidural	26	26
Elective Caesarean	13	10
Emergency Caesarean	12	13
Induction	20	21
Forceps	1	2
Ventouse	8	7
Episiotomy	10	10

Knighton · **Knighton Hospital**

Ffrydd Road, Knighton
Powys, LD7 1DF
Phone: 01547 528 633
Fax: 01547 520 522

Trust: Powys Healthcare
NHS Trust

Knighton Hospital is an isolated rural maternity unit providing home-from-home care for low-risk women. It has two labour beds, both in single rooms. The unit's emphasis is on providing an atmosphere conducive to a natural childbirth; the small team of midwives ensure you will be supported by midwives you get to know well. The hospital was the first in Wales to get Baby Friendly Initiative accreditation. Pain relief options at Knighton Hospital are limited to gas and air, opiate injections and TENS. However, unusually for a unit of this type, a full waterbirth service is offered, with midwives trained in this type of delivery available at all times and a birthing pool provided. In the event of an emergency midwives would arrange a transfer by ambulance to County Hospital, Hereford.

Midwife Unit

Number of beds	2
Births	28
Midwives	3
Home births	15%
Amenity Rooms, Price	-

Obstetrician 24 hours	No
Paediatrician 24 hours	No
Full Water Birth Service	Yes

Tests

Routine Triple Testing	No
Nuchal Fold Scan	Yes
Fetal Assessment Unit	No

Pain Relief

24 Hour epidural	No
Mobile epidural	No
Pethidine injections	Yes
Water (eg Bath)	Yes

Midwife-led units are adequately equipped to care for women whose pregnancy is progressing normally without complications. As a result, intervention tends to be low in these units. Basic pain relief will be offered, but any woman requesting an epidural during the delivery will need to be transferred to the nearest consultant-led unit. A woman will also be transferred to the obstetric unit if any complications develop during the delivery.

Llandrindod Wells · **Llandrindod Wells Hospital**

**Temple Street, Llandrindod Wells
Powys, LD1 5HF
Phone: 01597 822 951
Fax: 01597 822 951**

**Trust: Powys Healthcare
NHS Trust**

Llandrindod Wells Hospital has a small midwife-led maternity service. There is only one bed in the delivery suite and a small team of midwives which can provide a friendly personal service. The unit has a 'home-from-home' feel and it is a good choice if you have a low-risk pregnancy and wish to give birth with the minimum of intervention. There are no water birth facilities but home births are done. You will be offered a range of tests and scans, although double testing is done rather than triple testing. For most tests you will be referrred to another unit. For example, for ultrasound scans, you will be referred to Builth Hospital, seven miles away, for a nuchal fold scan to University Hospital of Wales, Cardiff and for an amniocentesis you would travel to Hereford Hospital.

Midwife Unit

Number of beds	4
Births	39
Midwives	3
Home births	7%
Amenity Rooms, Price	-
Obstetrician 24 hours	No
Paediatrician 24 hours	No
Full Water Birth Service	No

Tests

Routine Triple Testing	No
Nuchal Fold Scan	Yes
Fetal Assessment Unit	No

Pain Relief

24 Hour epidural	No
Mobile epidural	No
Pethidine injections	Yes
Water (eg Bath)	Yes

Midwife-led units are adequately equipped to care for women whose pregnancy is progressing normally without complications. As a result, intervention tends to be low in these units. Basic pain relief will be offered, but any woman requesting an epidural during the delivery will need to be transferred to the nearest consultant-led unit. A woman will also be transferred to the obstetric unit if any complications develop during the delivery.

Llanidloes · **Llanidloes War Memorial Hospital**

Eastgate street, Llanidloes
Powys, SY18 6HF
Phone: 01686 412 121
Fax: 01686 412 999

Trust: Powys Healthcare
NHS Trust

This maternity unit offers integrated care in home-from-home surroundings. All rooms are individual and have ensuite facilities. As a small facility, with 29 births last year, the unit has a friendly atmosphere. With a small team of midwives you are bound to get to know the midwives who look after you and get good continuity of care.

Home births are done regularly and there is a water birth service. You can also have home water birth if you supply your own pool.

If you want antenatal screens and tests the service is more limited. Triple testing is not done, although double testing is. To get a nuchal fold scan you will have to pay to have it arranged privately. There are people available to help you with breastfeeding if you need it.

Midwife Unit

Number of beds	3
Births	29
Midwives	3
Home births	12%
Amenity Rooms, Price	-

Obstetrician 24 hours	No
Paediatrician 24 hours	No
Full Water Birth Service	Yes

Tests

Routine Triple Testing	No
Nuchal Fold Scan	No
Fetal Assessment Unit	No

Pain Relief

24 Hour epidural	No
Mobile epidural	No
Pethidine injections	Yes
Water (eg Bath)	Yes

Midwife-led units are adequately equipped to care for women whose pregnancy is progressing normally without complications. As a result, intervention tends to be low in these units. Basic pain relief will be offered, but any woman requesting an epidural during the delivery will need to be transferred to the nearest consultant-led unit. A woman will also be transferred to the obstetric unit if any complications develop during the delivery.

Llantrisant · **Royal Glamorgan General Hospital**

Ynys Maerdy, Llantrisant
Mid Glamorgan CF72 8XR
Phone: 01443 443443
Fax: 01443 217213

Trust: Pontypridd and Rhondda NHS Trust

Maternity care at the Royal Glamorgan General Hospital is shared between consultants and midwives. Although the unit is high tech, if you have a low-risk pregnancy, you will receive most of your antenatal and postnatal care from midwives. Staffing levels at the unit are comparatively high, and midwives offer domino system deliveries, where a midwife who looks after you through pregnancy also cares for you through labour.

Should you wish to have your baby in water, the unit has a pool and midwives trained in water birth are available around the clock. Intervention rates are broadly average for this size unit overall, although the emergency caesarean rate is above average, while instrumental deliveries are relatively infrequent.

Consultant and Midwife Unit

Number of beds	52
Births per midwife	19.37
Births per bed	0.89
Home births	2%
Amenity Rooms, Price	-
Obstetrician 24 hours	Yes
Paediatrician 24 hours	Yes
Full Water Birth Service	Yes

Tests

Routine Triple Testing	No
Nuchal Fold Scan	No
Fetal Assessment Unit	Yes

Pain Relief

24 hour epidural	Yes
Mobile epidural	No
Pethidine injections	Yes
Water (eg bath)	Yes

Intervention Rates

	%	national average %
Epidural	29	26
Elective Caesarean	10	10
Emergency Caesarean	15	13
Induction	20	21
Forceps	3	2
Ventouse	3	7
Episiotomy	10	10

Merthyr Tydfil · **Prince Charles General Hospital**

Merthyr Tydfil
Mid Glamorgan, CF47 9DT
Phone: 01685 721721
Fax: 01685 388001

Trust: North Glamorgan NHS Trust

This is a medium sized unit with both obstetricians and midwives providing care. The domino system is not offered, but the midwives work in teams and over half of the women are cared for in labour by someone they know. If you need to go into hospital early, your partner would also be allowed come and stay with you in the early labour ward. Home births are very rarely done here, but the service is available. There are separate antenatal sessions for women only and classes for teenage mothers are also provided. Routine triple testing and nuchal fold scans are not available but the unit offers double tests and amniocentesis. Aromatherapy and TENS are additional options for pain management.

Consultant and Midwife Unit

Number of beds	29
Births per midwife	21
Births per bed	0.5
Home births	0.08%
Amenity Rooms, Price	-

Obstetrician 24 hours	Yes
Paediatrician 24 hours	Yes
Full Water Birth Service	No

Tests

Routine Triple Testing	No
Nuchal Fold Scan	No
Fetal Assessment Unit	Yes

Pain Relief

24 hour epidural	Yes
Mobile epidural	No
Pethidine injections	Yes
Water (eg bath)	Yes

Intervention Rates

	%	national average %
Epidural	33	26%
Elective Caesarean	10%	10%
Emergency Caesarean	14%	13%
Induction	21%	21%
Forceps	0%	2%
Ventouse	8%	7%
Episiotomy	7%	10%

Neath · **Neath General Hospital**

Briton Ferry Rd, Neath
SA11 2LQ
Phone: 01639 641161

Trust: Bro Morgannwg NHS Trust

The maternity unit provides a full range of midwifery and low-risk obstetric services. Women experiencing problems during the early stages of pregnancy have direct access to the early pregnancy assessment facility within the hospital. Women are usually cared for by midwives at home until they need to go into the unit. As part of its flexible policy, your partner may be allowed to stay with you if you have to go into the unit early. There are amenity beds for hire. Antenatal classes include sessions for grandmothers.

TENS machines, relaxation techniques and aromatherapy are all used to help control pain. Epidurals are available but not used as widely as in most hospitals. Inductions and use of forceps are also relatively infrequent.

Consultant and Midwife Unit

Number of beds	24
Births per midwife	30
Births per bed	0.71
Home births	2%
Amenity Rooms, Price	£24
Obstetrician 24 hours	Yes
Paediatrician 24 hours	Yes
Full Water Birth Service	No

Tests

Routine Triple Testing	Yes
Nuchal Fold Scan	Yes
Fetal Assessment Unit	No

Pain Relief

24 hour epidural	Yes
Mobile epidural	No
Pethidine injections	Yes
Water (eg bath)	Yes

Intervention Rates

	%	national average %
Epidural	14	26
Elective Caesarean	11	10
Emergency Caesarean	11	13
Induction	13	21
Forceps	1	2
Ventouse	8	7
Episiotomy	12	10

Newport · **Royal Gwent Hospital**

Cardiff Road, Newport
Gwent NP20 2UB
Phone: 01633 234234
Fax: 01633 221217

Trust: Gwent Healthcare NHS Trust

The unit offers a choice of midwife-led delivery on the ward area, or more traditional shared midwife and consultant care on the main delivery unit. This system allows you to be flexible about what sort of birth you want and what pain relief you have right up to the birth itself. Staffing levels are better than average, increasing the chance that you will receive one-to-one care throughout labour. There are three beds in the low risk area and a number of single rooms which can also be used for deliveries if the main unit it full.

The triple test is not routinely offered to all women, and you would have to look elsewhere for nuchal fold translucency scanning. Epidurals are available and are widely used but mobile epidurals are not offered.

Consultant and Midwife Unit	
Number of beds	68
Births per midwife	24
Births per bed	1.35
Home births	2%
Amenity Rooms, Price	-

Obstetrician 24 hours	Yes
Paediatrician 24 hours	Yes
Full Water Birth Service	No

Tests	
Routine Triple Testing	No
Nuchal Fold Scan	No
Fetal Assessment Unit	Yes

Pain Relief	
24 hour epidural	Yes
Mobile epidural	No
Pethidine injections	Yes
Water (eg bath)	Yes

Intervention Rates	%	national average %
Epidural	32	26
Elective Caesarean	10	10
Emergency Caesarean	13	13
Induction	21	21
Forceps	2	2
Ventouse	7	7
Episiotomy	12	10

Newtown · **Montgomery County Infirmary**

Llanfair Road, Newtown
Powys, SY16 2DW
Phone: 01686 627 722
Fax: 01686 626 652

Trust: Powys Healthcare NHS Trust

This unit provides shared midwife and GP-led services. It aims to provide a home-from-home atmosphere and women are encouraged to make their own decisions about the type of care they receive.

You will get to know the small team of midwives who look after you through your pregnancy and labour. You are free to bring whoever you wish to antenatal classes. Home births are offered and account for about one in ten of the births overseen by the unit.

Antental screens and tests such as nuchal fold scans are not always offered or available. Double testing is done rather than triple testing. Some later-pregnancy testing is done at Royal Shrewsbury Hospital.

Midwife and GP Unit

Number of beds	3
Births	97
Midwives	6
Home births	9%
Amenity Rooms, Price	0

Obstetrician 24 hours	No
Paediatrician 24 hours	No
Full Water Birth Service	No

Tests

Routine Triple Testing	No
Nuchal Fold Scan	No
Fetal Assessment Unit	No

Pain Relief

24 Hour epidural	No
Mobile epidural	No
Pethidine injections	Yes
Water (eg Bath)	Yes

Midwife-led units are adequately equipped to care for women whose pregnancy is progressing normally without complications. As a result, intervention tends to be low in these units. Basic pain relief will be offered, but any woman requesting an epidural during the delivery will need to be transferred to the nearest consultant-led unit. A woman will also be transferred to the obstetric unit if any complications develop during the delivery.

Penarth · **Llandough Hospital**

Penlan Road, Llandough, Penarth
Vale of Glamorgan CF64 2XX
Phone: 029 20711711
Fax: 02920 708 973

Trust: Cardiff and Vale NHS Trust

Care is provided by midwives and consultants. Most people are looked after by teams of midwives, but there are obstetricians and paediatricians on site to deal with more complex pregnancies. Epidurals are offered but the unit also provides alternative methods of pain relief.

Intervention rates are kept low and in particular elective caesareans are much less common than in other units. Water births may be provided in the home by special request. Staffing levels are more stretched than at many units in Wales and the unit reports that continuity of care has been eroded by staff vacancies. However in the past about half the women giving birth have known the midwife who delivered them.

Consultant and Midwife Unit

Number of beds	53
Births per midwife	30
Births per bed	0.77
Home births	1%
Amenity Rooms, Price	-

Obstetrician 24 hours	Yes
Paediatrician 24 hours	Yes
Full Water Birth Service	No

Tests

Routine Triple Testing	No
Nuchal Fold Scan	Yes
Fetal Assessment Unit	No

Pain Relief

24 hour epidural	Yes
Mobile epidural	No
Pethidine injections	Yes
Water (eg bath)	Yes

Intervention Rates

	%	national average %
Epidural	16	26
Elective Caesarean	7	10
Emergency Caesarean	14	13
Induction	18	21
Forceps	2	2
Ventouse	10	7
Episiotomy	3	10

Powys · **Bro Ddyfi Community Hospital**

Machynlleth
Powys, SY20 8AD
Phone: 01654 702266/7

Trust: Powys Healthcare NHS Trust

Bro Ddyfi Community Hospital is a small maternity unit where only 18 births took place here last year, and a quarter of all births were performed at home. Care is led by midwives and GPs, and the small scale of the service makes continuity of care excellent – you will of course, get to know the people who look after you in a way that is difficult in a large hospital. There are full water birth facilities and midwives are available around the clock to assist women who choose this option. For pain relief there is a TENS machine, water and the midwives can adminster pethidine injections. Antenatal classes take place only during the day. The unit does not offer triple testing or nuchal fold scans, but it does offer double testing.

Midwife and GP Unit

Number of beds	3
Births	18
Midwives	1
Home births	25%
Amenity Rooms, Price	0

Obstetrician 24 hours	No
Paediatrician 24 hours	No
Full Water Birth Service	Yes

Tests

Routine Triple Testing	No
Nuchal Fold Scan	No
Fetal Assessment Unit	No

Pain Relief

24 Hour epidural	No
Mobile epidural	No
Pethidine injections	Yes
Water (eg Bath)	Yes

Midwife-led units are adequately equipped to care for women whose pregnancy is progressing normally without complications. As a result, intervention tends to be low in these units. Basic pain relief will be offered, but any woman requesting an epidural during the delivery will need to be transferred to the nearest consultant-led unit. A woman will also be transferred to the obstetric unit if any complications develop during the delivery.

Pwllheli · **Bryn Beryl Hospital**

Caernarfon Road, Pwllheli
Gwynedd, LL53 6TT
Phone: 01758 701122
Fax: 01758 701295

Trust: North West Wales NHS Trust

This unit is currently closed, but will reopen in January 2002 as a one-bed home-from-home midwife-led facility. The unit will provide flexible care with a minimum of intervention, and you can expect a high level of personal service.

You will be able to book antenatal appointments on any day to suit you, and phone-in and drop-in facilities will be available throughout the week. With antenatal tests, triple testing is not routine, but the unit will refer you for a nuchal fold scan.

Pain relief, as is usual for a midwife-led unit, is fairly limited.

In the event of complications or an emergency, you would be transferred by ambulance to the large consultant-led unit in Bangor.

Midwife Unit

Number of beds	1
Births	-
Midwives	-
Home births	-
Amenity Rooms, Price	-

Obstetrician 24 hours	No
Paediatrician 24 hours	No
Full Water Birth Service	No

Tests

Routine Triple Testing	No
Nuchal Fold Scan	Yes
Fetal Assessment Unit	No

Pain Relief

24 Hour epidural	No
Mobile epidural	No
Pethidine injections	Yes
Water (eg Bath)	Yes

Midwife-led units are adequately equipped to care for women whose pregnancy is progressing normally without complications. As a result, intervention tends to be low in these units. Basic pain relief will be offered, but any woman requesting an epidural during the delivery will need to be transferred to the nearest consultant-led unit. A woman will also be transferred to the obstetric unit if any complications develop during the delivery.

Rhyl · **Glan Clwyd District General Hospital**

Bodelwyddan, Rhyl
Clwyd LL18 5UJ
Phone: 01745 583910
Fax: 01745 583143

Trust: Conwy and Denbighshire NHS Trust

At this maternity unit you will be looked after by a named midwife in your home or at local clinics with rapid access to the acute service if required. Staffing levels are good and you should get one-to-one care during labour – something that has been shown to improve women's experience of birth. For more complex deliveries there is a full obstetric service and intervention rates are a little above average with a particularly high induction rate. The unit is currently moving towards midwifery-led care, and operates a caseload midwifery system. You can arrange to have a water birth, although you will need to hire your own pool. Antenatal classes take place around the clock and include weekend, evening and women-only sessions.

Consultant and Midwife Unit

Number of beds	50
Births per midwife	26
Births per bed	0.91
Home births	1%
Amenity Rooms, Price	-

Obstetrician 24 hours	Yes
Paediatrician 24 hours	Yes
Full Water Birth Service	Yes

Tests

Routine Triple Testing	No
Nuchal Fold Scan	Yes
Fetal Assessment Unit	No

Pain Relief

24 hour epidural	Yes
Mobile epidural	Yes
Pethidine injections	Yes
Water (eg bath)	Yes

Intervention Rates

	%	national average %
Epidural	41	26
Elective Caesarean	11	10
Emergency Caesarean	12	13
Induction	28	21
Forceps	3	2
Ventouse	10	7
Episiotomy	16	10

Swansea · **Singleton Hospital**

Sketty Road
Swansea, SA2 8QA
Phone: 01792 205666
Fax: 01792 208647

Trust: Swansea NHS Trust

The purpose-built maternity unit at Singleton Hospital is operated as a shared midwife and consultant unit. It is a regional referral centre for higher risk pregnancies – a fact that is reflected in a relatively high caesarean rate. Other intervention rates, however, are broadly average and inductions are done less frequently than in other hospitals.

Epidural anaesthesia is available 24hrs a day, although use of this is slightly below average.

Midwife staffing levels are better than most UK hospitals and staff turnover is reported to be low.

There is a birthing pool and midwives are available around the clock to assist women who choose this option.

Consultant and Midwife Unit

Number of beds	62
Births per midwife	28
Births per bed	0.90
Home births	1%
Amenity Rooms, Price	£35

Obstetrician 24 hours	Yes
Paediatrician 24 hours	Yes
Full Water Birth Service	Yes

Tests

Routine Triple Testing	No
Nuchal Fold Scan	Yes
Fetal Assessment Unit	Yes

Pain Relief

24 hour epidural	Yes
Mobile epidural	No
Pethidine injections	Yes
Water (eg bath)	Yes

Intervention Rates

	%	national average %
Epidural	24%	26%
Elective Caesarean	12%	10%
Emergency Caesarean	15%	13%
Induction	19%	21%
Forceps	2%	2%
Ventouse	6%	7%
Episiotomy	11%	10%

Tywyn · **Tywyn & District War Memorial Hospital**

Tywyn
Gwynedd, LL36 9HH
Phone: 01654 710411
Fax: 01654 712206

Trust: North West Wales
NHS Trust

The maternity unit at Tywyn & District War Memorial Hospital is a small midwife-led service with just one delivery bed and only eight births last year. Antenatal care can be shared between your GP and midwife, but in practice most care is provided by a midwife at your home. There is a consultant clinic at the unit twice a month. The unit only takes one patient at a time and partners are allowed to stay for the duration of your time in hospital. You will usually get a booking ultrasound scan and a further scan at 18 weeks. But triple testing is not usually offered. You can get nuchal fold scans if you are prepared to pay to have it privately. If complications arise you may be referred to Aberystwyth.

Midwife Unit

Number of beds	2
Births	8
Midwives	1
Home births	0
Amenity Rooms, Price	-

Obstetrician 24 hours	No
Paediatrician 24 hours	No
Full Water Birth Service	No

Tests

Routine Triple Testing	No
Nuchal Fold Scan	No
Fetal Assessment Unit	No

Pain Relief

24 Hour epidural	No
Mobile epidural	No
Pethidine injections	Yes
Water (eg bath)	Yes

Midwife-led units are adequately equipped to care for women whose pregnancy is progressing normally without complications. As a result, intervention tends to be low in these units. Basic pain relief will be offered, but any woman requesting an epidural during the delivery will need to be transferred to the nearest consultant-led unit. A woman will also be transferred to the obstetric unit if any complications develop during the delivery.

Welshpool · **Victoria Memorial Hospital**

Salop Road, Welshpool
Powys, SY21 7DU
Phone: 01938 553 133
Fax: 01938 556821

Trust: Powys Healthcare
NHS Trust

This is a small midwife-led unit which can deliver you either in the 6 bedded unit or at home. The unit itself is small, with just two delivery beds. Whether you have your baby at home or in the hospital, you will receive far better continuity of care than you are likely to get in most large hospitals and will be looked after through pregnancy and labour by the small team of midwives at the unit. As a midwife-led unit, there are not the facilities for intervention in labour, although a few children have been delivered by forceps. You will not get an epidural here, but the unit does practice a range of alternative pain management techniques including homeopathy and reflexology. Antenatal classes are held on weekday evenings.

Midwife Unit

Number of beds	6
Births	90
Midwives	6
Home births	13%
Amenity Rooms, Price	35

Obstetrician 24 hours	No
Paediatrician 24 hours	No
Full Water Birth Service	No

Tests

Routine Triple Testing	No
Nuchal Fold Scan	No
Fetal Assessment Unit	No

Pain Relief

24 Hour epidural	No
Mobile epidural	No
Pethidine injections	Yes
Water (eg bath)	Yes

Midwife-led units are adequately equipped to care for women whose pregnancy is progressing normally without complications. As a result, intervention tends to be low in these units. Basic pain relief will be offered, but any woman requesting an epidural during the delivery will need to be transferred to the nearest consultant-led unit. A woman will also be transferred to the obstetric unit if any complications develop during the delivery.

Wrexham · **Wrexham Maelor Hospital**

Croesnewydd Road, Wrexham
Clwyd LL13 7TD
Phone: 01978 291100
Fax: 01978 290951

Trust: North East Wales NHS Trust

Maternity care at Wrexham Maelor Hospital is shared between consultants and midwives in both the hospital and in the community. Consultant clinics are held regularly in the towns of Mold, Deeside, Ruabon, Llangollen, Chirk, Corwen, Bala and Dolgellau.

There are no water birth facilities at the unit, but three delivery rooms have a corner bath if you wish to use water to help with pain relief. Midwives at the unit work provide domino system deliveries which are designed to ensure you get most of your care at home and that you are looked after in labour by someone you know.

Consultant and Midwife Unit

Number of beds	44
Births per midwife	27
Births per bed	0.89
Home births	1%
Amenity Rooms, Price	£40

Obstetrician 24 hours	Yes
Paediatrician 24 hours	Yes
Full Water Birth Service	No

Tests

Routine Triple Testing	No
Nuchal Fold Scan	Yes
Fetal Assessment Unit	No

Pain Relief

24 hour epidural	Yes
Mobile epidural	No
Pethidine injections	Yes
Water (eg bath)	Yes

Intervention Rates

	%	national average %
Epidural	17	26
Elective Caesarean	8	10
Emergency Caesarean	11	13
Induction	26	21
Forceps	4	2
Ventouse	8	7
Episiotomy	15	10

Northern Ireland

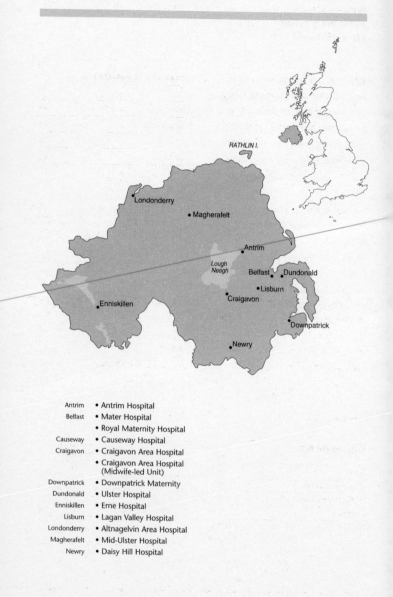

Antrim	• Antrim Hospital
Belfast	• Mater Hospital
	• Royal Maternity Hospital
Causeway	• Causeway Hospital
Craigavon	• Craigavon Area Hospital
	• Craigavon Area Hospital (Midwife-led Unit)
Downpatrick	• Downpatrick Maternity
Dundonald	• Ulster Hospital
Enniskillen	• Erne Hospital
Lisburn	• Lagan Valley Hospital
Londonderry	• Altnagelvin Area Hospital
Magherafelt	• Mid-Ulster Hospital
Newry	• Daisy Hill Hospital

Antrim · **Antrim Hospital**

Antrim
N.Ireland BT41 2RL
Phone: 028 94424000
Fax: 01849 424293

Trust: United Hospitals Group HSS Trust

Care here is shared between midwives and consultants, and the majority of patients give birth on the ward. Very few women have home births. The unit offers domino care, and staffing levels here are generally very good.

The unit supplies a full range of antenatal classes, including sessions for teenage mothers and multiple births. Note that induction rates are high at this unit; less than a third of women here last year gave birth without some kind of intervention.

The maternity unit at the hospital encourages new mothers to breastfeed. Unusually, the hospital will usually try to accommodate your partner if you have to go into hospital before your labour has started.

Consultant and Midwife Unit

Number of beds	49
Births per midwife	21
Births per bed	0.98
Home births	0.42
Amenity Rooms, Price	£23

Obstetrician 24 hours	Yes
Paediatrician 24 hours	Yes
Full Water Birth Service	No

Tests

Routine Triple Testing	No
Nuchal Fold Scan	Yes
Fetal Assessment Unit	Yes

Pain Relief

24 hour epidural	Yes
Mobile epidural	No
Pethidine injections	Yes
Water (eg bath)	Yes

Intervention Rates	%	national average %
Epidural	47	36
Elective Caesarean	13	10
Emergency Caesarean	11	13
Induction	35	30
Forceps	8	6
Ventouse	4	8
Episiotomy	22	22

Belfast · **Mater Hospital**

47-51 Crumlin Road, Belfast
N.Ireland BT14 6AB
Phone: 028 90741211
Fax: 01232 741342

Trust: Mater Hospital
HSS Trust

As with many hospitals in Northern Ireland, the Mater has relatively high rates of intervention in childbirth with almost one third of women having their labour induced and a quarter being delivered by caesarean section.

A new hospital building development is nearing completion and maternity outpatient clinics will be held in new ultra modern facilities. These will include antenatal and postnatal clinics as well as early pregnancy and baby assessment. There is a full range of medical facilities including a special care baby unit for babies who are born with complications. Breastfeeding counsellor facilitates a weekly breastfeeding support group and provides advice to a range of local community groups.

Consultant and Midwife Unit

Number of beds	35
Births per midwife	37.5
Births per bed	0.53
Home births	0%
Amenity Rooms, Price	£35

Obstetrician 24 hours	Yes
Paediatrician 24 hours	Yes
Full Water Birth Service	No

Tests

Routine Triple Testing	No
Nuchal Fold Scan	Yes
Fetal Assessment Unit	Yes

Pain Relief

24 hour epidural	Yes
Mobile epidural	No
Pethidine injections	Yes
Water (eg bath)	Yes

Intervention Rates

	%	national average %
Epidural	35	36
Elective Caesarean	12	10
Emergency Caesarean	13	13
Induction	32	30
Forceps	6	6
Ventouse	8	8
Episiotomy	20	22

Belfast · **Royal Maternity Hospital**

Grosvenor Rd, Belfast
N.Ireland BT12 6BB
Phone: 01232 894656

Trust: Royal Group of Hospitals
   HSS Trust

The Royal Maternity Hospital has one of the highest rates of caesarean deliveries in the UK with about one third of babies delivered this way. Northern Ireland hospitals tend to have higher caesarean rates and this hospital is a specialist referral centre for more comlex pregancies from across Northern Ireland. You can choose between consultant-led, midwife-led care or shared care with the GP. The unit offers both domino system and caseload midwifery – both designed to ensure you get continuous care from one or two midwives. Options for pain relief include alternative therapies as well as traditional methods. Epidurals are very widely used. After the birth you will be offered an outpatient review appointment as well as follow-up baby clinics.

Consultant and Midwife Unit

Number of beds	82
Births per midwife	18
Births per bed	0.97
Home births	0.5%
Amenity Rooms, Price	£60

Obstetrician 24 hours	Yes
Paediatrician 24 hours	Yes
Full Water Birth Service	Yes

Tests

Routine Triple Testing	No
Nuchal Fold Scan	Yes
Fetal Assessment Unit	Yes

Pain Relief

24 hour epidural	Yes
Mobile epidural	No
Pethidine injections	Yes
Water (eg bath)	Yes

Intervention Rates

	%	national average %
Epidural	60	36
Elective Caesarean	16	10
Emergency Caesarean	16	13
Induction	32	30
Forceps	6	6
Ventouse	5	8
Episiotomy	18	22

Causeway · **Causeway Hospital**

4, Newbury Road, Coleraine,
Co. Londonderry
Phone: 028 7032 7032
Fax: 028 7034 6125

Trust: Causeway HSS Trust

The Causeway Hospital's maternity service operates shared care between consultants and midwives. Almost a third of breech presentations at the unit are delivered vaginally rather than by caesarean section. This proportion is significantly higher than the national average and indicates that the service's consultant obstetricians are experienced in performing External Cephalic Version.

Staffing levels at the unit are also above average, increasing the likelihood that you will receive one-to-one care in labour.

Unlike most other high-tech units, availability of epidural anaesthesia at Causeway Hospital is not guaranteed 24 hours a day. However, other forms of pain relief such as opiate injections and TENS machines are available.

Consultant and Midwife Unit

Number of beds	22
Births per midwife	24
Births per bed	0.76
Home births	0.36%
Amenity Room, Price	£23

Obstetrician 24 hours	No
Paediatrician 24 hours	No
Water Birth Offered	No

Tests

Routine Triple Testing	No
Nuchal Fold Scan	Yes
Fetal Assessment Unit	Yes

Pain Relief

24 Hour epidural	No
Mobile epidural	No
Pethidine injections	Yes
Water (eg bath)	Yes

Intervention Rates

	%	national average %
Epidural	16	36
Elective Caesarean	9	10
Emergency Caesarean	8	13
Induction	21	30
Forceps	3	6
Ventouse	3	8
Episiotomy	18	22

Craigavon · **Craigavon Area Hospital**

68 Lurgan Road, Portadown,
Co Armagh, BT66 5QQ
Phone: 02838 334444

Trust: Craigavon Area Hospital Group
HSS Trust

As with many hospitals in Northern Ireland, intervention rates at Craigavon are very high. Twenty eight per cent of women attending the hospital are delivered by caesearean section. However, the hospital has set up a separate midwife-led unit which may encourage more natural childbirth. Epidurals are not guaranteed 24 hours a day although in practice a relatively high number of women do have epidurals suggesting that getting one if you want one is rarely a problem. Nuchal fold scans are available and although triple testing is not offered routinely it is available on request. Water births are not offered. Home births are organised separately by the local community midwife service which can also deliver you in the main hospital unit under a domino system.

Consultant and Midwife Unit

Number of beds	38
Births per midwife	32
Births per bed	1.00
Home births	-
Amenity Rooms, Price	£35

Obstetrician 24 hours	Yes
Paediatrician 24 hours	Yes
Full Water Birth Service	No

Tests

Routine Triple Testing	No
Nuchal Fold Scan	Yes
Fetal Assessment Unit	Yes

Pain Relief

24 hour epidural	No
Mobile epidural	No
Pethidine injections	Yes
Water (eg bath)	Yes

Intervention Rates	%	national average %
Epidural	58	36
Elective Caesarean	14	10
Emergency Caesarean	14	13
Induction	33	30
Forceps	3	6
Ventouse	6	8
Episiotomy	28	22

Craigavon · **Craigavon Area Hospital**

68 Lurgan Road, Portadown,
Co Armagh, BT66 5QQ
Phone: 02838 334444

Trust: Craigavon Area Hospital Group
HSS Trust

This is one of the rare midwife-led units in Northern Ireland and is unusual for being situated in a large hospital with a maternity unit that has a very high rate of medical intervention. The aim of the midwife-led unit is to provide a less medical environment for women with straightforward pregnancies who will be encouraged to give birth naturally. Water is used as a pain management technique in most labours along with relaxation and movement techniques. There are also full facilities for water birth – something that attracts women to Craigavon from other parts of Northern Ireland. The facilities are comfortable – single rooms with ensuite facilities – and women can be quickly transferred to the main unit in the hospital should complications arise.

Midwife Unit

Number of beds	9
Births	336
Midwives	67
Home births	0%
Amenity Rooms, Price	-

Obstetrician 24 hours	Yes
Paediatrician 24 hours	Yes
Full Water Birth Service	Yes

Tests

Routine Triple Testing	Yes
Nuchal Fold Scan	Yes
Fetal Assessment Unit	No

Pain Relief

24 Hour epidural	No
Mobile epidural	No
Pethidine injections	Yes
Water (eg Bath)	Yes

Midwife-led units are adequately equipped to care for women whose pregnancy is progressing normally without complications. As a result, intervention tends to be low in these units. Basic pain relief will be offered, but any woman requesting an epidural during the delivery will need to be transferred to the nearest consultant-led unit. A woman will also be transferred to the obstetric unit if any complications develop during the delivery.

Downpatrick · **Downpatrick Maternity Hospital**

Stuell Wells Road, Downpatrick
N.Ireland BT30 6RL
Phone: 028 4461 3311 ext 34
Fax: 028 4483 9809

Trust: Down Lisburn
   HSS Trust

This relatively small maternity unit has remarkably low intervention rates, particularly for Northern Ireland. Only one in six women gave birth by caesarean section last year and delivery by forceps is only in exceptional circumstances. There is a high level of midwife staffing which should enable a good level of personal attention, especially during labour. The unit operates the domino system which is designed to ensure you are cared for in labour by a midwife involved in your antenatal care. There is medical cover at the unit, with an obstetrician on site 24-hours a day, but very limited anaesthetic cover. Epidurals are not available as pain relief in labour. However opiate injections, gas & air and a TENS machine are all available.

Consultant and Midwife Unit

Number of beds	20
Births per midwife	22
Births per bed	0.46
Home births	0.2%
Amenity Rooms, Price	-

Obstetrician 24 hours	Yes
Paediatrician 24 hours	No
Full Water Birth Service	No

Tests

Routine Triple Testing	No
Nuchal Fold Scan	Yes
Fetal Assessment Unit	No

Pain Relief

24 hour epidural	No
Mobile epidural	No
Pethidine injections	Yes
Water (eg bath)	Yes

Intervention Rates	%	national average %
Epidural	6	36
Elective Caesarean	5	10
Emergency Caesarean	10	13
Induction	24	30
Forceps	0.8	6
Ventouse	8	8
Episiotomy	-	22

Dundonald · **The Ulster Hospital**

Upper Newtownards Road, Dundonald
Belfast, N.Ireland BT16 0RH
Phone: 028 9048 4511
Fax: 028 9048 1753

Trust: Ulster Community and Hospitals
HSS Trust

The unit offers consultant-led or midwife-led care and domino or home births although home births are extremely rare. Intervention rates are high – in particular the use of forceps.

There is 24hr anaesthetic and paediatric cover as well as a neonatal unit. The range of pain relief options include patient controlled systems which allow you to decide how much anaesthetic you receive. Epidurals are available and widely used. Low risk mothers who wish to use natural methods of pain relief can be accommodated in a family friendly room outside the main labour ward area. Water births are offered but the unit does not promise to have suitably trained midwives available all the time, so they may not be around when you go into labour.

Consultant and Midwife Unit

Number of beds	46
Births per midwife	25
Births per bed	1.08
Home births	0.08%
Amenity Rooms, Price	£46

Obstetrician 24 hours	Yes
Paediatrician 24 hours	Yes
Full Water Birth Service	No

Tests

Routine Triple Testing	No
Nuchal Fold Scan	Yes
Fetal Assessment Unit	Yes

Pain Relief

24 hour epidural	Yes
Mobile epidural	Yes
Pethidine injections	Yes
Water (eg bath)	No

Intervention Rates

	%	national average %
Epidural	58	36
Elective Caesarean	10	10
Emergency Caesarean	14	13
Induction	20	30
Forceps	8	6
Ventouse	8	8
Episiotomy	18	22

Enniskillen · **Erne Hospital**

Enniskillen, Co Fermanagh
N.Ireland BT74 6AY
Phone: 028 66 324711
Fax: 028 66 326131

Trust: Sperrin Lakeland
    HSS Trust

Care at the unit is shared midwife and consultant led, with a reasonably good staffing ratio of 30 births per year for every midwife. This can enable a better level of personal attention, especially during labour. There is a very good chance you will be looked after in labour by a midwife who already knows you from ante-natal care. Parent education sessions and antenatal classes are available during the daytime and in the evenings, with special for women only classes also available. You also have access to breastfeeding counsellors.

Intervention rates are a little below average for Northern Ireland. Epidurals for pain relief are not standardly available 24 hours.

Consultant and Midwife Unit

Number of beds	28
Births per midwife	30
Births per bed	0.62
Home births	0.37%
Amenity Rooms, Price	£17

Obstetrician 24 hours	No
Paediatrician 24 hours	No
Full Water Birth Service	No

Tests

Routine Triple Testing	No
Nuchal Fold Scan	No
Fetal Assessment Unit	No

Pain Relief

24 hour epidural	No
Mobile epidural	No
Pethidine injections	Yes
Water (eg bath)	Yes

Intervention Rates

	%	national average %
Epidural	9	36
Elective Caesarean	9	10
Emergency Caesarean	10	13
Induction	35	30
Forceps	3	6
Ventouse	11	8
Episiotomy	21	22

Lisburn · **Lagan Valley Hospital**

39 Hillsborough Road, Lisburn
Co Antrim, N.Ireland BT28 1JP
Phone: 028 92665141

Trust: Down Lisburn HSS Trust

The Lagan Valley Maternity Unit has recently been redecorated with a view to creating a more friendly, relaxing atmosphere. It has 24 maternity beds and five individual labour rooms furnished with homely furnishings such as reclining and rocking chairs, and birthing balls. There are three consultant obstetricians in the maternity unit in addition to a registrar and four senior house officers. The majority of care is delivered by midwives with an integrated service covering care during labour as well as care before and after the birth. One to one antenatal sessions are available. There is a qualified aromatherapist on staff. Epidurals for pain relief are not available 24 hours a day although there is a booked epidural service. Triple testing is not routinely offered but is available on request.

Consultant and Midwife Unit

Number of beds	26
Births per midwife	28.3
Births per bed	0.59
Home births	0.19%
Amenity Rooms, Price	-

Obstetrician 24 hours	No
Paediatrician 24 hours	No
Full Water Birth Service	No

Tests

Routine Triple Testing	No
Nuchal Fold Scan	Yes
Fetal Assessment Unit	Yes

Pain Relief

24 hour epidural	No
Mobile epidural	No
Pethidine injections	Yes
Water (eg bath)	No

Intervention Rates

	%	national average %
Epidural	32	36
Elective Caesarean	10	10
Emergency Caesarean	14	13
Induction	35	30
Forceps	8	6
Ventouse	5	8
Episiotomy	17	22

Londonderry · **Altnagelvin Area Hospital**

Gleshane Road, Londonderry
Londonderry, BT47 6SB
Phone: 028 71345171
Fax: 028 71611222

Trust: Altnagelvin Group HSS Trust

This is a shared-care unit between midwives and consultants. Most births take place within the unit; it does not frequently cater to home births. Water births can be made available if requested, although you will have to provide a pool if you want this option. Antenatal testing is done selectively. Triple testing is not routinely offered and alpha-feto protein is only done on request. Anomaly scans have recently been introduced.

Epidural rates are very low but episiotomies are higher than average, being given to almost one in three women. The unit has a dedicated lactation specialist and breastfeeding support team of midwives. The maternity department has been awarded the UNICEF UK Baby Friendly Initiative Accreditation.

Consultant and Midwife Unit

Number of beds	46
Births per midwife	20
Births per bed	1.00
Home births	0.8%
Amenity Rooms, Price	£25

Obstetrician 24 hours	Yes
Paediatrician 24 hours	Yes
Full Water Birth Service	Yes

Tests

Routine Triple Testing	No
Nuchal Fold Scan	No
Fetal Assessment Unit	Yes

Pain Relief

24 Hour epidural	Yes
Mobile epidural	No
Pethidine injections	Yes
Water (eg Bath)	Yes

Intervention Rates

	%	national average %
Epidural	27	36
Elective Caesarean	9	10
Emergency Caesarean	10	13
Induction	24	30
Forceps	5	6
Ventouse	10	8
Episiotomy	29	22

Magherafelt · **Mid-Ulster Hospital**

59 Hospital Road,
County Londonderry, BT35 8DR
Phone: 028 7963 1031
Fax: 028 7963 1674

Trust: United Hospitals Group
HSS Trust

This midwife and consultant unit shares antenatal care with local GPs in the community. The unit can arrange a domino midwife to care for you, and the majority of women know the midwife who delivers them. Water births are not available here. For more complex pregnancies, or in an emergency, women may be transferred to Antrim Hospital, though there is a general operating theatre adjacent to the labour ward.

Single rooms are available to hire, and partners may stay on the ward overnight.

Tests are not always routinely offered to all women: triple-testing is only routinely offered to women over the age of 35. Intervention rates are low, and the rate of epidurals administered here is far lower than average.

Consultant and Midwife Unit

Number of beds	16
Births per midwife	24
Births per bed	0.43
Home births	0%
Amenity Rooms, Price	£23
Obstetrician 24 hours	No
Paediatrician 24 hours	No
Water Birth Offered	No

Tests

Routine Triple Testing	No
Nuchal Fold Scan	No
Fetal Assessment Unit	No

Pain Relief

24 hour epidural	No
Mobile epidural	No
Pethidine injections	Yes
Water (eg bath)	Yes

Intervention Rates

	%	national average %
Epidural	12	36
Elective Caesarean	7	10
Emergency Caesarean	7	13
Induction	22	30
Forceps	5	6
Ventouse	4	8
Episiotomy	22	22

Newry · **Daisy Hill Hospital**

5 Hospital Road, Newry
County Down, N.Ireland BT35 8DR
Phone: 02830 835 000
Fax: 01693 250624

Trust: Newry and Mourne HSS Trust

Daisy Hill Hospital is unusual for the UK as a large hospital based maternity unit with limited medical and anaesthetic cover. There is neither an obstetrician nor a paediatrician on the hospital site most of the time, although junior doctors are always on hand and a consultant is on call 24 hours a day. Epidurals are only offered weekdays during office hours unless medically necessary. That said, a relatively large number of women in the unit do get epidurals. Caesarean rates are relatively low for Northern Ireland. Midwife staffing levels are good which should enable a good level of personal attention during labour. However home births are rare and water births are not offered. Amenity rooms are available for £30 and an en suite room can be hired for £50.

Consultant and Midwife Unit

Number of beds	27
Births per midwife	28
Births per bed	0.64
Home births	0.06%
Amenity Rooms, Price	£30
Obstetrician 24 hours	No
Paediatrician 24 hours	No
Full Water Birth Service	No

Tests

Routine Triple Testing	No
Nuchal Fold Scan	No
Fetal Assessment Unit	No

Pain Relief

24 hour epidural	No
Mobile epidural	No
Pethidine injections	Yes
Water (eg bath)	No

Intervention Rates	%	national average %
Epidural	39	36
Elective Caesarean	9	10
Emergency Caesarean	12	13
Induction	34	30
Forceps	6	6
Ventouse	10	8
Episiotomy	39	22

Methodology

This guide covers maternity units across the UK. Statistics for England have been adjusted, as described below, to take account of maternal age and social demographics.

Establishing scope of research and data collection

Questionnaires were sent to every maternity unit in the country. These were constructed using focus group research and then circulated to leading institutions and organisations including the Department of Health, the Royal College of Obstetricians and Gynaecologists, the Royal College of Midwives and the National Childbirth Trust, all of which approved the final version.

Because of gaps in nationally collected statistical data and possible concerns about data quality, statistical data was collected directly from maternity units and then compared to nationally collected data as a check. Figures were supplied for the more recent available complete year which in most cases was the year to March 2001 or the year to December 2000.

Definitions of staffing data

Staffing figures are based on number of whole time equivalent midwives at each unit, including community and ward based midwives, expressed as the number of births in the unit per year per midwife. Community hospitals tend to carry out antenatal and posnatal care for women who give birth elsewhere. As a result their staffing levels appear much higher with far fewer births per midwife per year. This accurately reflects the fact that these units are, in general, able to provide a more personal level of midwife care than consultant-led units. However caution should be taken comparing figures for one community unit with another on the basis of the staffing figures since the ratios will be influenced by what other duties the unit undertakes.

Intervention rates – adjustment for low-risk units

Figures for caesarean section rates, instrumental intervention rates (forceps and ventouse) and induction rates are usually given as the number of live births involving such an intervention as a percentage of all live births at the unit. An exception has been made for units with a high number of high-risk women requiring intervention caused by the proximity of alternative facilities for low-risk women. The first group of hospitals affected by this are the eight hospitals with two units on one site – one low risk midwife or GP-led unit and one consultant-led unit for higher risk deliveries. In these cases the intervention rates quoted for the consultant unit are the intervention rates for the hospital as a whole. In most cases there are no interventions in the midwife unit. The staffing ratio for the main unit is also a figure for the whole hospital.

A similar approach is used for the Princess Anne Wing of the Royal United Hospital in Bath which operates a service from teams of midwives operating from GP clinics, in addition to the consultant led unit at the hospital. The figures for these teams have been combined with the consultant unit at the Princess Anne Wing.

For hospitals where births in neighboring mid-wife led units (which would transfer emergencies to that hospital) come to 10 per cent of the births in the consultant unit, intervention rates are expressed as a percentage of births in both the hospital and the neighbouring community units. The hospitals affected by this are Princess Anne Wing at the Royal United Hospital, Bath; Poole Hospital; Royal Shrewsbury; Royal Devon and Exeter; Colchester General, the Cumberland Infirmary, Aberdeen Maternity Hospital, Scarborough General Hospital and the Prince Charles hospital in Merthyr Tydfil.

In the case of Scarborough General, the births figure used for Bridlington is the ONS figure for the year to September 2000.

Adjustment of English Data for demographics

The raw intervention rates and the rates of pain relief delivered for each hospital will be affected by outside factors. To understand how intervention rates and epidural rates are affected by external factors Imperial College of Science Technology and Medicine analysed the Hospital Episode Statistics (HES) database which is compiled by the Department of Health and records about 98% of births in England. Two factors outside the control of the hospital were found to be important: maternal age and social deprivation. We used the HES database to calculate average figures for these two variables for each hospital. Deprivation scores were based on postcode of residence.

Using four years of data from 1 April 1996 to 31 March 2000 we found that for combined emergency and elective caesarean rates, being older and more deprived were independently associated with a higher proportion of deliveries by caesarean section. Therefore, a hypothetical hospital with an actual caesarean rate of 27%, a high average age and high levels of deprivation would have an adjusted caesarean rate much lower than its unadjusted rate, in this case it might fall to 22%.

These adjustments were only made to consultant led units with significant intervention rates. For midwife-led units which do not do caesareans or which have very few interventions, no adjustment for social factors has been made.

Episiotomies

Rates of episiotomies are simply expressed by unit without any adjustment.

Averages

Intervention rates have been compared to the average for the relevant country. Separate averages have been calculated for England, Scotland, Wales and Northern Ireland. In each case the average is the total number of births involving the intervention covered by the survey divided by the total number of births covered by the survey.

Home Birth Rates

Home birth rates are the number of planned home births expressed as a percentage of live births at the unit plus planned home births. Where a hospital runs two units, the home birth rate is expressed as the number of home births as a percentage of all births at the hospital and the figure is given under the low-risk unit. No figure is given for the high risk unit.

Index of Hospitals

Aberdare General Hospital 467

Aberdeen Maternity Hospital 422

Addenbrooke's Hospital 163

Airedale General Hospital 273

Alexandra Hospital 406

Alnwick Infirmary 252

Altnagelvin Area Hospital 505

Andover War Memorial
  Community Hospital 292

Antrim Hospital 495

Arbroath Infirmary 424

Arran War Memorial Hospital 450

Ashington Hospital 254

Ayrshire Central Hospital 443

Balfour Hospital 449

Barnet Hospital 183

Barnsley District General Hospital
  373

Basildon Hospital 159

Bassetlaw District General Hospital
  392

Bedford Hospital 160

Belford Hospital 434

Berwick Infirmary 255

Billinge Hospital 249

Birmingham City Hospital 396

Birmingham Heartlands Hospitaol
  394

Birmingham Women's Hospital 395

Bishop Auckland General Hospital
  256

Blackbrook House Maternity Home
  307

Blackpool Victoria Hospital 224

Borders General Hospital 455

Bradford Royal Infirmary 257

Brecon War Memorial Hospital 471

Bridgnorth Hospital 397

Bridgwater Community Hospital
  342

Bridlington & District Hospital 258

Bro Ddyfi Community Hospital 487

Bronglais General Hospital 469

Bryn Beryl Hospital 488

Buckland Hospital 305

Burnley General Hospital 226

Buxton Hospital 375

Caithness General Hospital 464

Calderdale Royal (Midwife Unit)
  267

Calderdale Royal Hospital 266

Campbeltown Hospital 425

Castle Hill Hospital 260

Causeway Hospital 498

Central Middlesex Hospital 186

Chalmers Hospital 426

Chase Farm Hospital 192

Chelsea & Westminster Hospital
  203

Cheltenham General Hospital 346

Chesterfield & North Derbyshire
  Royal Hospital 376

Chippenham Community Hospital
  347

Chipping Norton Community
  Hospital 302

Chorley & South Ribble District
  General Hospital 229

Clacton & District Hospital 165

Clenoch Maternity Unit 462

Colchester General Hospital 166

Conquest Hospital 329

Countess of Chester Hospital 228

County Hospital, Hereford 400

Craigavon Area Hospital (Midwife Unit) 500

Craigavon Area Hospital 499

Cresswell Maternity Hospital 427

Crowborough War Memorial Hospital 303

Cumberland Infirmary 259

Daisy Hill Hospital 507

Darent Valley Hospital 304

Darlington Memorial Hospital 261

Derby City General Hospital 377

Derriford Hospital 358

Devizes Community Hospital 348

Dewsbury & District Hospital 262

Dolgellau & Barmouth Hospital 476

Doncaster Royal Infirmary 378

Dorset County Hospital 349

Downpatrick Maternity Hospital 501

Dr Gray's Hospital 431

Dr Mackinnon Memorial Hospital 446

Dunoon & District General 429

Ealing Hospital 191

East Surrey & Crawley Hospitals 327

Eastbourne District General 306

Edgware Birth Centre

Edgware Community Hospital 184

Elizabeth Garrett Anderson Hospital 188

Epsom General Hospital 193

Erne Hospital 503

Fairfield General Hospital 227

Falkirk Royal Infirmary 423

Farnborough Hospital, Bromley 187

Forth Park Hospital (Midwife Unit) 448

Forth Park Hospital 447

Fraserburgh Hospital 435

Friarage Hospital 280

Frimley Park Hospital 308

Furness General Hospital 222

George Eliot Hospital 404

Gilbert Bain Hospital 451

Gilchrist Maternity Unit 167

Glan Clwyd District General Hospital 489

Gloucestershire Royal Hospital (Midwife Unit) 353

Gloucestershire Royal Hospital 352

Good Hope District General 414

Gosport War Memorial Hospital 311

Grantham & District Hospital 379

Grimsby Maternity Hospital 380

Guisborough General Hospital 265

Guy's Hospital 211

Harold Wood Hospital 199

Harrogate District Hospital 268

Harwich & District Hospital 170

Heatherwood Hospital 293

Hexham General Hospital 270

Hillingdon Hospital 200

Hinchingbrooke Hospital 171

Homerton Hospital 195

Honiton Hospital 354

Hope Hospital 245

Hospital of St John & St Elizabeth 210

Huddersfield Royal Infirmary 271

Hull Maternity Hospital 272

Hythe Hospital 331

Insch & District War Memorial Hospital 441

Inverclyde Royal Hospital 439

Ipswich Hospital 172

Islay Hospital 445

James Cook University Hospital 276

James Paget Hospital 168

John Radcliffe Hospital 321

Jubilee Hospital 440

Kent & Cantebury Hospital 299

Kettering General Hospital 314

Kidderminster Hospital 401

Kincardine O'Neill War Memorial Hospital 463

King George Hospital 209

King's College Hospital 205

King's Mill Hospital 391

Kingston Hospital 204

Knighton Hospital 478

Lagan Valley Hospital 504

Leeds General Infirmary 274

Leicester General Hospital 381

Leicester Royal Infirmary 382

Leighton Hospital 203

Lichfield Victoria Hospital 402

Lincoln County Hospital 383

Lister Hospital 178

Liverpool Women's Hospital 233

Llandough Hospital 486

Llandrindod Wells Hospital 479

Llanidloes War Memorial Hospital 480

Lorn and Island District Hospital 456

Ludlow Hospital 402

Luton & Dunstable Hospital 174

Lymington Hospital 315

Macclesfield District General 235

Maidstone Hospital 316

Malmesbury Community 356

Malton Norton & District Hospital 277

Manor Hospital 416

Mater Hospital 416

Mayday Hospital 190

Medway Maritime Hospital 309

Mid Argyll Hospital 453

Mid Ulster Hospital 506

Milton Keynes General 318

Montgomery County Infirmary 485

Montrose Royal Infirmary 454

Neath General Hospital 483

Nevill Hall Hospital 468

New Cross Hospital 419

Newham General Hospital (Midwife Unit) 208

Newham General Hospital 207

Ninewells Hospital 428

Norfolk & Norwich Hospital 176

North Devon District Hospital 339

North Hampshire Hospital 296

North Manchester General 236

North Middlesex Hospital 197

North Staffordshire Hospital 411

North Staffordshire Hospital (Maternity Unit) 412

North Tyneside General 279

Northampton General Hospital 320

Northwick Park Hospital 198

Nottingham City Hospital 386

Okehampton & District Hospital 357

Ormskirk & District Hospital 241

Paulton Memorial Hospital 343

Pembury Hospital 322

Penrith Hospital 281

Perth Royal Infirmary 458

Peterborough District 177

Peterhead Hospital 459

Petersfield Hospital 323

Pilgrim Hospital 374

Pinderfields General 287

Pontefract General 282

Poole Hospital 359

Portree Hospital 460

Prince Charles General Hospital 482

Princess Alexandra Hospital 169

Princess Anne Hospital 332

Princess Margaret Hospital 364

Princess of Wales Hospital 472

Princess Royal Hospital, Hayward's Heath 312

Princess Royal Hospital, Telford 415

Princess Royal Maternity Hospital 436

Queen Charlotte's & Chelsea 196

Queen Elizabeth Hospital, Gateshead 264

Queen Elizabeth Hospital, King's Lynn 173

Queen Elizabeth Hospital, Greenwich 194

Queen Elizabeth II Hospital 180

Queen Elizabeth the Queen Mother Hospital 317

Queen Mary's Hospital 185

Queen Mother's Hospital 438

Queen's Hospital 398

Queen's Medical Center 387

Queen's Park Hospital 223

Raigmore Hospital 442

Robert Jones & Agnes Hunt Hospital 405

Rochdale Infirmary 244

Romsey Hospital 328

Rotherham District General Hospital 388

Royal Alexandra Hospital 457

Royal Berkshire & Battle Hospitals 326

Royal Bolton Hospital 225

Royal Bournemouth Hospital 341

Royal Cornwall Hospital 369

Royal Devon & Exeter Hospital 350

Royal Free Hospital 189

Royal Glamorgan Hospital 481

Royal Gwent Hospital 484

Royal Hallamshire Hospital 390

Royal Hampshire County Hospital 336

Royal Infirmary of Edinburgh 430

Royal Lancaster Infirmary 232

Royal London Hospital 214

Royal Maternity Hospital 497

Royal Oldham Hospital 240

Royal Shrewsbury Hospital (Maternity Unit) 408

Royal Shrewsbury Hospital 407

Royal Surrey County 310

Royal Sussex County Hospital 297

Royal United Hospital 340

Royal Victoria Infirmary 278

Ruth Lancaster James Cottage Hospital 253

Salisbury District Hospital 361

Sandwell General Hospital 418

Scarborough General Hospital 283

Scunthorpe General Hospital 389

Sharoe Green Hospital 243

Shepton Mallet Community Hospital 362

Singleton Hospital 490

Solihull Hospital 409

South Tyneside District Hospital 284

Southend Hospital 181

Southern General Hospital 437

Southmead Hospital 345

Southport & Formby District 246

St Austell Community Hospital 360

St George's Hospital 217

St Helier Hospital 212

St James's University Hospital 275

St John's Hospital at Howden 452

St John's Hospital 164

St Mary's Hospital (Midwife Unit) 325

St Mary's Hospital, Isles of Scilly 355

St Mary's Hospital, Manchester 237

St Mary's Hospital, Melton Mowbray 385

St Mary's Hospital, Newport, IoW 319

St Mary's Hospital, Portsmouth 324

St Mary's Hospital, Westminster 218

St Michael's Hospital 344

St Peter's Hospital, Maldon 175

St Peter's Hospital, Chertsey 300

St Richard's Hospital 301
Staffordshire General 410
Stepping Hill Hospital 247
Stirling Royal Infirmary 451
Stoke Mandeville Hospital 298
Stroud Maternity Hospital 363
Sunderland Royal Hospital 286
Tameside General Hospital 221
Taunton & Somerset Hospital 365
The Birth Centre 213
The Horton Hospital 295
The Portland Hospital 219
The Ulster Hospital 502
Tiverton & District Hospital 366
Torbay District General Hospital 367
Trafford General Hospital 238
Trowbridge Community Hospital 368
Tywyn & District War Memorial Hospital 491
University Hospital, Aintree 234
University Hospital, Lewisham 206
University Hospital of Hartlepool 269
University Hospital of North Durham 263
University Hospital of North Tees 285
University Hospital of Wales 474
Vale of Leven District General Hospital 423
Victoria Hospital, Frome 351
Victoria Hospital, Isle of Bute 444
Victoria Memorial Hospital 492
Wallingford Community Hospital 334

Walsgrave Hospital 399
Wantage Community Hospital 335
Warrington Hospital 248
Warwick Hospital 417
Watford General Hospital 179
Wessex Maternity Centre 333
West Cumberland Hospital 289
West Middlesex Hospital 201
West Suffolk Hospital 162
West Wales General Hospital 475
Westmorland General Hospital 231
Weston General Hospital 370
Wexham Park Hospital 330
Whipps Cross Hospital (Midwife Unit) 216
Whipps Cross Hospital 215
Whiston Hospital 242
Whitby Hospital 288
Whitehills Hospital 433
Whittington Hospital 202
Whitworth Hospital 384
William Harvey Hospital 294
William Julien Courtauld Hospital 161
Wirral Hospital 250
Wishaw General Hospital 465
Withybush General Hospital 477
Worcester Royal Infirmary 420
Wordsley Hospital 413
Worthing Hospital 337
Wrexham Maelor Hospital 493
Wycombe Hospital 313
Wythenshawe Hospital 239
Yeovil District Hospital 371
York District Hospital 290
Ysbyty Gwynedd 470

Index

Figures in **bold** indicate main references.

Abnormality Ultrasound Scan 32
abortion *see* termination 30
Active Birth Centre 23, 43
AFP *see* alpha-feto protein testing
afterpains 138
alcohol 120
allergies 28, 77, 79, 118
alpha-feto protein testing (AFP) 34, 36
amenity rooms 68-9
amnihook 89, 94
amniocentesis 29-30, 31, 33, 34, 35, **36-7**, 122
amnioscope 96
amniotic fluid 33, 80, 91, 96, 97, 123
anaemia 35, 91, 106, 116, 123
anaesthesia 14, 16, 69; spinal *see* spinal anaesthesia
anencephaly 32
antenatal care 21, 24; hospital 27-9; options 24-6
antenatal classes 24, 40, 44-5, 89, 140
antenatal clinics 21, 38-40
antenatal records 21
antenatal swimming classes 43
antenatal wards 21, 67, 68, 69, 74
anti-D 35, 36, 107
antibodies 35, 131, 135
Apgar score 61
aquanatal classes 24
Arden, Sarah 52-3
aromatherapist 42
aspirin 136, 138

assisted delivery 97-101
Association for Postnatal Illness (APNI) 146

baby: abnormalities 33; birth weight 91, 99; brain damage 105; breathing difficulties 115; checking after birth 86, 87; child health records 143, 146-7; cord around neck 60-61; crowning 41, 71, 141; engagement of head 39; head in unusual position 95; heartbeat 39, 67, 80, 88, 91, 93, 94, 109, 121, 140; resuscitation 83, 101; small-for-dates 83, 86; tagging 82
bacteria 46, 51, 86
bacterial vaginosis 51
bed capacity 15
biparietal diameter 32
birth centres *see* midwife-led units
birth partners 42-3
birth plan 23, **26-7**, 41, 42, 72, 103, 105
birthing pool 73
bleeding 27, 28, 39, 47, 54, 80, 91, 101, 111, 116
blighted ovum 46
blood clots 115, 142
blood clotting tests 62, 79
blood group 34-5
blood tests 21, 26, 29, **34-6**, 55
bottle-feeding 61, 126, 131, 139; *see also* formula milk
Braxton-Hicks contractions 67, 85

breastfeeding 61, 62, 126, **130-37**, 146
breastfeeding counsellors 42, 45
breathing 43, 73, 84, 85, 148, 149
breathing monitor 148
breech position 57, 69, 96, 98, 99, 100, 102, **106-9**, 111, 115, 116, 125
burial service 55, 58

caesarean section 9, 10-11, 60, 98-9, **109-15**, **118-19**; and baby's head 95; and breech delivery 107-8; death of baby in the womb 91; and domino delivery 81; elective 11, 13, 57, 68, 69, 79, 99, 100, 109, 111-14, **115**, 117, 122; emergency 11, 23, 98-101, 112, 125; epidurals 41; and failed induction 94; maternity units 16, 69; and the partner 98, 101, 118; previous 83, 91, 110, 115; rates 16, 97, 100, 109-10; and shape of womb 33; and twins 124, 125; wound care 137, 143
catheterisation 89, 98, 99, 104, 118, 119
CDH see congenital dislocation of the hip
cephalhaematoma 106
cervical smear tests 39, 40, 139
cervix: dilated see dilatation; previous surgery 40, 51, 95; stitch in 40
Changing Childbirth report (Cumberlege, 1992) 12, 80
chemotherapy 135
chignon 106
chorionic villus sampling (CVS) 29, 31, 32, 34, 35, 36, **37-8**, 122
chromosomal abnormalities 31, 37, 46, 51

chromosomes 38
cleft lip 33
colostrum 61, 135
combined pill 135
community-based midwifery 25, 84, 85, 99
cone biopsy 51, 95
congenital dislocation of the hip (CDH) 109
congenital heart disease 31
consultant-led units 14-16, 69, 80, 81
contraception 135-6, 139
contractions 66, 70, 72, 74, 75, 81, 92, 94, 95, 104, 105, 117, 140
cot death 147, 148-9
cracked nipples 134, 143
crowning 41, 71, 141
CTGs (Cardiotocogram; foetal heart monitoring) 62, 67, 80, 90, 91, 96, 97, 121
Cumberlege, Baroness Julia: Changing Childbirth report (1992) 12, 80
CVS see chorionic villus sampling
cystic fibrosis 28, 33, 143
cytomegalovirus 120

day care facilities 21
dehydration 80, 91, 149
delivery pack 86-7
delivery suite 40, 74, 140
depression 28; see also postnatal depression
Derriford Hospital, Plymouth 23
diabetes 28, 39, 46, 59, 86, 91
diarrhoea 149
diet 139
dilatation 67, 70, 72, 79, 80, 81, 85, 89, 91, 93, 95, 103, 107, 109, 111, 140
Director of Midwifery Services 25, 83

doctors 11, 14; *see also* GPs; obstetricians
domino (DOMiciliary IN and Out) system 22, 25, 80, **81**
doppler 39
double testing 29, 34
Down's Syndrome 16, 22, 29-30, 34, 36, 37, 38, 46
Dynan, Emily 74-5

Early Pregnancy Assessment Unit (EPAU) 47-8, 54
Early Pregnancy Ultrasound Scan 31
eclampsia 58-9
ectopic pregnancy 40, 47, 49-50
ECV *see* external cephalic version
Edinburgh Postnatal Depression Score 145
electronic tagging 82
empowerment 9, 12
endometritis 139
engagement of baby's head 39
engorgement 143
Entonox *see* gas and air
epidural 13-14, 16, 23, 25, 60, 62, 74-5, **77-9**, 81, 83, 88, 89, 95, 98, 101, 103-4, 105, 110, 112, 115, 116, 118, 124, 140
epilepsy 28
episiotomy 41, 75, **102-3**, 104, 106, 138
estimated date of delivery (EDD) 28, 90, 91, 94
ethnic minority groups 45
exercise 43, 84
external cardiotocograph 109
external cephalic version (ECV) 35, 107

fever 80, 91
fibroids 33, 46, 54, 95
Field, Emma 60-61
fluid retention 39, 58

foetal blood sampling 81, 91, 96-7
foetal distress 80, 91, 102, 103, 108, 111, 121
foetal monitoring 23
forceps delivery 10, 16, 69, 78, 81, 83, 97, 102, **103-5**, 106, 112, 116, 117
formula milk 61, 131, 135, 136-7; *see also* bottle-feeding

gas and air (Entonox) 41, 74, 75, **76**, 79, 86, 87, 94, 117, 140
gastroenteritis 51, 131
genetic mapping 38
genital herpes 110
German measles test 36
gestation 32
glucose in urine 39
Gold, Lorna 116-17
GPs 9, 11, 22, 23; and child health 150; and home birth 83, 84, 86, 87; home visits 150; and maternity units 11, 16, 20; postnatal visits 143; registering the baby 149, 150; shared care 24, 41
Guthrie test 143

HCG (human chorionic gonadotrophin) testing 36
health authorities 25
health visitor 89, 146-7
heart defects 33
heart disease 28, 31
heparin 115
hepatitis B or C 28
hepatitis B testing 36
high blood pressure (hypertension) 28, 38, 58-9, 62, 73, 80, 83, 91, 108, 120
High Dependency Unit 98
HIV 28, 36, 111, 135
home birth 10-13, 21, 22, 71, **82-7**, **90**, 117

Horn, Angela 90
hospital birth 9, **66-82**; amenity
    rooms 68-9; going into hospital
    66-7; pros and cons 69
hospitals: choosing 20, 21; first
    appointment 27-8; private 26;
    private wings in NHS hospitals
    26
Howarth, Dawn 22-3, 42-3
hypertension *see* high blood
    pressure
hypoglycaemia 135
hypospadias 33

ibuprofen 138
Imperial College, London:
    Faculty of Medicine 10
Independent Midwives
    Association 26
induction of labour 10, 40, 41,
    60, 68, 75, 88-9, 98, 121
infections 46, 51, 91, 115, 120,
    121, 131, 135, 138, 142
inherited conditions 28
instrumental vaginal delivery 81,
    91
internal examination 39-40
internal podalic version 125
intervention: avoiding 84; and
    caseload midwifery 25; high-
    tech 69; by obstetrician 80-81,
    91, 103, 107, 111; rates 13, 16,
    20
iodine 118
iron tablets 35
iso-immunisation 35, 36

Jarman, Professor Sir Brian 10
jaundice 143

kidney cysts 33
kidney disease 28, 62
kidney function 58

La Leche League 136
labetalol 62
labour 66, 67-8, 88-9; after 97;
    home birth 82-3, 85, 86, 87;
    pain relief 73, 76-9; positions
    23, 43, 73, 78; stages of 72-3
labour wards 54-5, 68, 79, 82
last menstrual period (LMP) 28
listeria 120
lithium 135
liver function 58
LMP *see* last menstrual period
lochia 138

massage 43
mastitis 143
maternity blues 144
maternity leave 58, 122, 125
maternity services: and home
    births 11, 13; postnatal care
    130
maternity units 10, 11-12;
    antenatal classes 24, 40, 44;
    capacity 15; comparing services
    11-12; consultant units 14-16,
    69, 99; data 10; intervention
    rates 16; midwife-run units 16-
    17; pain relief 16; profiles 14;
    staffing levels 15-16
meconium 61, 80, 91, **95-6**
medical card 149
medical history 28
medical insurance policies 26
meningitis 110
methotrexate 50
methydopa 62
midwife-led units 11, 16-17, 20,
    77, 101
midwife-per-mother statistics 23

midwives 9, 11; and breastfeeding 132, 133; community-based 25, 84, 85, 99, 133, 142-3; consultant units 14, 15; continuity of care 22, 24, 79-80, 84, 87; domino system 22, 25; group practice/caseload 25; home birth 21, 83, 84, 85; independent 25-6; midwife-led care 25-6; shared care 24; team 25; water birth 92, 93

mini-pill 135-6

miscarriage 29, 30, 33, 35-8, 40, **46-9**, 52-3, 56-7, 59; late 51, 54-5, 58

Miscarriage Association 58

mobile epidurals 78

morphine 113, 118

mother and baby unit 145-6

moxibustion 69

MRSA (methicillin-resistant staphyloccus aureus) 86

multiple pregnancy 32, 59, 69, 110, 115, **122-6**; *see also* twins

National Childbirth Trust (NCT) 22, 24, 40, 42, 43, **44-5**, 60, 90, 134, 136

National Health Service (NHS) 24, 26, 149

natural childbirth 9, 11, 13, 17, 100, 112

neonatal intensive care unit (NICU) 55, 57

neonatal units 69

neural tube disorders 34

NICE (National Institute for Clinical Excellence) guidelines on induction 90

nuchal fold scans 16, 29, **30-31**

nursery nursing students 126

nutrition 84

obstetric operating theatre 100-101

obstetricians 9, 20, 69; and caesarean birth 13; duty 104; female 21; involvement of 80-81, 91, 103, 107, 111; maternity units 14; obstetrician-led care 26

ovarian cyst 40, 92

oxygen saturation monitor 148-9

oxytocin drip 60

Oyeyi, Jackie 92-3

paediatrics 69, 87, 109, 142

pain relief 9, 10; avoiding 84, 85; birth plan 41; and choosing the hospital 20; in consultant units 16; forceps delivery 105; home birth 83-7; in midwife-run units 17; *see also* epidural; gas and air (Entonox); spinal anaesthesia

paracetamol 136, 138

parentcraft classes 22, 24, 42

partogram 80

pelvic floor 102, 103

pelvis: contracted 95; fracture 28; pelvic abscess 40; unusual shape 95

perineal damage 80, 91, 102, 103, 105, 110, 116, 143

pethidine 41, 75, **76**, 87, 94, 116

phenylketonuria 33

Pinard stethoscope 39, 67

placenta: after a miscarriage 54; and ECV 107; failure 51, 90, 120; position of 32, 39, 92; removal 72-3, 101, 104; retained 138, 139, 141, 142

placenta praevia 31, 110

placental abruption 91, 120

planning your pregnancy 20-21

platelet count 58

poisons 46

post-mortem examination 55
postnatal care 130
postnatal depression 139, 144-5, 146, 147
postnatal examination 119, 139
postnatal psychiatric illness 144-6
postnatal wards 97, 142
pre-eclampsia 58-62
pre-eclamptic toxaemia 58
preloading 77-8
previous pregnancies 28-9
private care 26
private medical insurance 26
progestogen-only pill 135-6
prolapse 102, 141
prostaglandin 94, 98
protein 58, 60, 62
Pseudomonas 86
psychiatric illness 28
puerperal psychosis 28, 146
puerperal sepsis 139

quadruple testing 34
Quamie, Sharon 84-5
Queen Charlotte's hospital, Chiswick, London 10-11, 88

raspberry leaf extract 103
'red book' 143
Register Office 149
relaxation techniques 43
resuscitation 83, 101
rhesus factor 34-5, 107
ritodrine 107
Royal College of Obstetricians and Gynaecologists 97, 100
rubella 120; test 36

St Mary's Hospital, Paddington 56
scans see nuchal fold scans; ultrasound scans
schizophrenia 28

screening 10, 16
selective foetal reduction 125
shared care 24, 41, 70
sickle cell disease 33, 35-6, 59, 143
SLE (systematic lupus erythematosus) 46
smoking 46, 51, 108, 120, 139, 148
Sonicaid 39, 67
spina bifida 29, 32, 33, 34, 36, 38
spinal anaesthesia 14, 16, 77, 79, 81, 101, 105, 110, 115
staffing levels 15-16
stillbirth 120-22
Stillbirth and Neonatal Death Society (SANDS) 122
stirrups, obstetric 75, 96, 104, 106
stitches: caesarean section 137; perineum 138, 143
students at the birth 23, 41, 75, 109, 118, 124
Syntocinon drip 81, 91, 94, 95, 104, 105, 125
Syntometrin 72, 73, 141
syphilis test 36

teenagers 45, 59
TENS (transcutaneous electrical nerve stimulation) machine 73, 76, 87, 92
termination 29, 30, 35, 40, 51, 59
thrombosis 28, 115, 142
thyroid disease 28, 46, 135, 143
toxoplasma 120
triple test 16, 29, 31, **34**
twins 29, 31, 32, 45, 73, 83, **122-6**, 148
Twins and Multiple Births Association (TAMBA) 126

UCH (University College
   Hospital), London 93
ultrasound scans 10, 21, 22, 26,
   28, 29, 62, 90; Abnormality
   Ultrasound Scan 32; and
   breech position 107; and
   caesarean section 116; CDH
   109; and community midwives
   33-4; Early Pregnancy
   Ultrasound Scan 31; and foetal
   heartbeat 121; information
   provided by 32-3; and twins
   123, 124; what the scan does
   not show 33
umbilical cord 41, 51, 71, 72, 73,
   108, 111
UNICEF baby friendly status 130
UNICEF breast accreditation 130
UNICEF UK Baby Friendly
   Hospital Initiative 134
urinary infection 27, 28, 38, 51

urine tests 62

vaginal breech delivery 107-9,
   111
varicose veins 39
venous thrombosis 142
ventouse delivery 16, 75, 83, 89,
   97, 102, 104, 105, **106**
vomiting 27, 28, 74, 97, 149

water birth 9, 20, 69, **73**, 86, 87,
   92-3, 112
waters broken 40, 54, 66, 67, 69,
   70, 74, 87, 89, 91, 94, 101, 140
Wolf, Diana 88-9
womb, shape of 32-3, 52
World Health Organisation 97,
   100, 134
wound care 137-9, 142

yoga classes 23, 43, 140

Dr Foster Q&A

What is Dr Foster?

Dr Foster is an independent organization which measures healthcare
standards through ongoing assessments of every major hospital, maternity
unit, care home, consultant, dentist and complementary therapist in the UK.
Information from government, hospitals and medical professionals is
analyzed with the help of leading universities such as Imperial College of
Science, Technology and Medicine, Exeter University and City University. An
ethics committee, made up of some of the most distinguished figures in
healthcare, ensures accuracy and impartiality. Supported by the government
and leading professional healthcare organizations, Dr Foster brings together
world-renowned academics, healthcare experts and media professionals.

What makes Dr Foster unique?

For the first time ever an independent body of experts has assessed the UK's
health services ranging from hospitals to maternity services, dentists and
complementary therapists. Their unique content derives from questionnaires,
statistical research and analysis, contributions from industry experts, individual
hospitals, the Department of Health and individual GPs and consultants. These
outstanding guides give you the public an unprecedented opportunity to find
out how and where to get the best possible care and service.

The Doctor Foster Guides

Available now:

0091883792   Dr Foster Good Birth Guide
0091883776   Dr Foster Good Hospital Guide
0091883784 Dr Foster Good Complementary Therapist Guide

Forthcoming titles:

0091883857   Dr Foster Good Care Home Guide
0091883822   Dr Foster Breast Cancer Guide
0091883806   Dr Foster Heart Disease Guide
0091883814   Dr Foster Infertility Guide
0091883830   Dr Foster Good Dentist Guide
0091883849   Dr Foster Good Consultant Guide

How can I order more Dr Foster titles?

To order copies of any of these books direct from Vermilion, an imprint of
the Random House group Ltd, call The Book Service credit card hotline on
01206 255800.

The Dr Foster guides are also available from all good booksellers.